Bioinformatics
Concepts, Skills & Applications
Second Edition

Bioinformatics
Concepts, Skills & Applications
Second Edition

S.C. RASTOGI
Former Professor of Biosciences, BITS, Pilani
Director, iBiosciences, New Delhi

NAMITA MENDIRATTA
Vice President, Information Technology
Invenio Biosolutions, New Delhi

PARAG RASTOGI
Consultant, iBiosciences, New Delhi

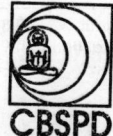

CBSPD

CBS Publishers & Distributors Pvt Ltd

New Delhi • Bengaluru • Chennai • Kochi • Kolkata • Lucknow • Mumbai
Hyderabad • Jharkhand • Nagpur • Patna • Pune • Uttarakhand

Bioinformatics
Concepts, Skills and
Applications
Second Edition

ISBN: 978-81-239-1482-4

Copyright © Publisher

Second Edition 2006

Reprint: 2007, 2008, 2009, 2011, 2014, 2016, 2017, 2018, 2019, 2023, 2024 , 2025

First Edition: 2003

Reprint: 2003, 2004, 2005

Published by Satish Kumar Jain and produced by Varun Jain for

CBS Publishers & Distributors Pvt Ltd

4819/XI Prahlad Street, 24 Ansari Road, Daryaganj, New Delhi 110 002, India
Ph: 011-23289259, 23266861   Website: www.cbspd.com
                                                    e-mail: delhi@cbspd.com

Corporate Office: 204 FIE, Industrial Area, Patparganj, Delhi 110 092
Ph: 011-4934 4934   Fax: 011-4934 4935   e-mail: publishing@cbspd.com
                                                    publicity@cbspd.com

Branches

- **Bengaluru:** Seema House 2975, 17th Cross, KR Road, Banasankari 2nd Stage, Bengaluru 560 070, Karnataka, India
  Ph: +91-80-26771678/79   Fax: +91-80-26771680   e-mail: bangalore@cbspd.com
- **Chennai:** 7, Subbaraya Street, Shenoy Nagar, Chennai 600 030, Tamil Nadu, India
  Ph: +91-44-26680620, 26681266   Fax: +91-44-42032115   e-mail: chennai@cbspd.com
- **Kochi:** 42/1325, 1326, Power House Road, Opp KSEB, Power House, Ernakulam 682 018, India
  Ph: +91-484-4059061–65   Fax: +91-484-4059065   e-mail: kochi@cbspd.com
- **Kolkata:** 147, Hind Ceramics Compound, 1st Floor, Nilgunj Road, Belghoria, Kolkata 700 056, West Bengal, India
  Ph: +91-9096713055/56   e-mail: kolkata@cbspd.com
- **Lucknow:** Basement, Khushnuma Complex, 7-Meerabai Marg (behind Jawahar Bhawan), Lucknow 226 001, India
  Ph: +91-522-4000032   e-mail: tiwari.lucknow@cbspd.com
- **Mumbai:** PWD Shed. Gala no. 25/26, Ramchandra Bhatt Marg, Next to JJ Hospital Gate no. 2, Opp. Union Bank of India
  Noorbaug Mumbai 400 009, Maharashtra, India
  Ph: +91-22-66661880/89   e-mail: mumbai@cbspd.com

Representatives

- **Hyderabad**   0-9885175004   • **Jharkhand**   0-9811541605   • **Nagpur**   0-8692091830
- **Patna**   0-9334159340   • **Pune**   0-9664372571   • **Uttarakhand** 0-9716462459

Printed at Neekunj Print Process, Sonipat, Haryana

Preface to the Second Edition

The second edition of **Bioinformatics : Concepts, Skills & Applications** is appearing exactly three years after the book was first published in 2003. This short span has provided ample opportunity for the text material to be class-tested in several institutions across the country. We feel encouraged by the wide readership it has gained.

Ever since the publication of the first edition, the field of bioinformatics has gained greater momentum and the biological database worldwide has grown exponentially. Currently, the ability to sequence the genome of whole organisms, including man, presents opportunities that could hardly be visualized ten years ago. Many technological advances have occurred that provide bioinformaticians with new tools to serve society better. We want the readers to remain excited about these advancements and new tools.

Particular attention has been paid to making this new edition stimulating and highly readable. The result is a text that is clear, focussed and designed to capture student interest. While our major goal continues to provide concepts, skills and applications of bioinformatics, efforts are made to provide most significant advances in the area that is important to biotechnologists, molecular biologists and the industry. To achieve this goal, most of the chapters have been revised, involving amalgamation, division or deletion without loss of crucial information, but with gain of knowledge and clarity.

New features

Some new features introduced include :

- The chapter 'Bioinformatics : An Overview' has been revised and updated. Obsolete websites are deleted and new ones added.
- A new chapter 'Relational Database for Biological Information' for storing biological information has been added as it is crucial for creating and managing databases.
- A new chapter 'Object-Oriented Databases' has been included as it scores over conventional languages for programming applications.
- Addition of a new chapter 'Managing Biological Databanks' forms one of the basic skills that a bioinformatician should possess.

- A new chapter 'Alignment of Pairs of Sequences' is needed for discovering information related to protein functions, structure and evolution.
- Chapter on 'RNA Structure Prediction' has been included as RNA is involved in important biological functions, hence prediction from sequence analysis forms an important part of bioinformatics.
- The chapter 'Proteomics' has been revised and expanded. Improvements in high-throughput methods for identification of therapeutic targets for mode of action of drugs have been discussed.
- A new chapter 'Analyzing Metabolic Pathways' is essential since information about metabolic network in biochemical pathways is the most challenging problem in bioinformatics.
- A new chapter 'Methods of Statistical Analysis' has been incorporated. Managing a deluge of biological data is quite laborious and difficult to handle, hence analytical methods have been discussed to reduce large data sets to a few parameters.

Finally, a chapter on problems for self-assessment has been added that will go a long way to instill confidence in students. It is hoped that the coverage of new areas of increasing importance to bioinformatics will widen the scope of this book.

S.C. Rastogi
Namita Mendiratta
Parag Rastogi

Preface to the First Edition

The study of bioinformatics broadly addresses challenges arising from high-throughput molecular technologies. Modern laboratory techniques like whole genome sequencing and expression analysis generate an enormous amount of data and information about the activities at molecular level.

There are three fundamental issues that directly impact our understanding of life at the molecular level : understanding of the structure and function of gene products; the regulation of gene expression; and the metabolic networks of molecular interactions. The basic laboratory technologies deal with high-throughput chemical synthesis and biological assays, which are themselves amenable to analysis using informatics techniques. There are all-together new opportunities highly dependent on the bioinformatics skills like manipulation, control and modification of the interface at the molecular level which have broad applications in disease gene discovery, molecular diagnostics, drug design, metabolic engineering, bioconversion and biosynthesis. Bioinformatics provides the essential analysis and interpretation component which is crucial to derive and synthesize results from the massive data of these high-throughput technologies.

Bioinformatics is an interdisciplinary approach requiring sophisticated computer science, mathematics, and statistical methods, with a functional understanding of the biological and chemical context at the molecular level. The approach for understanding bioinformatics field in this book reflects this philosophy, covering the three core areas of computational methods, biomolecular structure and function, and bioinformatics-driven applications like genomics and proteomics. The book is aimed at two types of researchers and students. The goal of the pedagogical approach is to prepare and train a new generation of bioengineers from either of the two streams - biosciences and informatics. The students of biology and biochemistry need to understand the new data-driven algorithms, such as neural networks and hidden Markov models, in the context of biological sequences and their molecular structure and function. The students with a primary background in physics, mathematics, statistics, or computer science need to know more about specific applications of their respective fields in molecular biology. While this book may not specifically meet the aspirations of all the groups of students, it is hoped that the students would become capable of using computational analysis to solve important problems arising from the new frontiers of biology and medicine at molecular level.

Purpose

While there are a few books available in the Indian markets on the subject, there is none widely available by Indian authors. Moreover, there are only a couple of books accessible to the student - both in terms of availability and price. One of such books available in the market covers a lot of ground, but gives an undue focus on the structure visualization. This book, although satisfactory as an introduction and in readability, oversimplifies the subject at some points and touches several important issues peri-pherally. There is another book that has appeared in the market very recently. It is a good "little introduction", but a serious student may find it a bit too inadequate.

The present book attempts to cover the gaps in availability and subject treatment. The purpose of this book is to provide a systematic overview of bioinformatics for biological students and health care professionals, and for students of computer science. The book describes the concepts and skills for becoming a bioinformatician and provides illustrations of the principal applications in bioinformatics. There are four main reasons that we have developed this book :

1. Informatics is becoming part of the cirriculum in an increasing number of universities and insti-tutions for the higher education of biology and health care professionals worldwide. This book may serve as an introduction to the field for these students.

2. Increasing numbers of information technology students are turning to biological informatics as a discipline for study and investigation. The book would help such IT students for understand-ing the bioinformatics applications.

3. Workers in the fields of biosciences, health care workers, pharmaceutical researchers and pro-fessionals in the allied fields are frequently confronted with information systems for research, data interpretation, the support of patient care, the assessment of the quality of care, manage-ment and planning. For these professionals, the book can serve as an orientation to the rapidly developing field of computers in these fields.

4. The more advanced chapters of this book provide comprehensive overviews of topics in bio-logical informatics that should be of value to specialists in the bioinformatics field.

Organization

Bioinformatics : *Concepts, Skills and Applications* will hence allow students, scientists, researchers, and even enthusiasts interested in the use of computers in biological research to better grasp this dy-namic and rapidly growing field. This book has taken an integrated view of the interdisciplinary nature of the subject.

The content has been organized systematically. The 16 chapters are grouped into five main clusters that represent different themes of discussion.

Cluster 1 deals with introduction to bioinformatics. This cluster would help the students in under-standing the broad spectrum of activities in this field.

Chapter 1 : Bioinformatics : an Overview

Chapter 2 : Molecular biology and bioinformatics

Clsuter 2 deals with important concepts in molecular biology. Molecular biology is the underlying basis for bioinformatics study. This cluster helps a non-biology student understand the key concepts in molecular biology. It would also provide a very good review for biology students. This cluster does not assume any knowledge except for some basic biology and chemistry, nowadays taught at senior sec-ondary level.

Chapter 3 : The information molecules and information flow

Chapter 4 : Proteins : their structural profiles and properties

Cluster 3 deals with the core computational skills required for bioinformatics. This cluster is principally for the non-informatics students to understand the basics of informatics - operating system, basics of programming and using databases.

Chapter 5 : Using the linux operating system

Chapter 6 : Programming with Perl

Chapter 7 : Understanding and using biological databases

Cluster 4 deals with sequence and phylogenetic analyses. Sequence analysis is one of the key applications of bioinformatics - this cluster details this crucial application. The computational algorithms have been kept to the minimum so that a student with minimal mathematical background can also understand without feeling lost.

Chapter 8 : Aligning pairs of sequences

Chapter 9 : Tools for sequence alignment

Chapter 10 : Alignment of multiple sequences

Chapter 11 : Phylogenetic analysis

Cluster 5 deals with genomics, proteomics and other bioinformatics applications. This cluster takes the reader beyond the usual sequence analysis applications. The last chapter provides some useful illustrations of the problem solving techniques in bioinformatics.

Chapter 12 : Gene prediction methods

Chapter 13 : Visualization and prediction of protein structure

Chapter 14 : Gene mapping, sequence assembly and gene expression

Chapter 15 : Proteomics

Chapter 16 : Problem solving in bioinformatics

As bioinformatics is an interdisciplinary subject, we have incorporated an extensive glossary drawn from the diverse fields at the end. We strongly suggest the use of glossary by the reader.

The field of biological informatics is too extensive to be covered by a single author. Therefore, this book has been written by three authors with extensive experience in their fields. The authors took much care that the book would not be merely a collection of separate chapters, but rather would offer a consistent and structured overview of the field. We are also aware that there is still considerable room for improvement and that certain elements of bioinformatics are not fully covered due to the constraints of space. We feel that many of the basic methods described in this book can be used profitably and students may only need to consult other sources for specific discussions of topics. Some of the selected references are provided at the end of the Chapter 16.

The authors are developing a companion web-site to the book for providing additional material and some practical exercises for the students. The students can contact the authors on the following e-mail address : biconcepts@hotmail.com.

New Delhi
October, 2002

S.C. Rastogi
Namita Mendiratta
Parag Rastogi

Contents

Preface to the Second Edition vii

Preface to the First Edition ix

1. Bioinformatics : An Overview 1–17

    1.1.   Introduction, *1*

    1.2.   Objectives of bioinformatics, *3*

    1.3.   What kind of data is used, *4*

    1.4.   Multiplicity of data and data mining, *5*

    1.5.   Major bioinformatics databases, *5*

    1.6.   Data integration, *11*

    1.7.   Data analysis, *12*

    1.8.   Careers in bioinformatics, *12*

    1.9.   Reference list of the major bioinformatics databases and tools, *14*

2. Molecular Biology and Bioinformatics 18–26

    2.1.   What is molecular biology, *18*

    2.2.   Systems approach in biology, *18*

    2.3.   Central dogma of molecular biology, *18*

    2.4.   Important definitions related to central dogma, *21*

    2.5.   Problems in molecular approach and the bioinformatics approach, *23*

    2.6.   Overview of bioinformatics applications, *23*

3. The Information Molecules and Information Flow 27–42

    3.1.   Introduction, *27*

    3.2.   Basic components, *27*

    3.3.   Basic chemistry of nucleic acids, *28*

3.4. Structure of DNA, *29*

3.5. Structure of RNA, *31*

3.6. DNA replication is semi-conservative, *32*

3.7. Denaturation and renaturation of DNA, *33*

3.8. Genes - the functional elements in DNA, *34*

3.9. Organisation of genes in eukaryotic chromosomes, *36*

3.10. Structure of bacterial chromosome, *37*

3.11. Analysing DNA, *37*

3.12. Cloning methodology, *38*

3.13. DNA sequencing and polymerase chain reaction (PCR), *39*

4. **Proteins—Their Structural Profiles and Properties** **43–54**

4.1. Introduction, *43*

4.2. Amino acids, *43*

4.3. Protein structure, *46*

4.4. Secondary structure elements, *48*

4.5. Tertiary structure, *50*

4.6. Quaternary structure, *51*

4.7. Protein folding, *51*

4.8. Protein function, *51*

4.9. Proteins - purification and characterisation, *52*

5. **Using the Linux Operating System** **55–73**

5.1. Introduction to linux, *55*

5.2. The basics of linux system, *56*

5.3. Using linux file system and directories, *58*

5.4. Text processing, *63*

5.5. Writing shell programs, *68*

6. **Programming with Perl** **74–108**

6.1. Introduction to Perl, *74*

6.2. Programming in Perl, *74*

6.3. Illustrations of programming in Perl, *86*

6.4. Operations with associative arrays (Hashes), *88*

6.5. File input and output, *91*

6.6. Perl applications for bioinformatics, *94*

6.7. Perl application for bioinformatics - Bioperl, *106*

7. **Relational Databases for Biological Information** **109–123**

7.1. Introduction, *109*

7.2. Types of databases, *110*

8. Object-Oriented Databases 124–131

    8.1.   Introduction, *124*

    8.2.   Object oriented databases, *125*

    8.3   Introduction to the Java clients, *128*

    8.4.   Common object request broker architecture (CORBA), *130*

    8.5.   Some projects, *131*

9. Managing Biological Databanks 132–147

    9.1.   Introduction, *132*

    9.2.   Submission of data, *132*

    9.3.   Curation of databases, *134*

    9.4.   Establishing databases on networks, *134*

    9.5.   Integration of databases, *137*

    9.6.   Mining of databases, *143*

    9.7.   Management of workflow, *146*

10. Alignment of Pairs of Sequences 148–172

    10.1. Introduction to sequence analysis, *148*

    10.2. Sequence Analysis of Biological Data, *149*

    10.3. Models for sequence analysis and their biological motivation, *150*

    10.4. Methods of alignment, *152*

    10.5. Applications of dot matrices, *157*

    10.6. Methods for optimal alignments, *160*

    10.7. Using gap penalties and scoring matrices, *165*

    10.8. Sensitivity and specificity, *169*

    10.9. Illustrative examples, *170*

11. Tools for Sequence Alignment 173–190

    11.1. Introduction, *173*

    11.2. Fasta, *173*

    11.3. Blast, *179*

    11.4. Filtering and gapped blast, *183*

    11.5. PSI-blast, *187*

    11.6. Comparison of running time for various programs, *190*

12. Alignment of Multiple Sequences 191–205

    12.1. Introduction, *191*

    12.2. Tools for MSA, *193*

    12.3. Considerations in conducting MSA, *199*

    12.4. Applications of multiple alignment, *201*

    12.5. Viewing MSA, *204*

    12.6. Sequence detection efficiency measures : Sensitivity and specificity, *204*

13. Phylogenetic Analysis **206–222**

    13.1. Introduction, *206*

    13.2. Concept of trees, *206*

    13.3. Phylogenetic trees and multiple alignments, *207*

    13.4. Distance matrix methods (MD), *209*

    13.5. Character based methods, *212*

    13.6. Methods of evaluating phylogenies, *215*

    13.7. Summary of the phylogenetic methods, *216*

    13.8. Steps in constructing alignments and phylogenies, *217*

    13.9. Considerations in choice of the method, *217*

    13.10. Working with phylogenetic trees - an illustration, *219*

14. Gene Prediction Methods **223–234**

    14.1. Introduction, *223*

    14.2. Using patterns to predict genes, *224*

    14.3. Methods of gene prediction, *225*

    14.4. Gene prediction tools, *232*

    14.5. Summary of tools for DNA/RNA structure and function analysis,

15. Understanding and Using Biological Databases **235–247**

    15.1. Introduction, *235*

    15.2. Overview of RNA secondary structure, *236*

    15.3. Overview of RNA tertiary structure, *237*

    15.4. Assumptions in RNA structure prediction, *237*

    15.5. Methods of RNA structure prediction, *238*

16. Visualization and Prediction of Protein Structure **248–285**

    16.1. Protein structure overview, *248*

    16.2. Different structural proteins, *250*

    16.3. Protein structure databases and visualization tools, *252*

    16.4. Protein classification, *256*

    16.5. Protein structure prediction, *257*

    16.6. Methods of structure prediction for known folds, *261*

    16.7. Methods of structure prediction for unknown folds, *266*

    16.8. Protein function prediction, *284*

    16.9. Accuracy of prediction, *284*

17. Gene Mapping, Sequence Assembly and Gene Expression **286–308**

    17.1. Introduction, *286*

    17.2. Gene mapping, *287*

    17.3. Application of mapping, *290*

17.4. DNA sequencing, *293*

17.5. Algorithm for alignment of sequencing fragments, *298*

17.6. DNA microarrays, *301*

17.7. Microarray experiment design and data analysis, *304*

18. Proteomics **309–331**

18.1. Introduction to proteomics, *309*

18.2. Proteome analysis, *311*

18.3. Tools for proteome analysis, *312*

18.4. Metabolic pathways, *321*

18.5. Genetic networks, *323*

19. Analyzing Metabolic Pathways **332–343**

19.1. Introduction, *332*

19.2. Gene transcription networks, *332*

19.3. Metabolic pathways, *333*

19.4. Signalling network, *338*

19.5. Simulation of cellular metabolism, *340*

20. Methods of Statistical Analysis **344–364**

20.1. Introduction, *344*

20.2. Fundamentals of probability and statistics, *345*

20.3. Applications of Statistical Tools, *355*

21. Problem Solving in Bioinformatics **365–393**

21.1. Introduction, *365*

21.2. Genomic analysis for DNA sequences, *365*

21.3. Genomic analysis for protein sequences, *366*

21.4. Strategies and options for similarity search, *366*

21.5. Practical considerations in sequence analysis, *368*

21.6. Flowchart for protein structure prediction, *372*

21.7. Illustrations : Some problems and solutions, *373*

22. Problems for Self Assessment **394–404**

Selected References **405–406**

Glossary **407–418**

Index **419–426**

Bioinformatics : An Overview

1.1 INTRODUCTION

Biological data is being produced at an unprecedented rate. Managing and interpreting this data is a challenge for biologists. As an example, consider the database EMBL. There have been 82 releases (updates) of the database till 24th February, 2005. During the last 2 years, the number of sequence entries has tripled – the growth rates have been actually similar over the last 4 years now (Table 1.1). Almost all the major databank repositories now have entries running into millions.

Table 1.1 Growth in EMBL data

Release Number	Date	Sequence Entries	Number of Nucleotides
62	21/3/2000	5,865,742	6,120,908,677
–	–	–	–
69	18/12/2001	14,366,182	15,383,451,165
70	15/3/2002	15,851,373	17,807,926,047
–		–	–
81	26/11/2004	46,105,397	79,271,300,840
82	24/2/2005	49,474,402	85,134,714,382

If we just consider the data from the myriad of related projects that study gene expression, determine the protein structures encoded by the genes, and detail how these products interact with one another, we can begin to imagine the enormous quantity and variety of information that is being produced.

What is Bioinformatics?

Bioinformatics is conceptualising biology in terms of molecules (in the sense of physical chemistry) and applying "*informatics techniques*" (derived from disciplines such as applied mathematics, computer science and statistics) to *understand* and *organise* the *information* associated with these molecules, on a *large scale*. Hence, bioinformatics is the management information system for molecular biology and has many practical applications in various fields.

The fundamental issue for bioinformatics is: how do we describe, analyse, simulate and predict the dynamics of various biological processes by using the information technology tools? The raison d'etre of Bioinformatics is the complexity of issues created by the massive amounts of data obtained through numerous biological experiments. The most well known example is the determination of the complete nucleotide sequence of the human genome – the project was completed in 2003.

Definition of Bioinformatics

Bioinformatics is the science of using information to understand biological phenomena. It is part of the larger science of *computational biology*, which is the application of quantitative analytical techniques in modeling and solving problems in the biological systems. Bioinformatics is the application of the statistical methods, pattern recognition and some of the computational methods.

The NIH Biomedical Information Science and Technology Initiative Consortium have given the following definitions of bioinformatics and computational biology.

Bioinformatics: Research, development, or application of computational tools and approaches for expanding the use of biological, medical, behavioural or health data, including those to acquire, store, organize, archive, analyze, or visualize such data.

Computational Biology: It involves development and application of data-analytical and theoretical methods, mathematical modeling and computational simulation techniques to the study of biological, behavioural, and social systems.

These definitions are not unique or accepted universally and they do not preclude any overlap between the two fields. They, however, provide a good definition to start with.

Study of Biomolecules is Complex

Most of the large biological molecules are polymers: ordered chains of simpler molecular modules called *monomers*. Monomers can be thought of as beads or building blocks that, despite having different colours and shapes, all have the same thickness and the same way of connecting to one another. Each monomer molecule is of the same general class, but each kind of monomer has its own well-defined set of characteristics. Many monomer molecules can be joined together to form a single, far larger, macromolecule which has exquisitely specific informational content and/or chemical properties. According to this scheme, the monomers in a given macromolecule of DNA or protein can be treated computationally as letters of an alphabet, put together in pre-programmed arrangements to carry messages or do work in a cell.

However, biomolecules are much more complex than typical organic molecules in the following ways :

1. Biomolecules are polymers consisting of a large number of covalently linked monomeric units, called *residues*. As a result, the number of atoms and covalent bonds in a macromolecule is much larger than in a typical organic molecule. For example, the chromosome 14 in human cells contains 87,410,661 base pairs, and a single polypeptide chain in β-galactosidase is 1023 amino acids long.

2. Biomolecules fold into distinct three-dimensional structures. The number of theoretically possible three-dimensional structures that any macromolecule can take is enormous. However, under physiological conditions, a biomolecule like a protein adopts a single low-energy conformation called the *native conformation*. Such macromolecules are active only when they are in their native conformation.

3. A biomolecule may associate with another similar macromolecule, or with other macromolecules to form even larger supramolecular assemblies that may have properties that their component mol-

ecules did not possess. Many proteins function as dimers, trimers, tetramers, or oligomers. Haemoglobin is a protein composed of four polypeptide chains.

What does Bioinformatics comprise of?

Bioinformatics is not just data analysis and includes many components :

Functional genomics : Large-scale methods of identifying gene functions and associations like DNA microarrays.

Structural genomics : attempts to crystallize and/or predict the structures of all proteins. Structural genomics is also known as proteomics.

Comparative genomics : Study of multiple whole genomes for understanding the differences and similarities between all the genes of multiple species. From such studies we can draw particular conclusions about species and general ones about evolution.

Sequence analysis : Sequence analysis of DNA and protein segments represented as alphabets are one of the most widely used bioinformatics tools.

Phylogenetics : Phylogenetics is used to study the evolutionary aspects.

Medical informatics : the management of biomedical experimental data associated with particular molecules. This includes methods from mass spectroscopy, and *in vitro* assays to study clinical side-effects.

As a result of the massive surge in data and its complexity, many of the challenges in biology have actually become challenges in computing.

1.2 OBJECTIVES OF BIOINFORMATICS

The fundamental objectives of bioinformatics are as follows :

Organizing biological data

At its simplest and basic level, bioinformatics organizes data in a way that allows researchers to access existing information and to submit new entries, as they are produced such as the Protein Data Bank for 3D macromolecular structures. While data-curation is an essential task, the information stored in these databases is essentially useless until analyzed. Thus the purpose of bioinformatics extends far beyond mere volume control of data.

Analysis of data

The second key objective is to develop tools and resources that aid in the analysis of data. For example, having sequenced a particular protein, it is of interest to compare it with previously characterised sequences. This requires more than just a straightforward database search. As such, programs such as FASTA and PSI-BLAST must consider what constitutes a biologically significant resemblance. Development of such resources requires extensive knowledge of computational theory, as well as a thorough understanding of biology.

Interpretation and application of data

The third objective is to use these tools to analyze the data and interpret the results in a biologically meaningful manner. Traditionally, biological studies examined individual systems in detail, and frequently compared them with a few that are related. In bioinformatics, we can also conduct global analyses of all the available data with the aim of uncovering common principles that apply across many systems and highlight features that are unique to some.

1.3 WHAT KIND OF DATA IS USED?

The data types used in bioinformatics analysis can broadly be divided into 5 types : raw DNA sequences, protein sequences, macromolecular structures, genome sequences, and other whole genome data. Raw DNA sequences are strings of the four base-letters comprising genes, each typically 1,000 bases long. Protein sequences comprise of strings of 20 amino acid letters. Macromolecular structural data represents a more complex form of information. For example, a typical PDB (www.rcsb.org/pdb/) file for a medium-sized protein contains the xyz coordinates of approximately 2,000 atoms.

The Table 1.2 lists the types of data that are analyzed in bioinformatics and the range of topics that we can consider to fall within the field.

Table 1.2. Types of data that are analyzed in Bioinformatics research

Data source	Bioinformatics analysis
Raw DNA sequence	Identification of genes
	Identification of introns and exons
	Gene product prediction
	Forensic analysis
Protein sequence	Sequence comparison algorithms
	Multiple sequence alignments algorithms
	Identification of conserved sequence motifs
Macromolecular structure	Secondary, tertiary structure prediction
	3D structural alignment algorithms
	Protein geometry measurements
	Surface and volume shape calculations
	Intermolecular interactions
	Molecular simulations
Genomes	Characterisation of repeats
	Structural assignments to genes
	Phylogenetic analysis
Gene expression	Genomic-scale census
	Linkage analysis relating specific genes to diseases
	Correlating expression patterns
	Mapping expression data to sequence, structural and biochemical data
Other data	Digital libraries for automated bibliographical searches
Literature	Knowledge databases of data from literature
Metabolic pathways	Pathway simulations

Scientific euphoria has recently centred on whole genome sequencing (Fig. 1.1 Human Genome Project at www.ornl.gov/sci/techresources/Human_Genome/home.shtml).

An important aspect of complete genomes is the distinction between coding regions and non-coding regions –'junk' repetitive sequences making up the bulk of base sequences, especially in eukaryotes. Other genomic-scale data include biochemical information on metabolic pathways, regulatory networks, protein-protein interaction data from two-hybrid experiments, and systematic knockouts of individual genes to test the viability of an organism.

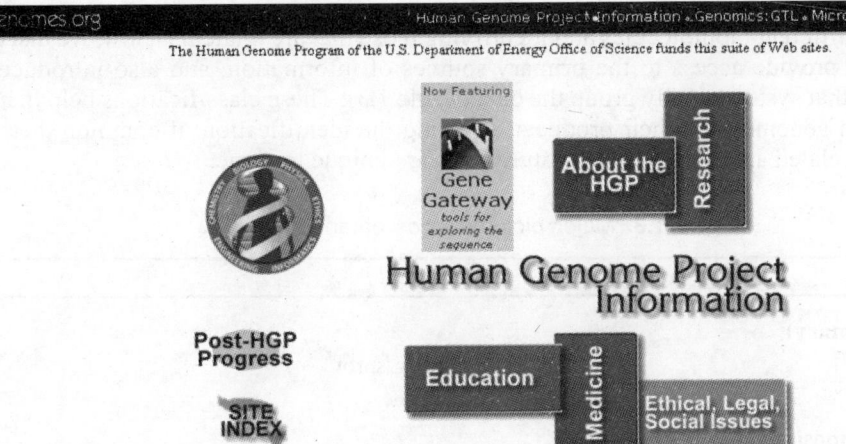

The Human Genome Program of the U.S. Department of Energy Office of Science funds this suite of Web sites.

Welcome! Explore this site for information about the Human Genome Project (1990-2003).

Completed in 2003, the Human Genome Project (HGP) was a 13-year project coordinated by the U.S. Department of Energy and the National Institutes of Health. During the early years of the HGP, the Wellcome Trust (U.K.) became a major partner; additional contributions came from Japan, France, Germany, China, and others. See our history page for more information.

Project goals were to

- *identify* all the approximately 20,000-25,000 genes in human DNA,
- *determine* the sequences of the 3 billion chemical base pairs that make up human DNA,
- *store* this information in databases,
- *improve* tools for data analysis,
- *transfer* related technologies to the private sector, and
- *address* the ethical, legal, and social issues (ELSI) that may arise from

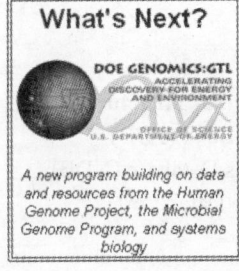

What's Next?

DOE GENOMICS:GTL
ACCELERATING
DISCOVERY FOR ENERGY
AND ENVIRONMENT
U.S. DEPARTMENT OF ENERGY

A new program building on data and resources from the Human Genome Project, the Microbial Genome Program, and systems biology

Fig. 1.1. Home page of Human Genome Project.

1.4 MULTIPLICITY OF DATA AND DATA MINING

During the last few years, bioinformatics has been overwhelmed with increasing floods of data, both in terms of volume and in terms of new databases and new types of data. In post-genomics era, in addition to complete genome sequences, we are learning about gene expression patterns and protein interactions on genomic scales. This poses new challenges and the traditional ways of dealing with data, item by item, are no longer feasible.

A concept that underpins most research methods in bioinformatics is that much of the data can be grouped together based on biologically meaningful similarities. It is necessary to explore data by *data mining*. Data mining is defined as "exploration and analysis by automatic and semi-automatic means, of large quantities of data in order to discover meaningful patterns and rules".

Data mining and the knowledge discovery process involve much more than the simple statistical analysis of data. For example, difficult-to-describe metrics, such as novelty, interestingness, and understandability, are often used to define data mining parameters for data discovery.

1.5 MAJOR BIOINFORMATICS DATABASES

An essential aspect of managing this large volume of data lies in developing methods for assessing similarities between different biomolecules and identifying those that are related. Below, we discuss the major databases that provide access to the primary sources of information, and also introduce some secondary databases that systematically group the data (Table 1.3). These classifications help in making comparisons between genomes and their products, allowing the identification of common themes between those that are related and highlighting features that are unique to some.

Table 1.3. Major bioinformatics databases

Database	Electronic address (URL)
Protein sequence (primary)	
SWISS-PROT	http://www.expasy.org/sprot/
PIR-International	pir.georgetown.edu/
Protein sequence (composite)	
OWL	http://umber.sbs.man.ac.uk/dbbrowser/OWL/
Protein sequence (secondary)	
PROSITE	http://www.expasy.org/prosite/http://www.expasy.org/prosite/
PRINTS	http://umber.sbs.man.ac.uk/dbbrowser/PRINTS/
Pfam	http://www.sanger.ac.uk/Software/Pfam/
Macromolecular structures	
Protein Data Bank (PDB)	www.rcsb.org/pdb/
Nucleic Acids Database (NDB)	http://ndbserver.rutgers.edu/
HIV Protease Database	http://mcl1.ncifcrf.gov/hivdb/
ReLiBase	http://relibase.ebi.ac.uk/reli-cgi/rll?/reli-cgi/general_layout.pl+home
PDBsum	http://www.biochem.ucl.ac.uk/bsm/pdbsum/
CATH	http://www.biochem.ucl.ac.uk/bsm/cath/
SCOP	http://scop.mrc-lmb.cam.ac.uk/scop/
FSSP	http://www.bioinfo.biocenter.helsinki.fi:8080/dali/index.html
Nucleotide sequences	
GenBank	http://www.ncbi.nlm.nih.gov/Genbank/
EMBL	http://www.ebi.ac.uk/embl/
DDBJ	http://www.ddbj.nig.ac.jp/
Genome sequences	
Entrez genomes	http://www.ncbi.nlm.nih.gov/entrez/query.fcgi?db=Genome
GeneCensus	http://bioinfo.mbb.yale.edu/genome/
COGs	http://www.ncbi.nlm.nih.gov/COG/
Integrated databases	
InterPro	http://www.ebi.ac.uk/interpro/
Sequence retrieval system (SRS)	http://www.expasy.ch/srs5
Entrez	http://www.ncbi.nlm.nih.gov/Entrez

1. Protein Databases

Protein sequence databases are categorised as primary and composite or secondary. These are discussed below.

Primary databases

Primary protein databases contain over 300,000 protein sequences and function as a repository for the raw data. Some more common repositories, such as SWISS-PROT and PIR-International, annotate the sequences as well as describe the proteins' functions, its domain structure and post-translational modifications.

The two major protein sequence databases SWISS-PROT and PIR are both curated. Groups of designated curators (scientists) prepare and annotate the entries from literature. SWISS-PROT strives to provide a high level of annotations (such as the description of the function of a protein, its domains structure, post-translational modifications, variants, etc.), a minimal level of redundancy and high level of integration with other databases. An entry from SWISS-PROT is shown in Fig. 1.2.

TrEMBL is a computer-annotated supplement of SWISS-PROT that contains all the translations of EMBL nucleotide sequence entries not yet integrated in SWISS-PROT.

PIR pir.georgetown.edu

The Protein Information Resource (PIR) grew out of Margaret Dayhoff's work in the middle of the 1960s. It strives to be comprehensive, well-organized, accurate, and consistently annotated.

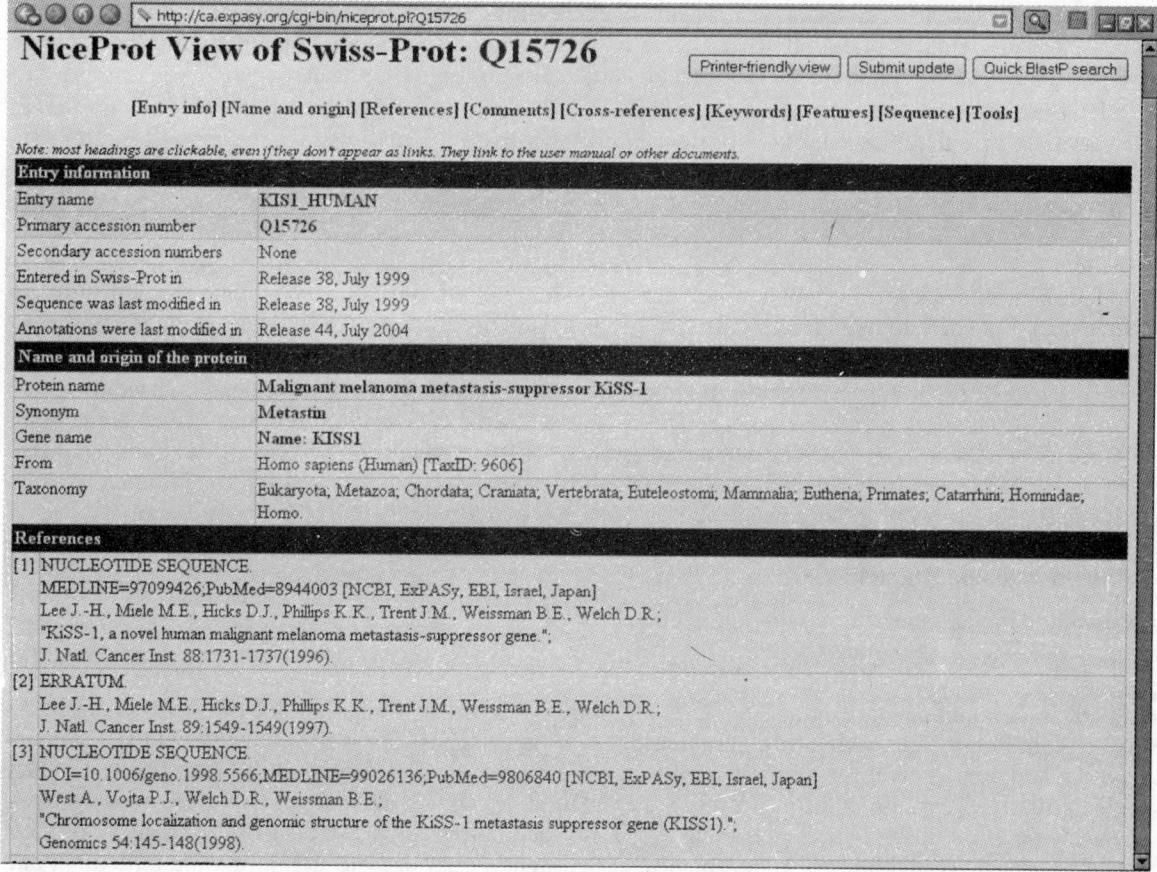

Fig. 1.2. A sample Swiss-Prot entry.

One can search for entries or do sequence similarity searches at the PIR site. The database can also be downloaded as a set of flat files. PIR also produces the PIR-NRL3D (http://pir.georgetown.edu/ pirwww/dbinfo/nrl3d.html), which is a database of sequences extracted from the three-dimensional structures in the Protein Databank (PDB). The PIR-NRL3D database makes the sequence information in PDB available for similarity searches and retrieval and provides cross-reference information for use with the other PIR Protein Sequence Databases.

Composite databases

Examples of such databases are OWL and PROSITE. These databases compile and filter sequence data from different primary databases to produce combined non-redundant sets that are more complete than the individual databases and also include protein sequence data from the translated coding regions in DNA sequence databases. Secondary databases contain information derived from protein sequences and help the user determine whether a new sequence belongs to a known protein family.

PROSITE www.expasy.ch/prosite/

PROSITE is a database of short sequence patterns and profiles that characterize biologically signifi-cant sites in proteins. PROSITE is a database of protein families and domains. It consists of *patterns* and *profiles* that help to reliably identify to which known protein family a new sequence belongs. It is part of SWISS-PROT system. The basis of it is regular expressions describing characteristic subsequences of specific protein families or domains. BLOCKS patterns without gaps in aligned protein families defined by PROSITE, found by pattern searching and statistical sampling algorithms

PRINTS expands on this concept and provides a compendium of protein fingerprints – groups of conserved motifs that characterize a protein family. Motifs are usually separated along a protein se-quence, but may be contiguous in 3D-space when the protein is folded. By using multiple motifs, finger-prints can encode protein folds and functionalities more flexibly than PROSITE.

Pfam http://www.sanger.ac.uk/Software/Pfam/

Pfam is a database of protein families defined as domains (contiguous segments of entire protein sequences). For each domain, it contains a multiple alignment of a set of defining sequences (the seeds) and the other sequences in SWISS-PROT and TrEMBL that can be matched to that alignment.

The alignments can be converted into Hidden Markov models (HMM), which can be used to search for domains in a query protein sequence. The software HMMER (http://hmmer.wustl.edu/) is the com-putational foundation for Pfam. The domain structure of protein sequences in SWISS-PROT and TrEMBL are available directly from the Pfam web sites, and it is also possible to search for domains in other sequences using servers at the web sites.

2. Structural databases

Structural databases pertain to macromolecular structures.

Protein Data Bank (PDB) www.rcsb.org/pdb/

PDB is the main primary database for 3D structures of biological macromolecules determined by X-ray crystallography and NMR. Structural biologists usually deposit their structures in the PDB on pub-lication, and some scientific journals require this before accepting a paper. PDB provides a primary archive of all 3D structures for macromolecules such as proteins, RNA, DNA and various complexes. Most of the ~13,000 structures are solved by x-ray crystallography and NMR, but some theoretical models are also available. It also accepts the experimental data used to determine the structures and homology models.

The PDB entries contain the atomic co-ordinates, and some structural parameters connected with the atoms, or computed from the structures (secondary structure). The annotation in PDB entries is not as comprehensive as in SWISS-PROT.

There are two major databases that classify proteins by structure in order to identify structural and evolutionary relationships: CATH and SCOP databases. Both comprise hierarchical structural taxonomy where groups of proteins increase in similarity at lower levels of the classification tree.

CATH www.biochem.ucl.ac.uk/bsm/cath/

The CATH database (Class, architecture, topology, homologous super-family) is a hierarchical classification of protein domain structures, which clusters proteins at four major structural levels.

SCOP scop.mrc-lmb.cam.ac.uk/scop/

The SCOP (Structural Classification of Proteins) database was started to classify protein 3D structures in a hierarchical scheme of structural classes. It is a curated database, all protein structures in the PDB are classified, and it is updated as new structures are deposited in the PDB. This is a typical secondary database - based on data in PDB, a primary database, but adds information through analysis. The analysis results in the classification of protein 3d structures into a hierarchical scheme of folds, super-families and families.

In addition, there are numerous databases that focus on particular types of macromolecules. These include the Nucleic Acids Database (NDB), for structures related to nucleic acids, the HIV protease database for HIV-1, HIV-2 and SIV protease structures and their complexes, and ReLiBase for receptor-ligand complexes.

3. Nucleotide and Genome sequences

The GenBank, EMBL and DDBJ databases contain DNA sequences for individual genes that encode protein and RNA products. These databases are the three primary nucleotide sequence databases and include sequences submitted directly by researchers and genome sequencing groups and sequences taken indirectly from literature and patents.

The entries in the EMBL, GenBank and DDBJ databases are synchronized on a daily basis and the accession numbers are managed in a consistent manner between these three. The nucleotide databases have reached such large sizes that they are available in subdivisions that allow searches or download that are more limited, and hence less time-consuming.

GenBank www.ncbi.nlm.nih.gov/Genbank/

The GenBank nucleotide database is maintained by the National Center for Biotechnology Information (NCBI), which is part of the National Institute of Health (NIH), a federal agency of the US government. It can be accessed and searched through the Entrez system at NCBI, or one can download the entire database as flat files.

EMBL www.ebi.ac.uk/embl/

The European Bioinformatics Institute (EBI) maintains the EMBL (European Molecular Biology Laboratory) nucleotide sequence database. It can be accessed and searched through the SRS system at EBI, or one can download the entire database as flat files.

DDBJ www.ddbj.nig.ac.jp

The DNA Data Bank of Japan began as collaboration with EMBL and GenBank.

Secondary nucleotide sequence databases contain subsets of the EMBL/GenBank databases. Some also contain more information or links than the primary ones, or have a different organization of the data to better some specific purpose. However, the nucleotide sequences themselves should always be available in the EMBL/GenBank databases.

UniGene www.ncbi.nlm.nih.gov/UniGene/

The UniGene system processes the GenBank sequence data into a non-redundant set of gene-oriented clusters. Each UniGene cluster contains sequences that represent a unique gene, as well as related information such as the tissue types in which the gene has been expressed and map location.

SGD genome-www.stanford.edu/Saccharomyces/

The Saccharomyces Genome Database (SGD) is a scientific database of the molecular biology and genetics of the yeast *Saccharomyces cerevisiae.*

EBI Genomes www.ebi.ac.uk/genomes/

This web site provides access and statistics for the completed genomes, and information about ongoing projects.

Ensembl www.ensembl.org

Ensembl is a joint project between EMBL-EBI and the Sanger Centre to develop a software system that produces and maintains automatic annotation on eukaryotic genomes.

As whole-genome sequencing is often conducted through international collaborations, individual genomes are published at different sites. The Entrez genome database brings together all complete and partial genomes in a single location and currently represents over 1,000 organisms. In addition to providing the raw nucleotide sequence, information is presented at several levels of detail including a list of completed genomes, all chromosomes in an organism, detailed views of single chromosomes marking coding and non-coding regions, and single genes. At each level there are graphical presentations, pre-computed analyses and links to other sections of Entrez. For example, annotations for single genes include the translated protein sequence, sequence alignments with similar genes in other genomes and summaries of the experimentally characterised or predicted function.

GeneCensus also provides an entry point for genome analysis with an interactive whole-genome comparison from an evolutionary perspective. The database allows building of phylogenetic trees based on different criteria such as ribosomal RNA or protein fold occurrence. The site also enables multiple genome comparisons, analysis of single genomes and retrieval of information for individual genes.

The COGs database classifies proteins encoded in 21 completed genomes on the basis of sequence similarity. Members of the same Cluster of Orthologous Group, COG, are expected to have the same 3D domain architecture and often, similar functions. An application of the database is to predict the function of uncharacterised proteins through their homology to characterised proteins, and also to identify phylogenetic patterns of protein occurrence.

4. Gene Expression data

The sources of genomic-scale data have been from expression experiments, which quantify the expression levels of individual genes. These experiments measure the amount of mRNA or protein products that are produced by the cell. There are three main technologies: the cDNA microarray, Affymetrix GeneChip and SAGE methods. The first method measures relative levels of mRNA abundance between different samples, while the last two measure absolute levels. Most of the effort in gene expression analysis has concentrated on the yeast and human genomes and till now there is no central repository for this data.

5. Other Databases

GeneCards bioinformatics.weizmann.ac.il/cards/

GeneCards is a database of human genes, their products and their involvement in diseases. It offers information about the functions of human genes. It is an example of a secondary database, which contains many links to other databases, and attempts to consolidate the information that is available for a specific class of entity.

KEGG www.genome.ad.jp/kegg/

The Kyoto Encyclopaedia of Genes and Genomes (KEGG) is an effort to computerize current knowledge of molecular and cellular biology in terms of the information pathways that consist of interacting molecules or genes and to provide links from the gene catalogues produced by genome sequencing projects.

1.6 DATA INTEGRATION

The most useful research in bioinformatics often results from integrating multiple sources of data. For instance, the 3D coordinates of a protein are more useful if combined with data about the protein's function, occurrence in different genomes, and interactions with other molecules. In this way, individual pieces of information are put in context with respect to other data. Unfortunately, it is not always straightforward to access and cross-reference these sources of information because of differences in nomenclature and file formats.

This problem is frequently addressed by providing external links to other databases, for example in PDBsum, web-pages for individual structures direct the user towards corresponding entries in the PDB, NDB, CATH, SCOP and SWISS-PROT. At a more advanced level, there have been efforts to integrate access across several data sources.

One is the Sequence Retrieval System (SRS), which allows any flat-file databases to be indexed to each other; this allows the user to retrieve, link and access entries from nucleic acid, protein sequence, protein motif, protein structure and bibliographic databases.

SRS is a system for integrating heterogenous databases. It is based on premade indexes of the items (words, entries, data fields, text etc.) found in a set of documents (database files). Apart from the database files themselves, the indexing procedure requires a grammar (Icarus) that describes what different words in the data files mean how they are to be indexed, and how they cross-reference to other items in other databases.

EBI runs an SRS service that can be used by anyone. It indexes a large number of databases, and it also provides a well-defined web interface that allows programs or web sites to create links that query SRS at EBI.

Another is the Entrez facility, which provides similar gateways to DNA and protein sequences, genome mapping data, 3D macromolecular structures and the PubMed bibliographic database. A search for a particular gene in either database will allow smooth transitions to the genome it comes from, the protein sequence it encodes, its structure, bibliographic reference and equivalent entries for all related genes.

The Entrez system is developed and accessible at the NCBI Entrez site. Similar to the SRS system, it provides search facilities for a large number of databases, and provides links between them. It provides a well-defined web interface that allows programs or web sites to define links that will query Entrez. However, the Entrez system is not available to set up at one's own server. It is purely a system for accessing and searching the databases at NCBI.

1.7 DATA ANALYSIS

Having examined the data, we can discuss the types of analyses that are conducted. As shown in Table 1.4, the broad subject areas in bioinformatics can be differentiated according to the sources of information that are used in the studies.

1. For raw DNA sequences, investigations involve separating coding and non-coding regions, and identification of introns, exons and promoter regions for annotating genomic DNA.
2. For protein sequences, analyses include developing algorithms for sequence comparisons, methods for producing multiple sequence alignments, and searching for functional domains from conserved sequence motifs in such alignments.
3. Investigations of structural data include prediction of secondary and tertiary protein structures, producing methods for 3D structural alignments, examining protein geometries using distance and angular measurements, calculations of surface and volume shapes and analysis of protein interactions with other subunits, DNA, RNA and smaller molecules.
4. These studies have lead to molecular simulation topics in which structural data are used to calculate the energetics involved in stabilizing macromolecular structures, simulating movements within macromolecules, and computing the energies involved in molecular docking.
5. The increasing availability of annotated genomic sequences has resulted in the introduction of computational genomics and proteomics – large-scale analyses of complete genomes and the proteins that they encode. Research includes characterization of protein content and metabolic pathways between different genomes, identification of interacting proteins, assignment and prediction of gene products, and large-scale analyses of gene expression levels.
6. Other subject areas of interest are development of digital libraries for automated bibliographical searches, knowledge bases of biological information from the literature, DNA analysis methods in forensics, prediction of nucleic acid structures, metabolic pathway simulations, and linkage analysis – linking specific genes to different disease traits.
7. In addition to finding relationships between different proteins, much of bioinformatics involves the analysis of one type of data to infer and understand the observations for another type of data. An example is the use of sequence and structural data to predict the secondary and tertiary structures of new protein sequences. These methods, especially the former, are often based on statistical rules derived from structures, such as the propensity for certain amino acid sequences to produce different secondary structural elements. Another example is the use of structural data to understand a protein's function; here studies have investigated the relationship different protein folds and their functions and analysed similarities between different binding sites in the absence of homology. Combined with similarity measurements, these studies provide us with an understanding of how much biological information can be accurately transferred between homologous proteins.

1.8 CAREERS IN BIOINFORMATICS

What skills are needed to pursue a career in bioinformatics? The answer is not quite easy, but broadly the prospective bioinformatics professional needs to have the following skill-sets:

1. Background in aspects of molecular biology - biochemistry, cell biology, molecular physics etc.
2. Understand the central dogma of molecular biology - how information is used in the biological systems
3. Basic comfort levels in using computers. You need to be familiar with Unix operating systems and Internet.
4. Understanding of the basic mathematical modeling techniques including statistical methods, probability and algorithms for sequence searching, pattern recognition etc.

Table 1.4 Illustration of analysis of data

Function	Types	Tools
Text based query of sequence databases	Search multiple databases like GenBank, SwissProt etc. Search DNA Sequence Databases Search Protein Sequence Databases Search 3D Structure Databases	Entrez Sequence Retrieval System GenBank SwissProt PIR PDB
Sequence Format Conversion Tools	Utilities which convert between several different sequence formats	SEQIO READSEQ
Database Similarity/ homology Searches	Integrated interfaces for the comparison of DNA and Protein sequence to existing DNA and Protein sequence databases and the rapid retrieval of the full database entries matched.	Basic Local Alignment Search Tool (BLAST) Parallel Fasta for Proteins Fasta3
Sequence Alignments	Compare two DNA or Protein Sequences Compare Multiple DNA or Protein Sequences	Dot Plot Clustal W
Determine DNA sites	Determine Restriction Enzyme Cut Sites in DNA	TACG2
Protein sequencing	Protein Sequence Analysis Tools	SAPS -Statistical Analysis of Protein Sequences ExPASy
Nucleic acid sequencing	Nucleic Acid Sequence Analysis Tools	BCM Gene Finder
Gene modeling	Predict Splice sites, Protein coding exons and Gene model construction	ProteinProspector
Protein structure prediction	Protein Secondary structure prediction	nnPredict PHD - Predict Protein Secondary Structure ProDom - A Protein Domain Database Pfam
Pattern Searches	Search for matches against "pattern databases"	Prosite database Signal Scan

5. If you are interested in development, you need to learn a programming language like C++ and Java. Perl and XML are the software most useful for working on the Web for the biologist. A grasp of these is essential for a lot of the Web/database work being done by many bioinformaticists.

How are these skills put to use? The tasks range from simple to highly complex, covering the cutting edge technology. The simplest tasks concern the creation and maintenance of databases of biological information. Nucleic acid sequences (and the protein sequences) comprise the majority of such databases. While the storage and organization of millions of nucleotides is far from trivial, designing a database and developing an interface whereby researchers can both access existing information and submit new entries is only the beginning.

The most common tasks in bioinformatics involve the analysis of sequence information, with applications like the following :

1. Finding the genes in the DNA sequences of various organisms
2. Developing methods to predict the structure and/or function of newly discovered proteins and structural RNA sequences.

3. Clustering protein sequences into families of related sequences and the development of protein models.
4. Aligning similar proteins and generating phylogenetic trees to examine evolutionary relationships.
5. The process of evolution has produced DNA sequences that encode proteins with very specific functions. It is possible to predict the three-dimensional structure of a protein using algorithms that have been derived from our knowledge of physics, chemistry and most importantly, from the analysis of other proteins with similar amino acid sequences.

1.9 CLASSIFICATION OF BIOINFORMATICS DATABASES AND TOOLS

Some important databases used widely are given here. The classification of various tools can be done on the following basis :

1. Databases

(i) Generalized databases (DNA, proteins and carbohydrates, 3D-structures)
(ii) Specialized databases (EST, STS, SNP, RNA, genomes, protein families, pathways, microarray data etc.)

2. Database search

(i) Text-based database search (SRS, Entrez etc.)
(ii) Sequence-based database search (sequence similarity search) (BLAST, FASTA etc.)
(iii) Motif-based database search (ScanProsite, eMOTIF)
(iv) Structure-based database search (structure similarity search) (VAST, DALI etc.)

3. Analysis tools

(i) DNA sequence analysis tools
(ii) RNA analysis tools
(iii) Protein sequence and structure analysis tools (primary, secondary, tertiary structure)

4. Tools for function analysis

(i) Phylogeny
(ii) Microarray analysis tools
(iii) Bioinformatics centers and servers

5. Other tools and resources

The description and examples of the tools/databases are listed below:

1. Databases

(i) **Generalized DNA, protein and carbohydrate databases**
   (a) **Primary sequence databases**
       EMBL http://www.ebi.ac.uk/embl/
       GenBank http://www.ncbi.nlm.nih.gov/Genbank/
       DDBJ http://www.ddbj.nig.ac.jp/

(b) **Protein sequence databases**
SWISS-PROT/TrEMBL http://www.expasy.org/sprot/
PIR pir.georgetown.edu/
(c) **Carbohydrate databases**
CarbBank (http://bssv01.lancs.ac.uk/gig/pages/gag/carbbank.htm)
(d) **3D structure databases**
PDB (www.rcsb.org/pdb/)

(ii) **Specialized databases**
(a) **Specialized sequence databases**
dbEST (www.ncbi.nlm.nih.gov/dbEST/)
HGBASE (www.fccc.edu/research/labs/ dunbrack/sauder/biolinks/hgbase.html)
(b) **RNA databases**
European Ribosomal RNA Database (http://www.psb.ugent.be/rRNA/index.html)
(c) **Genome databases**
GOLD (www.genomesonline.org/)
TIGR Database (www.tigr.org/tdb/)
(d) **Model organism databases**
E. coli Genome Project http://www.genome.wisc.edu/
TIGR *Arabidopsis thaliana* Database http://www.tigr.org/tdb/e2k1/ath1/
HGP www.sanger.ac.uk/HGP/
(e) **Specific protein family databases**
TRANSFAC (Transcription Factor Database) http://www.gene-regulation.com/
G-Protein Coupled Receptor Database www.**gpcr**.org/7tm/
The restriction enzyme database **ebase**.neb.com/**rebase/rebase**.html
(f) **Protein classification databases**
Pfam ww.sanger.ac.uk/Software/Pfam/
SCOP (Structural Classification of Proteins according to familiy, superfamily, common fold, and class) scop.mrc-lmb.cam.ac.uk/scop/
CATH (Protein structure classification based on Class, Architecture, Topology, and Homologous superfamilies) www.biochem.ucl.ac.uk/bsm/cath/
(g) **Specialized structure databases**
Protein-Nucleic Acid Recognition Database www.rtc.riken.go.jp/jouhou/3dinsight/recognition.html
3DInSight www.rtc.riken.go.jp/jouhou/3dinsight/3dinsight.html
MolMovDB molmovdb.mbb.yale.edu/molmovdb/
(h) **Pathway databases**
KEGG www.genome.jp/kegg/
EcoCyc www.ecocyc.org/
(i) **Microarray databases**
ArrayExpress www.ebi.ac.uk/**arrayexpress/**

2. Database Search

(i) **Text-based database search**
ENTREZ www.ncbi.nlm.nih.gov/**entrez**/query.fcgi

SRS6 http://srs6.ebi.ac.uk/srsbin
DBGET www.genome.jp/**dbget**/
(ii) Sequence-based database search (sequence similarity search)
FASTA http://www.ebi.ac.uk/fasta33/
BLAST www.ncbi.nlm.nih.gov/Education/ BLASTinfo/information3.html
PSI BLAST www.ncbi.nlm.nih.gov/Education/BLASTinfo/**psi**1.html
(iii) Protein Motif-based database search
ScanProsite www.expasy.org/tools/**scanprosite**
(iv) Structure-based database search (structure similarity search)
VAST http://www.fccc.edu/research/labs/dunbrack/sauder/biolinks/vast.html
DALI http://www.ebi.ac.uk/dali/

3 Analysis Tools

(i) **DNA sequence analysis tools**
  (a) **Restriction; Detect repeats and unusual patterns**
    Webcutter http://www.firstmarket.com/cutter/cut2.html
    LALIGN fasta.bioch.virginia.edu/fasta_www/**lalign**.htm
  (b) **Align sequences**
    ClustalW www.ebi.ac.uk/**clustalw**/
  (c) **Find genes**
    ORF Finder bioinformatics.org/sms/**orf**_find.html
    GeneMark www.ebi.ac.uk/**genemark**/
    GRAIL http://compbio.ornl.gov/Grail-1.3/
  (d) **Find transcriptional elements**
    SignalScan http://www-bimas.cit.nih.gov/molbio/signal/
  (e) **Find tRNA**
    tRNAscan-SE www.genetics.wustl.edu/eddy/tRNAscan-SE/
  (f) **Other tools**
    CountCodon www.kazusa.or.jp/codon/**countcodon**.html
  (g) **PCR primer selection**
    Primer3 www.genome.wi.mit.edu/cgi-bin/primer/**primer3**_www.cgi
(ii) **RNA analysis tools**
  MFOLD www.bioinfo.rpi.edu/applications/**mfold**/
  RNA World www.imb-jena.de/RNA.html
(iii) **Protein sequence and structure analysis tools**
  (a) **Physicochemical properties**
    ProtParam www.expasy.org/tools/**protparam**.html
  (b) **Analyse primary sequence**
    SAPS (Statistical Analysis for charge clusters, repeats, hydrophobic regions, compositional domains etc.) www.ebi.ac.uk/**saps**/
  (c) **Predict secondary structure**
    TMpred www.microbiology.adelaide.edu.au/learn/**tmpred**.htm
    PredictProtein www.embl-heidelberg.de/ **predictprotein/predictprotein**.html
    PairCoil theory.lcs.mit.edu/**paircoil**

(d) **3D viewers**
RasMol www.umass.edu/microbio/**rasmol/**
Cn3D ww.biosino.org/mirror/ www.ncbi.nlm.nih.gov/Structure/**cn3d/**

(e) **3D analysis**
TOPS www3.ebi.ac.uk/**tops/**

(f) **3D homology modeling**
Swiss-Model www.expasy.org/swissmod/SWISS-MODEL.html

(g) **Search for patterns, motifs, profiles, domains, families**
ScanProsite www.expasy.org/tools/**scanprosite/**
PFSCAN www.isrec.isb-sib.ch/software/PFSCAN_form.html
MEME **meme**.sdsc.edu/

(h) **Search and computation of pathways**
KEGG www.genome.jp/**kegg**

(i) **Protein-protein interactions**
DIP http://dip.doe-mbi.ucla.edu/

4. Tools for function analysis

(i) **Phylogenetic Analysis**
(a) **Multiple sequence alignment**
ClustalW www.ebi.ac.uk/**clustalw/**
(b) **Organism classification**
NCBI Taxonomy www.**ncbi**.nlm.nih.gov/entrez/query.fcgi?db=Taxonomy

(ii) **Microarray Data Analysis**
ClustArray www.cbs.dtu.dk/services/DNAarray/

5. Other tools and resources

(i) **Literature search**
PubMed www.ncbi.nlm.nih.gov/entrez/query.fcgi

(ii) Bioinformatics centers and servers
Biology Workbench **workbench**.sdsc.edu/
EBI www.**ebi**.ac.uk/
ExPASy www.**expasy**.org/

2

Molecular Biology and Bioinformatics

2.1. WHAT IS MOLECULAR BIOLOGY?

Molecular biology is the understanding of biological processes at the molecular level, (i.e) via physico-chemical laws. Molecular biology grew out of Genetics and Biochemistry. Biological processes involve molecules that can form complex biological structures (organelles, membranes, tissues, and organs). These structures interact via molecules. These molecules are present in the organism ultimately due to expression of information residing in the genetic material. Molecular biology fundamentally looks at the molecular understanding of inheritance or heredity.

Molecular biology deals with the biological activity at the molecular level - the other levels of abstraction of biological activity are the atomic at the basic level and the network level at a higher level than the molecular level. Hence, while it is important to study the atomic basis of biological activity, the approach taken by molecular biologists is to "reduce" it to a molecular level. The interaction between the various macro-molecules and their transformation within the cell is part of the pathway or network study.

2.2 SYSTEMS APPROACH IN BIOLOGY

The systems approach is useful to understand the complex systems like biological systems. The basic building blocks of biological systems are molecules like nucleic acids and proteins. The systems view gives the ease of integration of various approaches to understand their structure and function. While the traditional approach is "experimental" - performing various experiments in the laboratory to understand the molecular biology; bioinformatics offers a "synthetic" approach. The synthetic approach is much faster and in certain cases, is as reliable as the experimental approach.

2.3 CENTRAL DOGMA OF MOLECULAR BIOLOGY

The basic molecular biology (and in a way the living organisms) are governed by the central dogma of molecular biology. Central dogma of molecular biology is basically as follows : DNA makes RNA makes Protein. The processes related to central dogma are as follows:

- DNA makes DNA: *replication*
- DNA makes RNA: *transcription*
- RNA makes Protein: *translation*

18

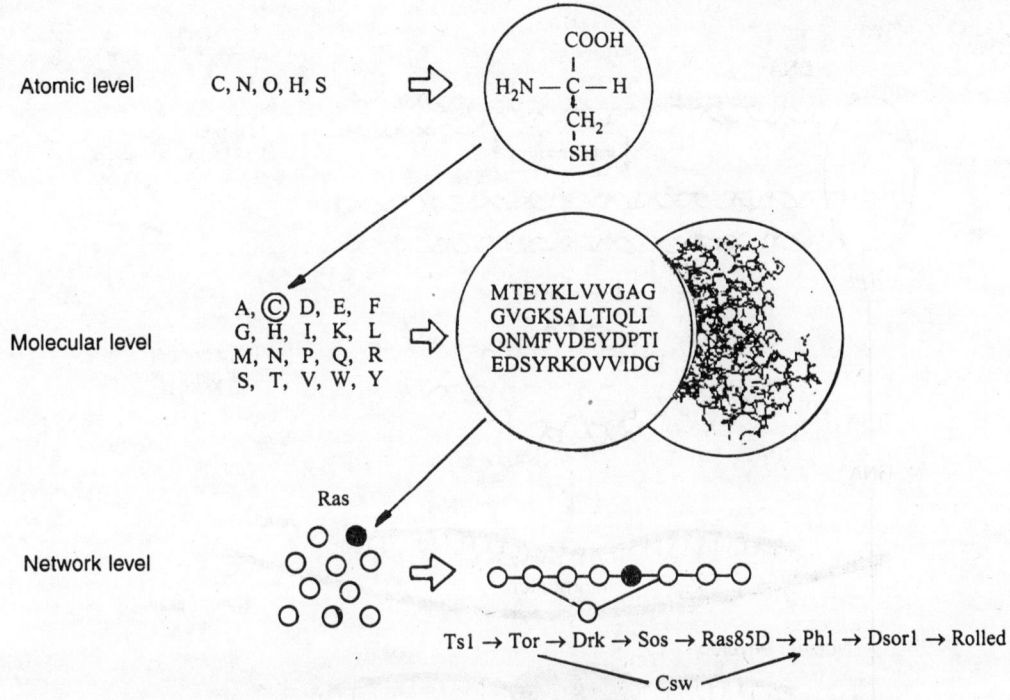

Fig. 2.1. The concept of level of abstraction - molecular level does not consider the atomic level activities.

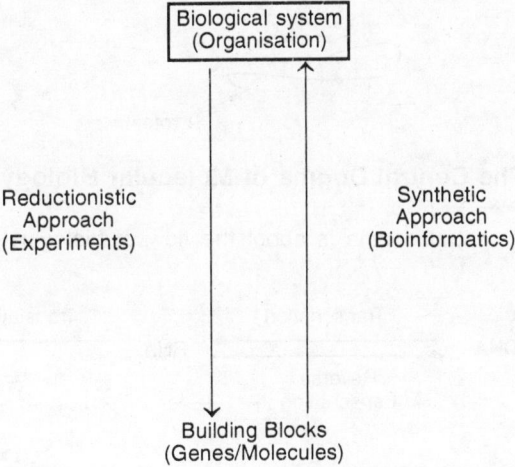

Fig. 2.2. Bioinformatics approach to the understanding of the biological systems.

Chromosomal Theory of Inheritance

There is a correlation of genetic maps with physical organelles called Chromosomes. Chromosomes contain the genetic material. Chiasmata is observed during meiosis (recombination). Gross mutational aberrations (translocations, etc) result in physical change in chromosome.

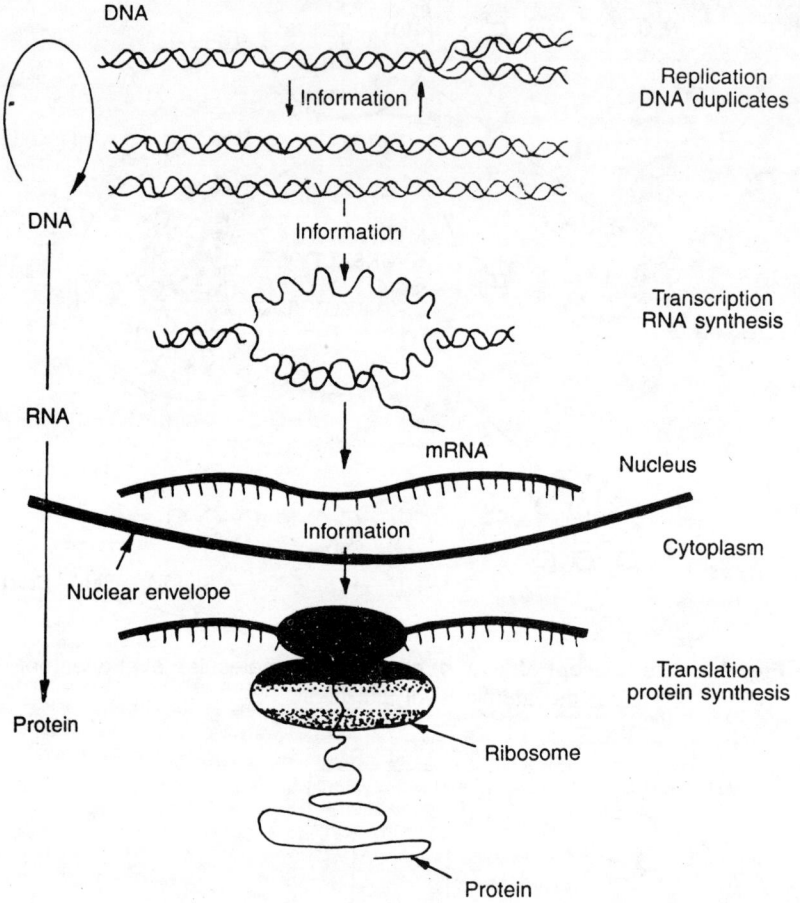

The Central Dogma of Molecular Biology

Fig 2.3. The central dogma is about the flow of biological information

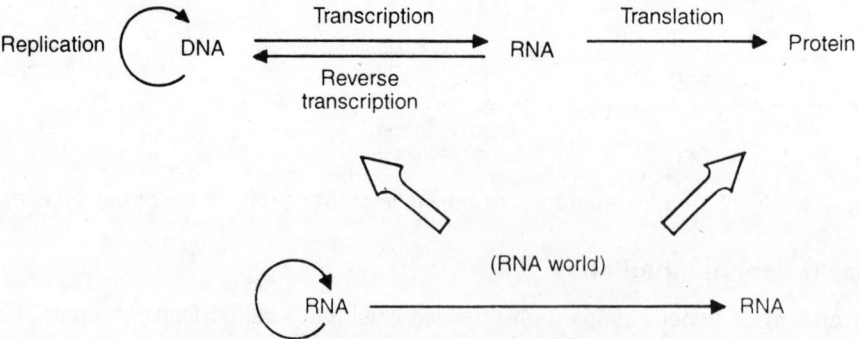

Fig 2.4. The systems view of the central dogma

Table 2.1. Molecules participating in information flow and the functional sites

Molecule	Processing	Functional sites	Interacting molecules
DNA	Replication transcription	Replication origin Promotor Enhancer Operator and other prokaryotic regulators	Origin recognition complex RNA polymerase Transcription factor Repressor, etc
RNA	Post-transcriptional processing Translation	Splice site Translation initiation site	Spliceosome Ribosome
Protein	Post-translational processing Protein sorting Protein function	Cleavage site Phosphorylation and other modification sites ATP binding sites Signal sequence, localization signals DNA binding sites Ligand binding sites Catalytic sites	Protease Protein kinase, etc. Signal recognition particle DNA Ligands Many different molecules

Table 2.2. Description of entities related to the central dogma and their principal function

Entity	Definition	Molecular Mechanisms
Genome	Unit of information transmission	DNA replication
Gene	Unit of information expression	Transcription to RNA Translation to protein

Table 2.3. The basics of the biological macromolecules

Macromolecule		Backbone	Repeating unit	Length	Role
Nucleic acid	DNA	Phosphodiester bonds	Deoxyribonucleotides (A, C, G, T)	10^3-10^8	Genome
	RNA	Phosphodiester bonds	Ribonucleotides (A, C, G, U)	10^3-10^5 10^3-10^4 10^2-10^3	Genome Messenger Gene product
Protein		Peptide bonds	Amino acids (A, C, D, E, F, G, H, I, K, L, M, N, P, Q, R, S, T, V, W, Y)	10^2-10^3	Gene product

2.4 IMPORTANT DEFINITIONS RELATED TO CENTRAL DOGMA

Genome

Genome is the total genetic material of an organism. The human genome is highly complex and contains about three billion nucleotides. The first draft of the human genome has revealed only between 30,000 to 40,000 genes which differs from the earlier much larger estimates.

DNA

All plants, bacteria, some viruses and animals contain genetic information in the form of DNA within their cells. A characteristic of living organisms is that DNA is reproduced and passed on to the next generation. DNA consists of two strands, which are in the form of a double helix.

DNA is a macromolecule composed of linear array of nucleotides, each of which comprises a base plus a deoxyribose sugar and phosphate. Four nucleotide bases form DNA: cytosine (C), thymine (T), adenine (A) and guanine (G). The information content of the DNA is embodied in the sequential arrangement of nucleotides. DNA contains the instructions for making proteins.

RNA

RNA is the other major nucleic acid and unlike DNA, it is single-stranded. It contains ribose instead of deoxyribose in its sugar-phosphate backbone, and uracil (U) instead of thymine (T) in its pyramidine bases. It can be assembled from nucleotides using DNA sequence as a template and RNA polymerase. Transcription preserves the whole information content of the DNA sequence that is transcribed on to RNA, since RNA has the same base-pairing characteristics. There are three major classes of RNA: messenger RNA (mRNA), transfer RNA (tRNA) and ribosomal RNA (rRNA).

Genes

A gene is a sequence of chromosomal DNA that is required for the production of a functional protein or a functional RNA molecule. Genes range in size from small (1.5 kb for globin gene) to large (approximately 2000 kb for Duchenne muscular dystrophy gene). A gene includes not only the actual coding sequences but also adjacent nucleotide sequences required for the proper expression of genes. Mature mRNA is about one-tenth the size of the gene from which it is transcribed. The same DNA strand of a gene is always translated into mRNA so that only one kind of mRNA is made for each gene. Genes are often described as blueprints of life and transmit inherited traits from one generation to another. Pseudo-genes are very similar to genes in terms of their structure, but do not do any protein synthesis.

Gene expression

Gene expression is the process in which DNA is used as a blueprint to produce a specific protein. Not all the genes are expressed in a typical human cell and those that are expressed vary from one cell to another. Patterns in which a gene is expressed provide clues to its biological role. Malfunctioning of genes is involved in most diseases, not only inherited ones. All functions of cells, tissues and organs are controlled by differential gene expression. For example, RBCs contain large amounts of the haemoglobin protein that is responsible for carrying oxygen throughout the body. The abundance of haemoglobin in RBCs reflects the fact that its encoding gene (the haemoglobin gene), is actively transcribed in the precursor cells that eventually produce red blood cells. In all other cells of the body, the hemoglobin does not express itself. It is this phenomenon that differential gene expression results in the carefully controlled (or regulated) expression of functional proteins, such as hemoglobin and insulin.

Gene expression is used for studying gene function. Genes are expressed in cultured cell lines by using viral vectors carrying cDNA, the transcription of which yields the gene's mRNA. The protein produced from mRNA may confer specific and detectable function on the cells used to express the gene. It is also possible to manipulate cDNA so that proteins are expressed in a soluble form fused to polypeptide tags. This allows purification of large amounts of proteins that can be used to raise antibodies or to probe protein function in vivo in animals. It is generally believed that a gene's protein-coding information is contained in only one of its two DNA strands, with this strand serving as a template for transcription of the precursor RNA that is eventually translated into protein.

Gene regulation

Mammalian cells possess the genetic instruction to make 50,000 to 100,000 different proteins but only 10-20% of these are found in any single cell. Therefore, a gene must contain instructions for the regulation of the production of protein in correct amount and at the correct time for each cell type. Gene regulation is one of the most complex molecular processes known, involving up to 10% of the proteins that our cells produce. Gene regulation can occur at a number of stages between DNA and the production of a particular protein-translational control and alternate splicing. Regulatory proteins that bind to specific sites on DNA can control gene expression. These are called activators or repressors depending on whether they increase or decrease transcription. Eukaryotes may have two systems for regulating genes- one using protein and the other using RNA.

Transcription factors

Gene regulation is mediated by a class of proteins termed "transcription factors" which bind to regulatory sequences of genes to increase or decrease the rate at which those genes are transcribed. Each gene has a unique set of transcription factors that regulates its activity. Gene is switched on during transcription. Protein factories (ribosomes) in the cell read the message from this RNA copy to manufacture the appropriate protein. The enzyme complex RNA polymerase unzips the DNA double helix and puts the RNA building blocks together. A single transcription factor can affect several genes in different ways. However, what regulates the transcription factors themselves, is unclear. They may respond to signals from the environment or other cells. The regulatory region of a gene can be considerably longer than the coding region. Small nucleotide sequences along the regulatory region serve as targets for specific transcription factors, which, in turn, are regulated in the cell in response to extracellular signals.

Chromatin

The complex of DNA and proteins of a chromosome is called chromatin and consists of histones and non-histone proteins. The basic structural unit of chromatin is a nucleosome, which is a complex of DNA with a core of histones.

Nucleosomes are further compacted to form solenoids, which are packed into loops, and each of these contains about 100,000 base pairs of DNA. The loops are the fundamental units of DNA replication and/or gene transcription. The protein machine that copies the chromosomes also plays a direct role in preserving the developmental state of cells. Chromatin is also reproduced for each gene to remain active or inactive as it was in the mother cell. The same complex of proteins that copies the DNA also transfers at least some of the special marks to the new chromosome as well.

2.5. PROBLEMS IN MOLECULAR APPROACH AND THE BIOINFORMATICS APPROACH

The information flow in the cell as understood by central dogma is fairly simple. However the complexity is enormous and gives rise to several problems for the biologist to resolve.

Some of the problems and their bioinformatics approach are summarised in the following table. (Table 2.4)

2.6. OVERVIEW OF BIOINFORMATICS APPLICATIONS

What are the kinds of problems bioinformatics can address and what is the approach? Some of these are illustrated in the discussion below:

Table 2.4.

Problems in Biological Science			Bioinformatics Method

Similarity search		Pairwise sequence alignment
		Database search for similar sequences
		Multiple sequence alignment
		Phylogenetic tree reconstruction
		Protein 3D structure alignment
			Optimization algorithms
			• Dynamic programming (DP)
			• Simulated annealing (SA)
			• Genetic algorithms (GA)
			• Markov Chain Monte Carlo
			  (MCMC: Metropolis and
			  Gibbs samplers)

Structure/function prediction	ab initio prediction	RNA secondary structure prediction RNA 3D structure prediction Protein 3D structure prediction	
	Knowledge based prediction	Motif extraction Functional site prediction Cellular localization prediction Coding region prediction Transmembrane domain prediction Protein secondary structure prediction Protein 3D structure prediction	Pattern recognition and learning algorithms 1. Discriminant analysis 2. Neural networks 3. Support vector machines 4. Hidden Markov models (HMM) 5. Formal grammar 6. CART
Molecular classification		Superfamily classification Ortholog/paralog grouping of genes 3D fold classification	Clustering algorithms Hierarchical, k-means, etc PCA, MDS, etc Self-organizing maps, etc

(i) DNA level

1. *Routine re-sequencing of megabase regions of genomic DNA* : Understanding the disease suscepti-bilities and predisposition - basically sequence affected and unaffected people. For example, isolate cancer cells, sequence tumour and normal tissue and get genotyping. Massively parallel DNA arrays are new sequencing technologies under development.

2. *Systematic identification of common variants in genes* : Usually, there are a small number of common variants per locus. Variants provide clues to susceptibilities, e.g. 3 variants of apolipoprotein E in Alzheimer's. Major applications include understanding of cardiovascular disease, thrombosis, heart disease, obesity, HIV resistance. The approach is to get most such variant sequences from sequences of 100 random individuals and move from Family-based Linkage Analyses to Associa-tion Analyses. This is usually done by testing disease susceptibility against all common variants simultaneously by genotyping a well-characterized clinical group with a comprehensive DNA ar-ray. This is done by characterizing the SNPs (Single Nucleotide Polymorphisms) associated with a given human disease. (Use of DNA array technology for human SNP analysis is already under-way with the availability of the Affymetrix GeneChip® and others.) This aids in identification of the susceptible genes.

3. *Rapid sequencing of other organisms* : Comparative whole genome analysis can provide clues about molecular evolution. While a conserved sequence provides information about key motifs; the sequence differences provide information about diversity of form and function. Bioinformatics provides facilities for sequencing - storage and automation of the analysis.

4. *DNA sequence assembly* : The problem : with given DNA sequence fragments of 200-700 base pairs length from a sequencing project, the objective is to assemble them into the original DNA sequence from which the fragments were derived. One approach is the Pairwise Sequence Alignment. For a given pair of sequences (DNA or protein) and a method for scoring similarity of sequences, one has to determine how similar the two sequences are (best similarity score) and show where the two sequences match (best alignment).

5. *Repetitive Sequences in DNA* : In the DNA domain, a motivation for multiple sequence alignment arises in the study of *repetitive sequences*. These are sequences of DNA, often without clearly understood biological functions, that are repeated many times throughout the genome. The repetitions are generally not exact, but differ from each other in a small number of insertions, deletions, and substitutions. As an example, the *Alu* repeat is approximately 300 bp long, and appears over 600,000 times in the human genome. It is believed that as much as 60% of the human genome may be attributable to repetitive sequences without known biological function. In order to highlight the similarities and differences among the instances of such a repeat family, one would like to display a good multiple sequence alignment of its constituent sequences.

(ii) RNA level

1. *Simultaneous Monitoring of Expression of all Genes* : mRNA levels define state of the cell. The approach is to monitor all mRNAs at quantitative sensitivity level of 1 molecule per cell and a qualitative sensitivity level sufficient to distinguish alternative splicing. Use of DNA microarrays can help in this. This information can be used for :
    1. Description: catalogs of proteins present in different cells, different stages, and different environments
    2. Classification: classify proteins re-susceptibilities, disease, and population subtypes
    3. Circuitry: Genetic Networks and gene expression circuits for development, response pathways

(iii) Monitoring Level and Modification State of all Proteins

It is important to monitor post-translational proteins and genetic network modifications, e.g. Phosphorylation State. It is possible to do a 2D Protein gel analyses of proteins, followed by Mass Spectrometry analysis. Mass Spectrometry analysis of peptide fragments helps in identification of Protein "signatures"

(iv) Identification of All Basic Protein Shapes

Most probably, there are limited number of protein shapes and hence a limited number of protein families. One can analyse amino acid sequences against database of protein shapes. Some of the bioinformatics databases are being used :

Pfam - protein multiple sequence alignments and common protein domains

SCOP - Structural Classification of Proteins

CATH - protein classification by Class, Architecture, Topology, and Homology

(v) Multiple Sequence Alignment of proteins

An important motivation for studying the similarity among multiple strings is the fact that protein databases are often categorized by protein families. A *protein family* is a collection of proteins with similar structure (i.e., three-dimensional shape), similar function, or similar evolutionary history. When we have a newly sequenced protein, we would like to know to which family it belongs, as this provides hypotheses about its structure, function, or evolutionary history. The new protein might not be particularly similar to a single protein in the database, yet might still share considerable similarity with the collective members of a family of proteins. One approach is to construct a representation for each protein family, for example a good multiple sequence alignment of all its members. Then, when we have a newly sequenced protein and want to find its family, we only have to compare it to the representation of each family. Common structure, function, or origin of a molecule may only be weakly reflected in its sequence. For example, the three-dimensional structure of a protein is very difficult to infer from its sequence, and yet is very important to predict its function. Multiple sequence comparisons may help highlight weak sequence similarity, and shed light on structure, function, or origin.

(vi) Determining Gene function

Much of Bioinformatics is focused on helping the biologist determine gene function. To do this, we need to:

- Find genes in a genome
- Predict the gene product
- Predict the gene function

Approaches to finding genes

- Search by sequence similarity: find genes by looking for matches to sequences that are know to be related to genes
- Search by signal: find genes by identifying the sequence signals involved in gene expression
- Search by content: find genes by statistical properties that distinguish protein-coding DNA from non-coding DNA

Evidence for genes can consist of matches to :

- Known proteins
- Protein motifs (e.g. zinc finger, ATP and GTP-binding motifs, etc.)
- Expressed sequence tags (ESTs)

Searching for matches to known proteins :

- Translate DNA sequence in all reading frames
- Search against protein database
- High-scoring matches suggest the presence of homologous genes in the DNA

3

The Information Molecules and Information Flow

3.1. INTRODUCTION

Nucleic acids are macromolecules present in all living cells, either in free state or in combination with proteins. Their main function is storage and transmission of genetic information. There are two types of nucleic acids, deoxyribonucleic acid (DNA) and ribonucleic acid (RNA). Both DNA and RNA are heteropolymers. The monomer units of DNA are deoxyribonucleotides and the monomer units of RNA are ribonucleotides.

3.2. BASIC COMPONENTS

Deoxyribonucleotides and ribonucleotides are comprised of three groups:

Bases

 a. The purines adenine and guanine are found in both DNA and RNA.
 b. The pyrimidines cytosine and thymine are found in DNA, while the pyrimidines cytosine and uracil are found in RNA.

Sugars

 a. DNA contains deoxyribose
 b. RNA contains ribose

Phosphate

DNA is a polymer of deoxyribonucleotides. Deoxyribonucleotides consist of :
 - A nitrogen-containing based from the purines (adenine or guanine) or pyrimidines (thymine or cytosine),
 - A sugar (deoxyribose in DNA - ribose missing the 2'-OH group), and
 - One or more phosphate groups .
   RNA is a polymer of ribonucleotides. Ribonucleotides consist of :
 - Nitrogen-containing bases from the purines (adenine or guanine) or pyrimidines (uracil or cytosine),

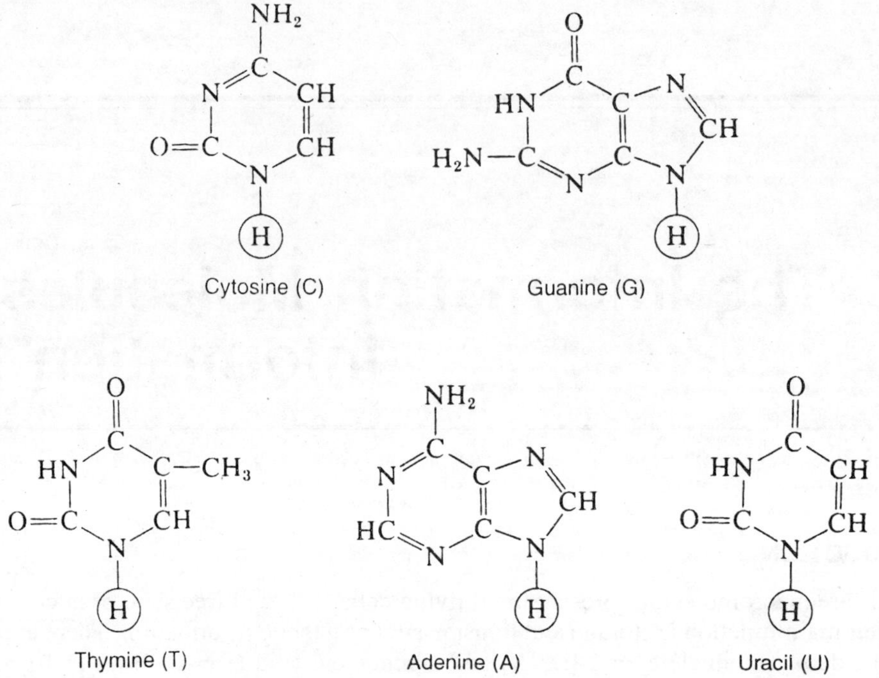

Fig. 3.1. Structure of the bases

- A sugar (deoxyribose in DNA, ribose in RNA), and
- One or more phosphate groups.

   DNA/RNA chains have polarity: the backbone is linked 5'-OH —> phosphate group —> 3'-OH in both RNA and DNA.

3.3. BASIC CHEMISTRY OF NUCLEIC ACIDS

In DNA, the bases are linked by an N-1'-glycosidic bond to 2' -deoxyribose to form a deoxynucleoside. In RNA, the bases are linked by an N-1'-glycosidic bond to ribose to form a nucleoside. Deoxyribonucleotides are 5' -monophosphate ester derivatives of deoxynucleosides. Ribonucleotides are 5' -

Table 3.1. Nomenclature of nucleosides and nucleotides

Nucleoside	Nucleotide	Scientific Name	Abbreviation
Adenosine	Adenylic acid	Adenosine-5'-monophosphate	AMP
Guanosine	Guanylic acid	Guanosine-5'-monophosphate	GMP
Cytidine	Cytidylic acid	Cytidine-5'-monophosphate	CMP
Ribosylthymine	Thymidylic acid	Thymine-5'-monophosphate	TMP
Uridine	Uridylic acid	Uridine-5'-monophosphate	UMP
Deoxyadenosine	Deoxyadenylic acid	Deoxyadenosine-5'-monophosphate	dAMP
Deoxyguanosine	Deoxyguanylic acid	Deoxyguanosine-5'-monophosphate	dGMP
Deoxycytosine	Deoxycytidylic acid	Deoxycytosine-5'-monophosphate	dCMP
Thymidine	Deoxythymidylic acid	Deoxythymidine-5'-monophosphate	dTMP

monophosphate ester derivatives of nucleosides. Nucleic Acids are Polymers of Nucleotide Phosphates. Phosphodiester bonds between the 5' hydroxyl of one nucleotide and the 3' hydroxyl of the next form the DNA or RNA polymers. The nucleotides are strong acids: the two pKa's of the phosphomonoester are between 0.7 and 1.0 and between 6.1 and 6.3. Thus, in RNA and DNA the sugar phosphate backbone is negatively charged. The bases all absorb light strongly in the near ultraviolet (~ 260 nm).

The phosphodiester bonds in nucleic acids are thermodynamically unstable (ΔG for hydrolysis is about –25 kJ/mol), but in the absence of a catalyst (enzyme) the polymers are quite stable.

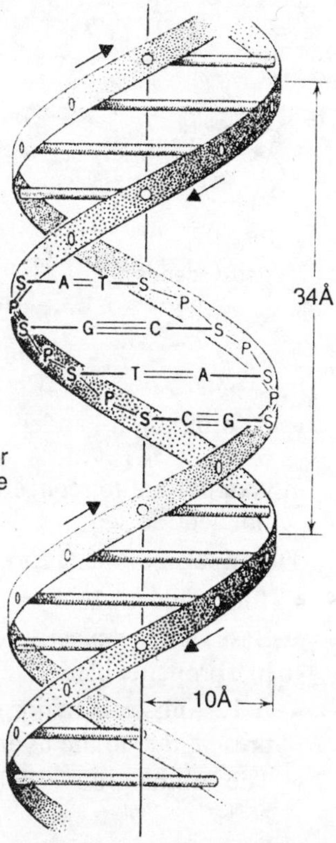

3.4. STRUCTURE OF DNA

Primary Structure

Nucleic acids have a primary structure -the sequence of bases along the polymer - and directionality with a free 5' hydroxyl at one end and a free 3' hydroxyl at the other end. By convention, nucleic acid sequences are written starting from the free 5' hydroxyl and ending at the free 3' hydroxyl. In this convention, the phosphodiester bonds run in β (1-4).

Fig. 3.2. DNA structure

Secondary Structure

The secondary structure of DNA is the well-known double helix. This structure was deduced from the analysis of the x-ray diffraction pattern of fibers of DNA. Fiber diffraction patterns do not contain the molecular information found in single crystal diffraction patterns, but the fiber diffraction patterns and the properties of the fibers provided the essential information to deduce the double helix structure. The diffraction pattern showed the presence of a helix. The spacing between the spots showed that there are 10 bases per turn of the helix. The density of the fibers indicated two molecules of DNA per helix. Watson and Crick proposed that the double helix is stabilized by hydrogen bonding between bases on the opposite strands - A-T base pair. G-C base pair. In their model the hydrophilic sugar-phosphate backbone are on the outside, in contact with water, and the hydrophobic bases are stacked perpendicular to the axis of the helix on the inside. The two strands of DNA are complementary and run in the opposite directions i.e. they are antiparallel. Although the bases are on the inside, they can be approach through two deep spiral groves called the major and minor grooves. This model also accounted for the fact that in the composition of DNA the % A=%T and %G=%C. (This is known as Chargaff's rule).

Double Helix Structures

Three major types of DNA structures are there :
- B form as described by Watson and Crick; probably the only important biological form.
- A form, a partially dried (75% humidity) form, in which the bases are not perpendicular to the helical axis.

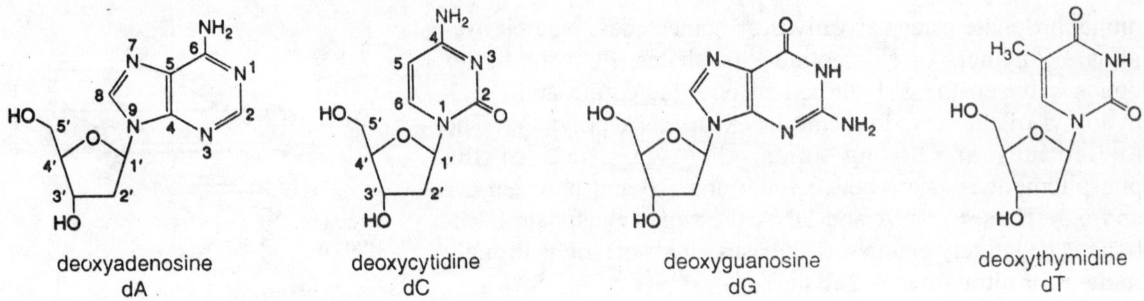

Fig. 3.3. Structure of the 4 bases with deoxy bonding

- Z form, a left-handed, formed by rotating the bases 180 degrees at the deoxyribose bond.

It is important to realize that DNA secondary structure is not rigid, but flexible, and depends on the exact nucleotide sequence and could be changed by interactions with proteins or other molecules.

Description of the B form of DNA:

- Ten residues (10.4 or approximately 10 base pairs) form one turn around the helix.
- Bases are not exactly coplanar or perpendicular to the molecular axis. They are "twisted" 1 degree, like propeller blades.
- A 12 Angstrom major groove and a 6 Angstrom minor groove are present due to the hydrogen bonding relationships.
- The minor groove contains the pyrimidine O-2 and the purine N-3.
- The major groove is on the opposite side from the minor groove.
- Each groove has potential hydrogen bonding sites for enzyme recognition.

A-DNA is a dehydrated (75% humidity) form of DNA:

- Strands are still antiparallel.
- The A helix is shorted, wider and the bases are more steeply angled (~19 degrees) to the axis, affecting the A-T and G-C base pairing.
- Puckering of the deoxyribose is thought to cause the shape change.
- The minor groove is almost completely gone.
- Double-stranded RNA and DNA-RNA hybrids form A-DNA-like structures. (The 2'-OH sterically interferes with assuming a B-DNA form.)

Z-DNA is a left-handed, antiparallel DNA structure:

- The phosphodiester backbone is "zigzagged," with altered A-T and G-C base pairing.
- Only short oligonucleotides with alternating sequences of pyrimidine and purines assume the Z-DNA form.
- High salt concentrations are required to minimize electrostatic repulsions and assume a Z form.

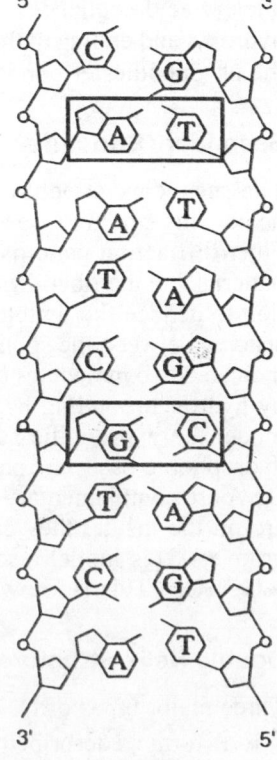

Fig 3.4. The double helix structure

Most DNA in most organisms is doubled-stranded and most doubled-stranded DNA is in the B form. The molecular structure suggests that the B form is found naturally because it, but not the A form, can accommodate a spine of water molecules lying in the minor groove. The hydrogen bonds contributed by the water give added stability to the B form. In some organisms the DNA is circular (no free 3' or 5' ends) and in others linear.

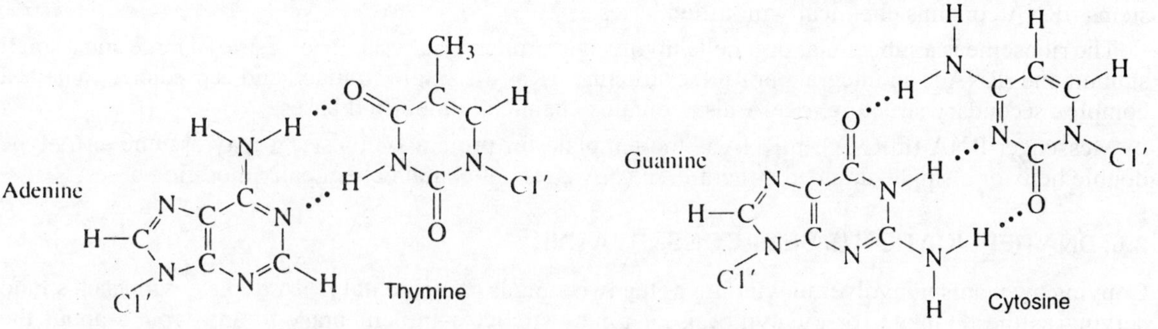

Fig. 3.5. DNA base pair structures

3.5. STRUCTURE OF RNA

There are three major types of RNA :

- Transfer RNA (tRNA)
- Ribosomal RNA (rRNA)
- Messenger RNA (mRNA).

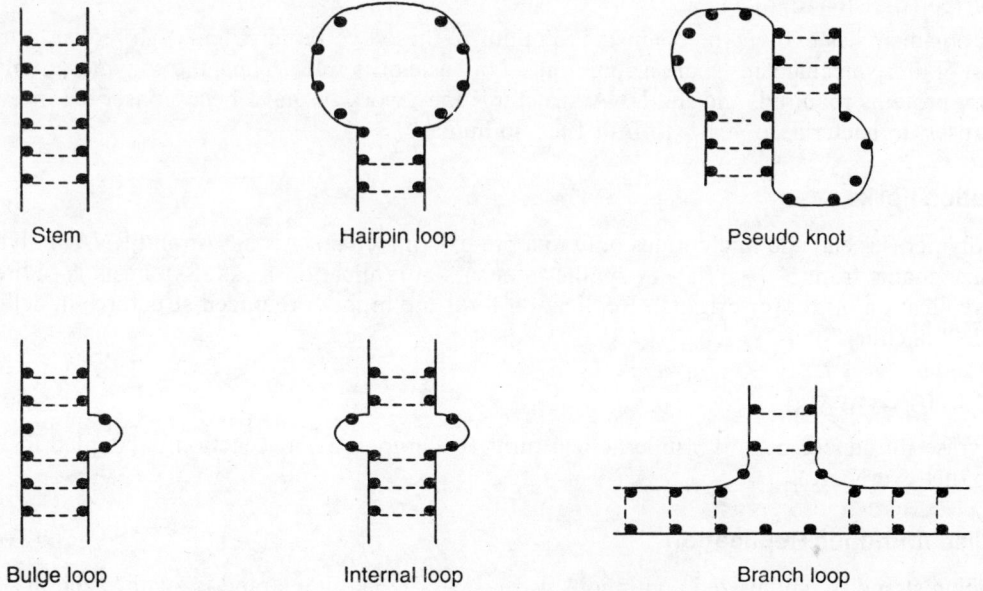

Fig. 3.6. Secondary RNA structures

mRNA is about 5% of the total RNA, tRNA is about 15%, and rRNA is about 80%. Other minor forms of RNA are important for splicing for functions such as splicing and telomere synthesis.

tRNAs are small with 73-94 nucleotides - they function in protein synthesis. Single-stranded DNA ard RNA have a tendency to adopt a random coil structure. However, such single-stranded molecules contain regions of self-complementary sequences (tRNA) where the molecule can form double-stranded stems. tRNA contains chemically modified bases.

The ribosome is a subcellular organelle involved in protein synthesis. It consists of a large and a small subunit and rRNA is an integral part of the structure. rRNA is single stranded and is predicted to have a complex secondary structure. rRNA also contains chemically modified bases.

Messenger RNA (mRNA) mRNA is the template for protein synthesis. It may assume an A-type double helix or a single-stranded structure. mRNA does not contain chemically modified bases.

3.6. DNA REPLICATION IS SEMI-CONSERVATIVE

Copying mechanism involves unwinding of the two strands of a parental DNA duplex, with each strand serving as the template for the synthesis of a new strand, complementary to and wound about the parental strand. At each base of the new strand, the complementary base to the parental strand is present and is held in position during polymerization by base pairing.

Expression of the genetic information in DNA involves transcription of the DNA sequence into RNA (messenger RNA, mRNA), then translation of the mRNA sequence into the protein sequence. In formation of the mRNA, complementary base pairing between ribonucleotides and the DNA sequence is involved. In the formation of proteins, each amino acid is specified by a sequence of the three bases (the codon) to which a transfer RNA, which carries the activated amino acid, binds.

Much of the complexity found in DNA replication (compared, say to transcription) derives from the requirements in all organisms for:
- High accuracy in duplicating the primary genetic information;
- High speed and processivity, so as to complete a copy of the genome in less than one cell generation (cell division time).

Each organism has evolved mechanisms to optimize these two requirements. Moreover, it turns out that most of these mechanisms share a common set of basic principles. Thus, the enzymes involved, the accessory proteins required, and the DNA structures they work on have been conserved in evolution from viruses, to bacteria, to yeast, to fruit flies, to humans.

Replication Forks

DNA polymerases can add nucleotides only to a pre-existing chain. All DNA (and RNA) polymerases synthesize chains from 5' → 3'. DNA synthesis occurs at replication forks. Synthesis is bidirectional from a replication origin (or origins). Replication forks are highly organized structures in cells (DNA synthesis "machines").

Role of DNA Gyrase

DNA gyrase introduces negative superhelical turns (endergonic). The reaction is coupled to ATP hydrolysis (net exergonic).

Semi-discontinuous Replication

The leading strand is synthesized continuously, 5' → 3'. The lagging strand is synthesized in segments using RNA as primers (and as always, only in the 5' → 3' direction).

RNA primers

Synthesized on the lagging strand template by DNA primase. Synthesized by RNA polymerase on the leading strand during replication initiation at the origin.

Table 3.2. Some examples of DNA polymerases

Enzyme	Template	Primer	Other activities	Other features
E. coli DNA pol I	DNA	DNA/RNA	3'-5' exo, 5'-3' exo	Monomeric
E. coli DNA pol I (Klenow fragment)	DNA	DNA/RNA	3'-5' exo	C-terminal fragment
E. coli DNA pol III	DNA	DNA/RNA	3'-5' exo (on a separate subunit)	Multimeric structure
Taq pol	DNA	DNA/RNA	extendase (adds 3'-A overhangs)	Thermostable, used in PCR
Reverse transcriptase	DNA/RNA	DNA/RNA	(ribonuclease H)	Used to make cDNA will synthesize DNA in non-templated reaction
Terminal transferase	None required	DNA		

3.7. DENATURATION AND RENATURATION OF DNA

Induction of Denaturation

Although the double helix is relatively stable under physiological conditions, the loss of secondary structure, denaturation, can be induced by:
- Enzymes, for example, RNA polymerase, helicases.
- High pH, which leads to electrostatic repulsion of the negatively charged phosphate, groups.
- These charges can be partially neutralized by ions or proteins.
- A change in the concentration of these "charge neutralizing" factors can lead to chain separation.
- Chemicals, such as formamide, which decrease the base stacking energy of the double helix.
- Another factor controlling denaturation is temperature due to the fact that the entropy of the denatured state (random coil) is higher than that of the helical state.

Nucleases

- Nucleases are enzymes that hydrolyze the phosphodiester bonds in nucleic acids. Some are specific for DNA, DNases, and others for RNA, RNases and still others show no specificity.
- Exonucleases remove nucleotides from the ends, either from the 5'- or 3'- ends.
- Endonucleases cleave internal phosphodiester bonds.

Nucleic Acids Hybridize by Base Pairing

- A crucial property of the double helix is the ability to separate the two strands without disrupting covalent bonds. This makes it possible for the strands to separate and reform under physiological conditions. The specificity of the process is determined by complementary base pairing. Hybridization refers to the formation of double stranded nucleic acids.
- It is often used to describe the formation of a DNA-RNA hybrid. But annealing of DNA is also hybridization.

Table 3.3. The genetic code

		Second Position of Codon				
		T	**C**	**A**	**G**	
	T	TTT Phe [F]	TCT Ser [S]	TAT Tyr [Y]	TGT Cys [C]	T
		TTC Phe [F]	TCC Ser [S]	TAC Tyr [Y]	TGC Cys [C]	C
		TTA Leu [L]	TCA Ser [S]	TAA *Ter* [end]	TGA *Ter* [end]	A
		TTG Leu [L]	TCG Ser [S]	TAG *Ter* [end]	TGG Trp [W]	G
	C	CTT Leu [L]	CCT Pro [P]	CAT His [H]	CGT Arg [R]	T
		CTC Leu [L]	CCC Pro [P]	CAC His [H]	CGC Arg [R]	C
		CTA Leu [L]	CCA Pro [P]	CAA Gln [Q]	CGA Arg [R]	A
		CTG Leu [L]	CCG Pro [P]	CAG Gln [Q]	CGG Arg [R]	G
	A	ATT Ile [I]	ACT Thr [T]	AAT Asn [N]	AGT Ser [S]	T
		ATC Ile [I]	ACC Thr [T]	AAC Asn [N]	AGC Ser [S]	C
		ATA Ile [I]	ACA Thr [T]	AAA Lys [K]	AGA Arg [R]	A
		ATG Met [M]	ACG Thr [T]	AAG Lys [K]	AGG Arg [R]	G
	G	GTT Val [V]	GCT Ala [A]	GAT Asp [D]	GGT Gly [G]	T
		GTC Val [V]	GCC Ala [A]	GAC Asp [D]	GGC Gly [G]	C
		GTA Val [V]	GCA Ala [A]	GAA Glu [E]	GGA Gly [G]	A
		GTG Val [V]	GCG Ala [A]	GAG Glu [E]	GGG Gly [G]	G

(First Position — T, C, A, G — labels the left margin; Third Position — T, C, A, G — labels the right margin.)

- Hybridization is also critical for:
  a. The Polymerase Chain Reaction (PCR).
  b. Southern Blotting, which involved DNA-DNA hybridization.
  c. Northern Blotting, which involves DNA-RNA hybridization.
  d. Assaying DNA Micro arrays.

3.8. GENES - THE FUNCTIONAL ELEMENTS IN DNA

Each chromosome is a single DNA molecule in all cases yet determined. Genetic information is encoded in units along this DNA molecule, each of which encodes a protein. These functional units are genes. Genes are hence the fundamental unit of function. Genetic mutants are usually because of changes in the nucleotide sequence in a Gene. A Gene can be taken as a region of a DNA molecule (or chromosome) that encodes a protein or structural RNA molecule (tRNA, rRNA or snRNA).

A Cistron is the basic or smallest unit of function, based on genetic cis-trans complementation test (it is structurally same as a gene). A recon is the basic unit of recombination in genetic crosses (it is structurally same as a Nucleotide. A muton is the basic unit of mutation.

Prokaryotic Genes

Genes encoding proteins involved catalytically in the same process are often found immediately adjacent to each other, e.g. *trp* biosynthetic and *lac* catabolic genes. Control of expression of these genes is such that they are all turned on or turned off together; such groups of genes that show coordinate expression, together with their control elements, are called Operons. An Operon is often expressed using a single mRNA molecule for all of its genes, e.g. the *trp* Operon. In bacteria and prokaryotes, most of the DNA is used to comprise Genes. DNA not used for a gene is called Intergenic DNA.

Eukaryotic Genes: Introns and Exons

Eukaryotic genes are often very different from prokaryotic genes. DNA encoding a gene is found in "pieces" on the total DNA molecule: regions encoding the gene are called exons (Expressed regions) and regions between the exons are called introns (Intervening sequences).

Exon comprises a few bp to a few hundred bp and an intron comprises a few 10s of bp to a few thousand bp. While exons are those regions of the DNA that are encoded in the final mRNA, usually not all of the mRNA is translated into the resulting protein. The region of the DNA (or mRNA) actually encoding amino acids found in the protein is called the coding sequence. Thus, the initial RNA made from the DNA contains introns. This RNA is enzymatically "processed" to yield the final mRNA, the RNA used during translation for protein biosynthesis. In some of these processing events, the introns are "spliced out" of the initial RNA.

Pseudo-genes are DNA regions that arose in evolution via tandem duplication recombination events of existing genes that subsequently mutated sufficiently extensively that they lost their original function (the original function, e.g. beta-globin function, is still provided by the original gene that was duplicated).

A gene then includes all DNA sequences found in the initial RNA transcript. This definition of genes is sometimes expanded to include all DNA Control Elements. These control elements comprise of protein binding sites on the DNA where proteins involved in control of expression of the gene bind, usually to "turn on" expression in eukaryotes (Activator Proteins). These binding sites can be as far as 50,000 bp (50 kb) either upstream or downstream from the exons and introns of the gene. (Upstream is in the direction 5' from the Exon-Intron region and downstream is in the direction 3' from the Exon-Intron region.) These binding sites are often found clustered in regions called enhancers.

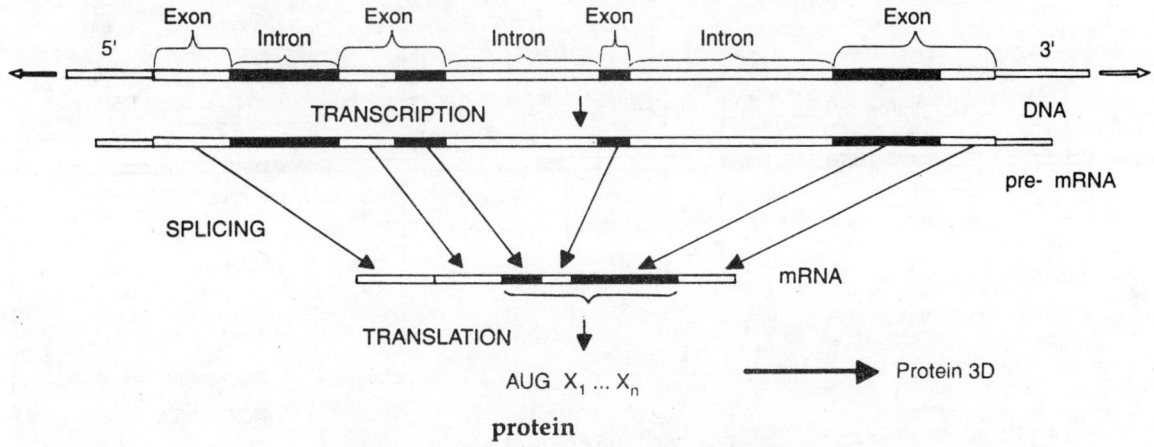

Fig. 3.7. The process of gene expression

Eukaryotic genes are usually expressed as monocistronic units: one mRNA for each gene. This is in contrast to the operon structure of expression of clusters of genes found in prokaryotes. Some eukaryotic genes can yield more than one protein, due to alternative splicing sites for processing of the initial RNA transcript.

3.9. ORGANISATION OF GENES IN EUKARYOTIC CHROMOSOMES

Higher eukaryotic DNA contains much DNA that does not encode protein or RNA, and thus does not comprise genes. Function of this DNA is unknown and may be nonfunctional DNA that is "going along for the ride", and is thus sometimes called Junk DNA or Selfish DNA. Consistent with this observation of nonfunctional DNA, amount of DNA (haploid content is called the C-value) does not always correlate with complexity of the organism, e.g. amphibians and some plants, e.g. lilies, have much more DNA than humans; this non-correlation is known as the C-value paradox.

1. *Classes of Eukaryotic DNA* : Solitary genes versus Gene Families, which mostly arise by tandem duplication mutational events. Pseudogenes are nonfunctional, mutated tandem duplications of functional genes.

2. *Repetitious DNA* : Discovered through reannealing or reassociation experiments. Reannealing, reassociation, renaturation, hybridization - all mean the same thing. Complementary ssDNA strands finding each other and forming H-bonds and dsDNA

Although eukaryotic chromosomes contain a single DNA molecule, this molecule is so large that it is nearly always fragmented into many fragments upon isolation from cells. So one always deals with populations of many DNA fragments. The size of these fragments depends on the severity of the isolation procedure, and varies usually from a few hundred kb to up to a megabase (1,000,000 bp; mb) of DNA (Fig. 3.8).

There are three types of DNA, as classified by repetitive structure:

1. Highly repetitive (simple sequence) DNA
2. Moderately repetitive (intermediate repeat) DNA
3. Single copy DNA

The number of tandem repeats in STRs (Short Tandem Repeats) often varies from one human to another, and hence has application to forensic science.

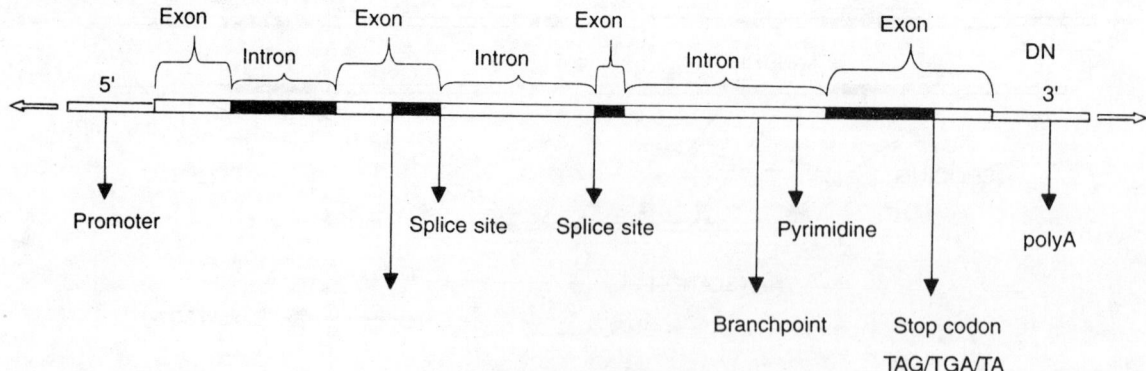

Fig. 3.8. Structure of gene

3.10. STRUCTURE OF BACTERIAL CHROMOSOME

In the bacterial cell, there is a nucleoid region, there is no distinct nuclear membrane and DNA is highly condensed (> 10 mg/ml) in a region less than 1 μm in diameter. When isolated in the presence of high salt (1 M NaCl), the bacterial chromosome is isolated as the bacterial nucleoid or folded chromosome. When isolated from cells very gently in the absence of high salt, proteins are removed from the nucleoid and the chromosome has then been "seen" (using tritium Autoradioaugraphy technique) as a circle with two forks (known as Replication Forks). When isolated from cells using typical isolation procedures, proteins are removed from the nucleoid and the chromosome (a single large circular DNA molecule of 4.5 million bp, diameter ~ 1 millimeter) is broken into linear fragments of size 5-500 kb.

Structure of eukaryotic DNA

Chromatin is the DNA-protein complex present in Interphase cells. Euchromatin consists of all chromatin except Heterochromatin. Euchromatin has chromatin regions that are relatively open, less condensed - where gene expression occurs. Heterochromatin consists of genome or chromatin regions that are always highly condensed- there is little gene expression in these regions. Heterochromatin is of two types. Constitutive heterochromatin is the specific genome regions, often containing short repeated sequences and facultative heterochromatin is the entire chromosomes that are transcriptionally inactivated. A key example is inactive X Chromosome in females. Only one of the two X chromosomes is active in gene expression

Structure of Chromatin

The major components are the expected DNA, RNA, nascent transcripts includes proteins: histones, which are small, basic proteins that bind DNA in sequence-independent manner and non-histones, which are various sized proteins (including many acidic proteins). There are also many DNA functional proteins: RNA polymerases, transcription factors etc.

Nucleosomes are approximately 200 bp DNA wrapped around 8 (octamer) histone proteins - bead-like 10 nm particles, with equal mass of DNA and protein. Assembly of nucleosomes occur during DNA replication / chromatin duplication. Nucleosome and other structures must be flexible enough to permit DNA function: replication and transcription. Replication occurs at forks where the 2 DNA strands separate. Many proteins are involved, forming large protein complex at the forks. Nucleosomes must be displaced for this to occur - they must then reassemble.

3.11. ANALYSING DNA

Digestion of a well-defined DNA molecule, e.g. viral DNA, with a restriction enzyme yields set of well-defined DNA restriction fragments. For example: EcoRI cleaves phage lambda DNA at 5 sites, yielding 6 fragments.

Gel Electrophoresis technique: when "loaded" as a "band" at top of a gel matrix, and subjected to an electric field, DNA migrates through the gel at rate inversely proportional to its size. Thus it can separate and purify individual restriction fragments from a gel and one can then analyse for presence and size of restriction fragments. One can use DNA Markers for size determination.

Uses of restriction enzymes, restriction sites and restriction fragments

Physical Map of Genome or DNA molecule

Genetic Map is colinear with physical placement of genes on DNA but quantitation is difficult due to variations of recombination processes between organisms (more rare in eukaryotes than in prokaryotes)

and due to dependence on DNA sequence (hot spots for recombination). The physical map of genome consists of placement of genes and sites on nucleotide sequence of DNA, i.e. on the physically real genetic material.

Restriction Map as a Physical Map

Given a large DNA molecule :

1. Digest it with a restriction enzyme, measure sizes via Agarose Gel
2. Repeat with additional restriction enzymes. You would only get sizes, but would not know which fragments are adjacent to each other.
3. Do double digests with the same enzymes as above, two at a time. Purify singly digested restriction fragments and digest with the 2nd restriction enzyme to get ordering of both sets of fragments.
4. Alternatively, one can also do partial digests with single restriction enzyme. This is particularly useful for end labelled DNA. One can also use hybridization of a radioactive 'probe' ssDNA or oligonucleotide to one end or the other of the DNA in a Southern gel analysis of the partial digests.

Cloning of DNA fragments

There are two essential parts of cloning: Cloning Vehicle and DNA of interest. The cloning vehicle is usually a DNA molecule with all elements for self-duplication (called a Replicon), (e.g.), Polylinker or Multiple Cloning Region (MCR). DNA of interest can be restriction fragments of complete genome, restriction fragments from Chimeric DNA, e.g from YAC for Plasmids, R.fragments purified from a gel, from a purified chromosome, etc and genome fragments made by shearing genomic DNA, followed by creating blunt ends by limited exonuclease digestion.

3.12. CLONING METHODOLOGY

The general steps in cloning method are :

1. Cut the cloning vehicle with R.enzyme of choice, e.g. EcoRI
2. Cut DNA of interest with same R.enzyme
3. Mix the restricted cloning vehicle and DNA of interest R.fragments together
4. Ligate fragments together: DNA ligase
5. Insert ligated DNA into host of choice, e.g. transformation of *E. coli*
6. Grow host cells under restrictive conditions.

Types of Cloning Vehicles

Examples of Cloning Vehicles: Plasmids, Lambda phage and Cosmids

1. Plasmids are used for routine cloning of relatively small inserts: 100 bp - 15 kb. Plasmid cloning vehicles must have 1) origin, 2) cloning sites, and 3) selection marker. Plasmids are extrachromosomal elements or replicons. They are self-replicating DNA molecules. The only genetic requirement for a DNA molecule to be self-replicating is that it contains an origin of DNA replication appropriate for the host in which it would propagate. For plasmids to function as cloning vehicles or vectors, they must also have cloning sites and selection locus
2. Viral DNA, e.g. Phage Lambda derivatives, e.g. lambda gt10 and lambda gt11. Lambda phages are used for cloning of same size to larger inserts than plasmids. Phage lambda is a bacteriophage or phage, i.e. bacterial virus that uses *E. coli* as host. Its structure is that of a typical phage: head, tail, tail fibers, head contain the genome. In this phase, DNA replication occurs and progeny lambda heads and tails are made. Lambda as a cloning vehicle: most lambda cloning experiments require

only the lytic phase of the lambda life cycle. (Lytic phase - progeny lambda DNA molecules are inserted into empty lambda heads and tails are joined, yielding progeny, infective lambda phage particles.A phage encoded lysozyme enzymatically lyses the *E. coli* host "from within", breaking apart the cell surface, and releasing the progeny phage.) Hence the lambda genes required for the Lysogenic Phase as "dispensable" for cloning. These "dispensable" genes constitute the replaceable region in lambda cloning.

3. Cosmids are Plasmid Cloning Vehicle with lambda sites. They are used to clone large inserts of DNA: size ~ 45 kb.

Few Examples of Types of Cloning Experiments

Gene Isolation: "Probe" with radioactive short DNA molecule of sequence from the gene. Obtain short DNA sequence, e.g, from amino acid sequence of purified protein. Thus go from protein to gene with no previously isolated mutations (Reverse Genetics). Often use such a short DNA oligonucleotide probe to partially purify R.fragments for further cloning.

Genomic Cloning : Genomic cloning is used to obtain library of complete genome.

*cDNA Cloning :*cDNA cloning is used to purify a messenger RNA of interest. The process is to "Reverse transcribe" the RNA into DNA, get a "complementary DNA strand".

3.16. DNA SEQUENCING AND POLYMERASE CHAIN REACTION (PCR)

DNA sequencing is the key technology for studying genes. Automated DNA sequencing in many labs is performed by Perkin-Elmer (provided by Applied Biosystems) DNA sequencing systems. These instruments automate the electrophoresis, detection, and data collection steps of the Sanger dideoxynucleotide termination sequencing method. The system uses fluorescently labeled primers or dideoxy terminators instead of radioactivity. Sequencing reactions prepared by thermocycle sequencing are resolved and read in a single lane, rather than four separate lanes, enabling a much higher throughput of DNA sequence data. With a high quality template, users should routinely receive DNA sequencing reads of over 900 bases in length, with 98% accuracy well beyond 600 bases. The quality of the sequence data obtained with the automated system depends heavily on the quality of the DNA template put into the sequencing reactions.

There are three DNA sequencing techniques, two of which use DNA polymerases.

1. Sanger dideoxy DNA Sequencing

Dideoxy sequencing (also called chain- termination or Sanger method) uses an enzymatic procedure to synthesize DNA chains of varying lengths, stopping DNA replication at one of the four bases and then determining the resulting fragment lengths. Each sequencing reaction tube (T, C, G, and A) contains a DNA template, a primer sequence and a DNA polymerase to initiate synthesis of a new strand of DNA. This happens at the point where the primer is hybridized to the template. The four deoxynucleotide triphosphates (dATP, dTTP, dCTP, and dGTP) extend the DNA strand. There is one labeled deoxynucleotide triphosphate (using a radioactive element or dye); and one dideoxynucleotide triphosphate which terminates the growing chain wherever it is incorporated.

Process is as follows :

1. Have a DNA template and a DNA primer. Cloning vehicles often have universal primers for sequencing into DNA cloned into one of the MCS (Multiple Cloning Sites) sites.

2. Execute 4 separate polymerization reactions containing each of the 4 dNTPs and one each of the four dideoxynucleoside TPs: ddGTP, ddATP, ddTTP, ddCTP. To assay the product DNA, one of the 4 dNTPs is radioactively labeled or the Primer is labeled, radioactively or fluorescently or the ddNTP is labeled fluorescently.

Dideoxy means 3'-H as well as 2'-H. When a ddNTP is incorporated, it acts as a chain terminator: DNA synthesis stops since the DNA primer no longer has a 3'-OH Primer Terminus

3. Thus, get as reaction products, a nested set of fragments, each terminated at one of the four bases: G in the ddGTP reaction, A in the ddATP reaction etc.
4. When "run" on a DNA sequencing gel (polyacrylamide, with DNA denatured), the "nested set" of fragments forms a ladder of DNA bands corresponding to the positions of the bases.
5. Read the DNA sequence by reading the 4 lanes, one for each base, from bottom up, to correspond to 5' -> 3' sequence

2. Maxam-Gilbert Chemical Sequencing

Process is as follows :

1. Use DNA, ds or ss, with radioactive label at one end ONLY
2. In at least 4 separate reactions, treat the DNA with base specific chemicals that result in cleavage of the DNA strand at that base.
3. Again get a nested set of DNA fragments.
4. Analyse as a ladder on a DNA sequencing gel as for Sanger DiDeoxy Sequencing.

The two basic sequencing approaches, Maxam- Gilbert and Sanger, differ primarily in the way the nested DNA fragments are produced. Both methods work because gel electrophoresis produces very high-resolution separations of DNA molecules; even fragments that differ in size by only a single nucleotide can be resolved.

Almost all steps in these sequencing methods are now automated. Maxam- Gilbert sequencing uses chemicals to cleave DNA at specific bases, resulting in fragments of different lengths. A refinement to the Maxam- Gilbert method known as multiplex sequencing enables investigators to analyze about 40 clones on a single DNA sequencing gel.

These first-generation gel-based sequencing technologies are now being used to sequence small regions of interest in the human genome. Although investigators could use existing technology to sequence whole chromosomes, time and cost considerations make large- scale sequencing projects of this nature impractical. The smallest human chromosome (Y) contains 50 Mb; the largest (chromosome 1) has 250 Mb.

3. PCR - Polymerase Chain Reaction

This is a combination of polymerization with denaturation-renaturation hybridization

PCR procedure is as follows:

1. Have two primers to a DNA fragment, one to each strand, which hybridize 500-2000 bp apart from each other.
2. Concentration of primers is very high compared with DNA
3. Denature the DNA (95°C, 1 min)
4. Hybridize the primers (e.g. 67·C, 2 min)
5. Extend the primers via DNA synthesis using a heat-resistant DNA polymerase
6. Now have doubled the DNA present.
7. Repeat steps 2-5 for 20-30 times ("cycles") via a heat-to-95°C : cool-to-67·C procedure

Each cycle doubles the amount of DNA present. Thus, the number of DNA molecules increases exponentially with numbers of cycles of PCR.. Nearly all of these molecules (> 99% after 12 cycles) are target DNA molecules, i.e. contains only primer nucleotides and nucleotides found between the primers.

PCR can be used for many purposes, e.g. DNA sequencing:

1. Use ONLY one Primer, with enough initial DNA for sequencing
2. Extend with DNA polymerase in presence of ddNTPs

Only one strand in made, and made as a Nested Set of chain terminated fragments. PCR can also be used for amplification of mRNA.

DNA Cloning. In order to study a specific sequence within a complex DNA population, the sequence fragment can be selectively amplified so that the population is purified to near-homogeneity. The amplification step involves a controlled increase in the number of copies of the fragment, and is achieved with the help of a *vector*, a molecule that is capable of self-replication in a suitable host. Vectors such as bacterial plasmids occur in nature, while others, such as yeast artificial chromosomes (YAC's), are genetically engineered. The cell-based DNA cloning essentially involves three steps:

1. The vector molecule is joined to the DNA insert
2. The resulting molecule is inserted into a suitable host cell (often a bacterial or yeast cell)
3. The host cell replicates to produce a colony of identical cell clones, each containing one or more copies of both the vector and the DNA insert. There are many different cloning vectors available, allowing for many different sizes of DNA inserts to be amplified (Table 3.4).

Table 3.4. Cloning vectors

Cloning Vector	Insert Size
Bacteriophage M13	= 1.5 kb
Plasmid	= 5 kb
Bacteriophage λ	= 25 kb
Cosmid	= 40 kb
BAC (bacterial artificial chromosome)	= 150 kb
YAC (yeast artificial chromosome)	= 500 kb

Hybridization

In molecular hybridization, the DNA fragment of interest is not amplified, but is instead specifically detected within a complex DNA population. Based on complementarity, hybridization involves mixing single-stranded DNA (or RNA) molecules, which can then pair with each other to form double helices. The process of splitting double-stranded molecules into single strands is called *denaturation* and the process of pairing is called *renaturation* or *annealing*. In the mix of DNA, the presence of a particular target DNA sequence can be tested for by constructing a fluorescently or radioactively labeled *probe* consisting of the complementary sequence, and observing whether it hybridizes to form a double-stranded molecule. An advantage of this method is that complementary strands will anneal even if they are from different organisms.

Polymerase Chain Reaction (PCR)

Besides cell-based DNA cloning, there exists a cell-free method to selectively amplify a fragment of target DNA. PCR-based cloning is used for amplifying short fragments (< 15 Kb, say), and requires that a *primer sequence*, often only 15-30 nucleotides long, is known at each end of the target DNA. When added to denatured DNA and cooled, the primers will bind to complementary sequences, and, under suitable experimental conditions, initiate the synthesis of new DNA strands complementary to both strands of the target DNA. A heat-stable DNA polymerase is used during the synthesis step, since one iteration of the reaction is composed of three temperature dependent steps. PCR is called a "chain reaction" because both newly synthesized strands act as templates for synthesis in future iterations. Therefore, if a particular sequence exists in a complex DNA population, then the number of copies of the sequence doubles with every iteration of PCR.

Restriction Enzymes

Type II restriction endonucleases are enzymes that cleave DNA at locations containing a specific recognition sequence, usually 4-8 bp long. If an enzyme cleaves both strands of a DNA molecule at the same point, then the resulting restriction fragments will have *blunt ends*. In most cases, however, the resulting fragments will have overhangs, or *sticky ends*, so called because they have a tendency to form base pairs with similar complementary overhangs from different fragments.

Complete digestion of a target DNA molecule with a restriction enzyme may produce very small fragments. With *partial digestion* of the molecule (i.e., low enzyme concentration, short time of incubation etc.), cleavage occurs only at a small number of the potential restriction sites, resulting in larger fragments.

Gel Electrophoresis

The final technique we discuss is one that separates DNA fragments by applying an electric field to samples in solution. During electrophoresis, DNA fragments are attracted, through a porous gel, to the positive electrode of the field. The velocity with which they move through the gel is related to both size and charge; for single-stranded DNA molecules, charge is approximately proportional to size. The net effect is that smaller fragments migrate faster than larger ones, and the gel can be "read" to estimate the fragment sizes that are present in the solution.

4

Proteins—Their Structural Profiles and Properties

4.1. INTRODUCTION

Proteins are macromolecules (heteropolymers) made up from 20 different L-α-amino acids, also referred to as residues. A certain number of residues is necessary to perform a particular biochemical function, and around 40-50 residues appears to be the lower limit for a functional domain size. Protein sizes range from this lower limit to several hundred residues in multi-functional proteins. Very large aggregates can be formed from protein subunits, for example many thousand actin molecules assemble into an actin filament. Large protein complexes with RNA are found in the ribosome particles, which are in fact 'ribozymes'.

Proteins usually contain thousands of atoms precisely arranged in a 3-D structure that is unique for each type. As a protein is made, it "folds" itself into a complex, 3-D shape, like a piece of ribbon that has been crumpled up. Each protein has one folded shape, and consistently folds into it, usually in less than a second. That complicated folded shape dictates how the protein works, and also how it interacts with other entities. The specific sequence of amino acids that make up each protein is coded by a gene in the DNA of living cells. A protein cannot be synthesized without its mRNA being present, but a protein can persist in the cell when its mRNA is no longer present. However, mRNA may be present in abundance but the message is not translated into proteins. There is, thus, no good correlation between mRNA and protein in a cell at any given time. Protein synthesis is a very complicated process. Ribosomes are the cell's protein factories. RNA bridges in the ribosomes are not just support structures but also a part of the protein forming machinery.

4.2. AMINO ACIDS

The basic structure of an a-amino acid is quite simple. R denotes any one of the 20 possible side chains (Table 4.1, Fig. 4.1). We notice that the Cα-atom has 4 different ligands (the H is omitted in the drawing) and is thus chiral. An easy trick to remember the correct L-form is the CORN-rule: when the Cα-atom is viewed with the H in front, the residues read "CO-R-N" in a clock-wise direction.

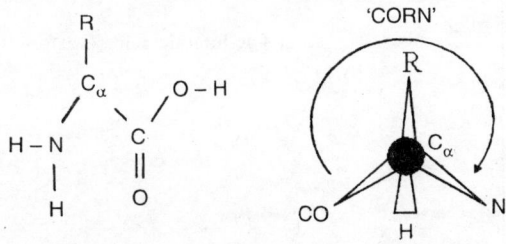

Fig. 4.1. Amino acid structure

Aliphatic amino acids.

  1. *Monoamino-monocarboxylic acids.*

      Glycine (Gly)

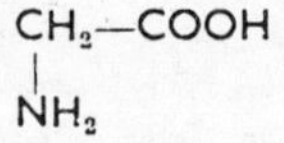

$$CH_2-COOH$$
$$|$$
$$NH_2$$

      L(+)Alanine (Ala)

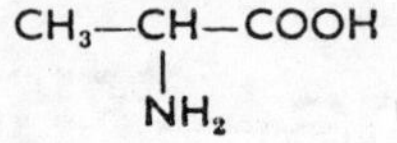

$$CH_3-CH-COOH$$
$$|$$
$$NH_2$$

      L(–)Serine (Ser)

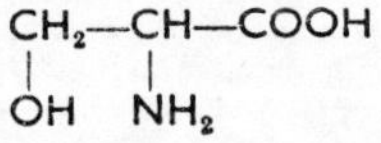

$$CH_2-CH-COOH$$
$$|\quad\quad|$$
$$OH\quad NH_2$$

      L(+)Threonine (Thr)

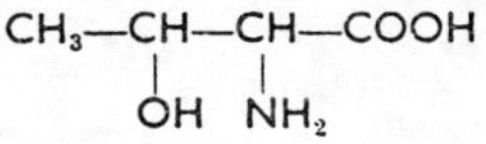

$$CH_3-CH-CH-COOH$$
$$|\quad\quad|$$
$$OH\quad NH_2$$

      L(+)Valine (Val)

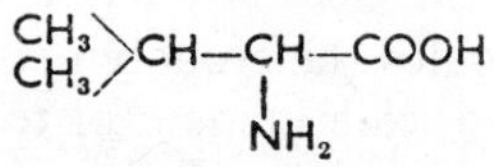

$$CH_3{\Large\diagdown}$$
$$CH_3{\diagup}CH-CH-COOH$$
$$|$$
$$NH_2$$

      L(–)Leucine (Leu)

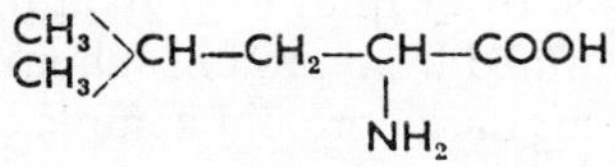

$$CH_3{\Large\diagdown}$$
$$CH_3{\diagup}CH-CH_2-CH-COOH$$
$$|$$
$$NH_2$$

      L(+)Isoleucine (Ileu)

$$CH_3{\Large\diagdown}$$
$$C_2H_5{\diagup}CH-CH-COOH$$
$$|$$
$$NH_2$$

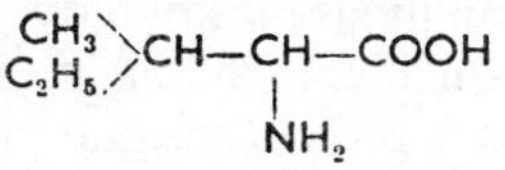

  2. *Monoamino-dicarboxylic acids.*

      L(–)Aspartic acid (Asp)

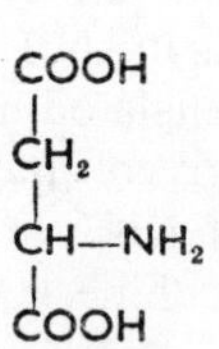

COOH		CONH$_2$
CH$_2$	and its	CH$_2$
CH—NH$_2$	amide asparagine (Asp(NH$_2$))	CH—NH$_2$
COOH		COOH

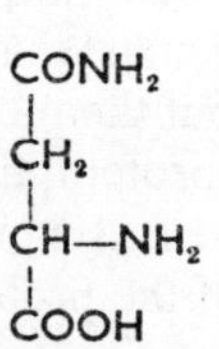

      L(+)Glutamic acid (Glu)

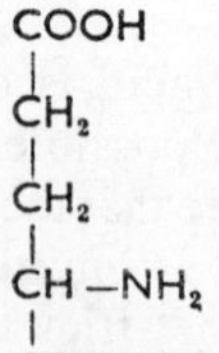

COOH		CONH$_2$
CH$_2$	and its	CH$_2$
CH$_2$	amide glutamine (Glu(NH$_2$))	CH$_2$
CH—NH$_2$		CH—NH$_2$
COOH		COOH

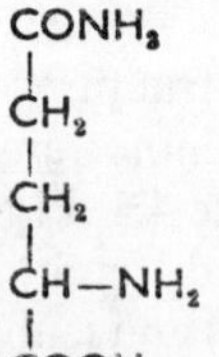

(Contd.)

Fig. 4.2.

3. *Diamino-monocarboxylic acids.*

L(+)Arginine (Arg)

(α-amino-δ-guanido-valeric acid)

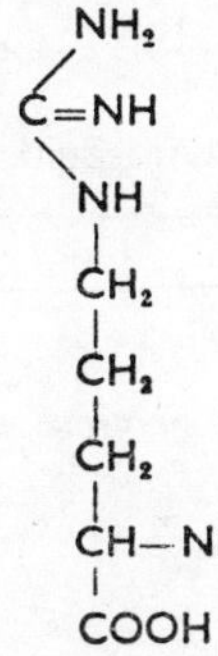

$$
\begin{array}{c}
NH_2 \\
| \\
C=NH \\
| \\
NH \\
| \\
CH_2 \\
| \\
CH_2 \\
| \\
CH_2 \\
| \\
CH-NH_2 \\
| \\
COOH
\end{array}
$$

L(+)Lysine (Lys)

(α, ε-diamino-caproic acid)

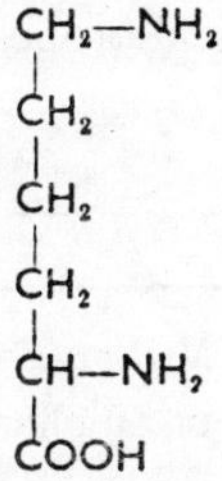

$$
\begin{array}{c}
CH_2-NH_2 \\
| \\
CH_2 \\
| \\
CH_2 \\
| \\
CH_2 \\
| \\
CH-NH_2 \\
| \\
COOH
\end{array}
$$

4. *Sulphur-containing amino acids.*

L(−)Cysteine (α-amino-β-thiol-propionic acid) (CySH) and L(−)Cystine (dicysteine) (CySSCy)

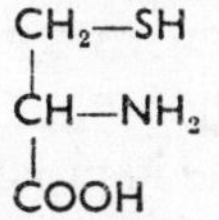

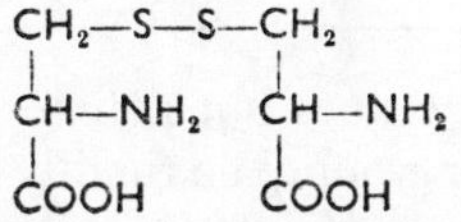

$$
\begin{array}{c}
CH_2-SH \\
| \\
CH-NH_2 \\
| \\
COOH
\end{array}
\qquad
\begin{array}{ccc}
CH_2-S-S-CH_2 \\
| \qquad\qquad | \\
CH-NH_2 \quad CH-NH_2 \\
| \qquad\qquad | \\
COOH \qquad COOH
\end{array}
$$

L(−)Methionine (Met)

(α-amino-γ-methylthio¹-butyric acid)

$$
\begin{array}{c}
CH_2-S-CH_3 \\
| \\
CH_2 \\
| \\
CH-NH_2 \\
| \\
COOH
\end{array}
$$

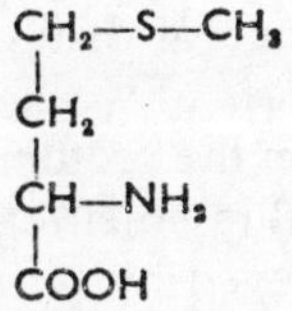

Aromatic and heterocyclic amino acids.

L(−)Phenylalanine (Phe)

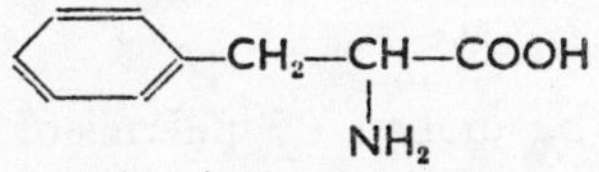

$$\langle\!\bigcirc\!\rangle-CH_2-\underset{\underset{NH_2}{|}}{CH}-COOH$$

L(−)Tyrosine (Tyr)

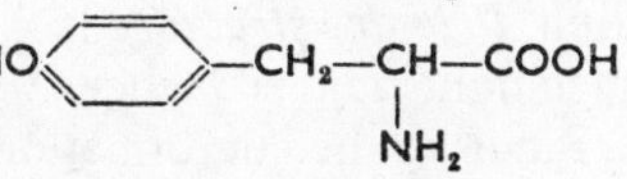

$$HO\langle\!\bigcirc\!\rangle-CH_2-\underset{\underset{NH_2}{|}}{CH}-COOH$$

L(−)Histidine (His)

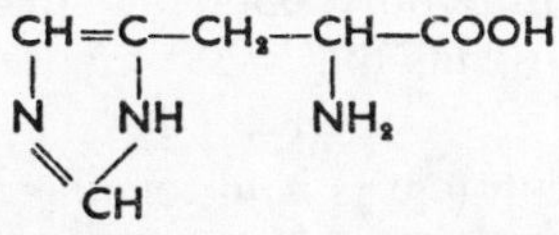

$$
\begin{array}{c}
CH=C-CH_2-\underset{\underset{NH_2}{|}}{CH}-COOH \\
| \qquad | \\
N \quad\; NH \\
\backslash \quad / \\
CH
\end{array}
$$

L(−)Tryptophan (Try)

$$
\begin{array}{c}
-CH_2-\underset{\underset{NH_2}{|}}{CH}-COOH \\
\end{array}
$$

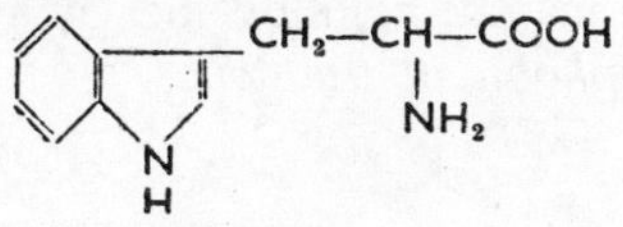

L(−)Hydroxyproline (Hypro)

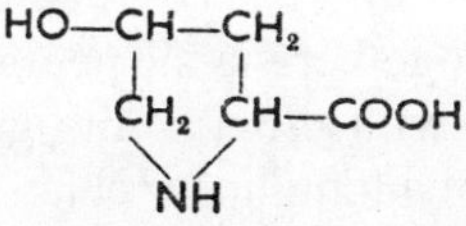

$$
\begin{array}{c}
HO-CH-CH_2 \\
| \qquad\quad | \\
CH_2 \;\; CH-COOH \\
\backslash \quad / \\
NH
\end{array}
$$

L(−)Proline (Pro)

$$
\begin{array}{c}
CH_2-CH_2 \\
| \qquad\quad | \\
CH_2 \;\; CH-COOH \\
\backslash \quad / \\
NH
\end{array}
$$

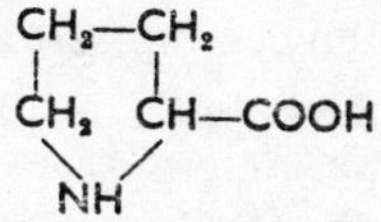

Fig. 4.2.

The different side chains R determine the chemical properties of the amino acid or residue (the residue is the amino acid side chain plus the peptide backbone) (Fig. 4.2). There is a wide diversity in the chemical properties of amino acid side chains, but they can be grouped into 6 classes (Table 4.1)

Table 4.1. Classification of Amino acids based on side chains

Side Chain	Amino Acids
Aliphatic (*Non-polar R groups*)	glycine, alanine, valine, leucine, isoleucine
Hydroxyl- or Sulphur-Containing (*Polar, uncharged R groups*)	serine, cysteine, threonine(hydroxyl), methionine (sulphur)
Aromatic	phenylalanine, tyrosine, tryptophan
Basic (*Positively Charged R groups*)	histidine, lysine, arginine
Acidic (*Negatively Charged R groups*) and Their Amides	aspartic acid, glutamic acid (acidic) and aspargine, glutamine (amides, having polar, uncharged R groups)
Cyclic	proline

Proline does not fit into any class because it is cyclic. Proline shares many properties with the aliphatic group. The rigidity of the ring plays a critical role in protein structure. The side chain sulphydryl groups of cysteine can undergo a reversible oxidation reaction to form cystine, which contains a disulphide bond. The presence of disulphide bonds in proteins is often a critical structural feature. Proteins contain several classes of weak acid groups. The ionization state of the side chain weak acid groups controls the charge on the protein. The aromatic amino acids, tryptophan, tyrosine and phenylalanine absorb light in the ultraviolet region of the spectrum (250-300 nm). Tryptophan has the highest molar absorptivity, followed by tyrosine, with phenylalanine making only a small contribution (Table 4.2).

4.3. PROTEIN STRUCTURE

The function of a protein can only be understood in terms of its structure. Protein structure is discussed in terms of four levels of organization. *Primary structure* is the amino acid sequence of its polypeptide chain(s). Every protein has a unique amino acid sequence. *Secondary structure* is the spatial arrangement of the polypeptide backbone, ignoring the conformation of the side-chains. *Tertiary structure* is the three dimensional structure of the entire polypeptide. *Quaternary structure* refers to the three dimensional structure of proteins that are composed of two or more polypeptide chains, called sub-units.

Whereas the primary sequence of a protein is held together by *covalent peptide bonds*, the three-dimensional structure of a protein may be held together by a variety of bonds: *hydrogen bonds, ionic bonds, covalent bonds, and hydrophobic interactions.*

The peptide bond

In proteins, amino acids are joined together via the peptide bond that is formed by the reaction of the α-carboxyl group of one amino acid with the a-amino group of another amino acid (Fig. 4.3). If this process is repeated many times, then a long linear chain of amino acids is produced -a polypeptide. By convention the sequence of the polypeptide is written beginning with the residue containing the free α-amino group (the N-terminal or amino terminal) and ending with the residue containing the free α-carboxyl group (the C-terminal or carboxyl terminal), e.g. NH_2-Glu-Gly-Ala-Lys-COOH. Due to the partial double bond character of the peptide bond, the O, C, N and H atoms are nearly planar and there

Table 4.2. Physical properties of major amino acids

Name (Residue)	Single code	Relative abundance	MW	pK	VdW volume ($Å^3$)	Charged, polar, hydrophobic Hydrophobic
Alanine	A	13.0	71		67	H
Arginine	R	5.3	157	12.5	148	C^+
Asparagine	N	9.9	114		96	P
Aspartate	D	9.9	114	3.9	91	C^-
Cysteine	C	1.8	103		86	P
Glutamate	E	10.8	128	4.3	109	C^-
Glutamine	Q	10.8	128		114	P
Glycine	G	7.8	57		48	-
Histidine	H	0.7	137	6.0	118	P,C^+
Isoleucine	I	4.4	113		124	H
Leucine	L	7.8	113		124	H
Lysine	K	7.0	129	10.5	135	C^+
Methionine	M	3.8	131		124	H
Phenylalanine	F	3.3	147		135	H
Proline	P	4.6	97		90	H
Serine	S	6.0	87		73	P
Threonine	T	4.6	101		93	P
Tryptophan	W	1.0	186		163	P
Tyrosine	Y	2.2	163	10.1	141	P
Valine	V	6.0	99		105	H

is no rotation about the peptide bonds. The planarity of these elements has important consequences for the three dimensional structure of proteins.

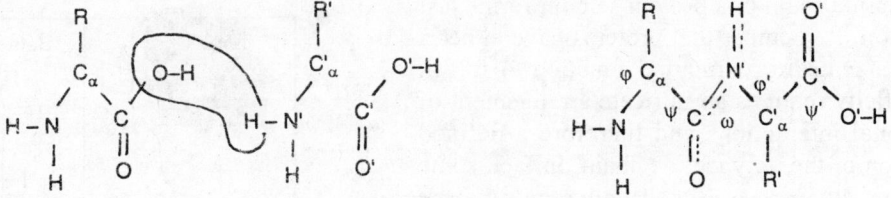

Fig. 4.3. Primary structure of proteins

The polypeptide chain

Two amino acids are combined in a condensation reaction. Notice that the peptide bond is in fact planar due to the delocalization of the electrons. The sequence of the different amino acids is considered the primary structure of the peptide or protein. Counting of residues always starts at the N-terminal end (NH_2-group).

In contrast to the rather rigid peptide bond angle w (always close to 180 deg), the bond angles phi ϕ and psi ψ can have a certain range of possible values. They are restrained by geometry to allow ranges typical for particular secondary structure elements, and represented in a Ramachandran plot (Fig. 4.4). A few important bond lengths are given in the table 4.3 below.

Table 4.3. Peptide bonds

Peptide bond	Average length	Single Bond	Average length	Hydrogen Bond	Average (±0.3)
Cα – C	1.53 (Å)	C - C	1.54 (Å)	O-H — O-H	2.8 (Å)
C – N	1.33 (Å)	C - N	1.48 (Å)	N-H — O=C	2.9 (Å)
N – Cα	1.46 (Å)	C - O	1.43 (Å)	O-H — O=C	2.8 (Å)

Amino Acid Sequence

Each amino acid in a protein is unique and determination of the amino acid sequence is an important part of characterizing proteins. Most protein amino acid sequences are deduced from the sequence of its gene, because sequencing DNA is much easier than sequencing proteins. However, determination of protein sequences is still an important tool in biochemistry. An automated process based on the Edman reaction and chromatographic techniques are used to identify the phenyl thiohydantoin(PTH)-derivative. Although these reactions proceed to > 90%, eventually (about 25 cycles) it becomes difficult to detect the newly released product. So a single Edman degradation is not able to determine the entire sequence of a protein. What is needed is a new amino terminal. This is accomplished by degrading the protein with a proteolytic enzyme, such as trypsin, which generates a number of peptides that can be separated and sequenced. Trypsin cleaves peptide bonds at the carboxyl of Lys or Arg residues, chymotrypsin cleaves peptide bonds at the carboxyl of Phe, Trp or Tyr residues. Other proteases have different specificities, which allow one a variety of ways to fragment the protein under investigation. The problem, of course, is that once the proteolysis has been accomplished and the peptides separated, you don't know how they are ordered in the original protein. Reestablishing the order is the big problem in protein sequencing.

4.4. SECONDARY STRUCTURE ELEMENTS

The polypeptide chain of a protein seldom forms just a random coil. Remember that proteins have either a chemical (enzymes) or structural function to fulfill. High specificity requires an intricate arrangement of 3-dimensional interactions and therefore a defined conformation of the polypeptide chain. In fact, some neuro-degenerative diseases like Huntington's may be related to random coil formation in certain proteins. The two most common secondary structure arrangements are the right-handed α-helix and the β-sheet, which can be connected into a larger tertiary structure (or fold) by turns and loops of a variety of types. These two secondary structure elements satisfy a strong hydrogen bond network within the geometric constraints of the bond angles ω, φ and φ. The β-sheets can be formed by parallel or, most common, antiparallel arrangement of individual β-strands.

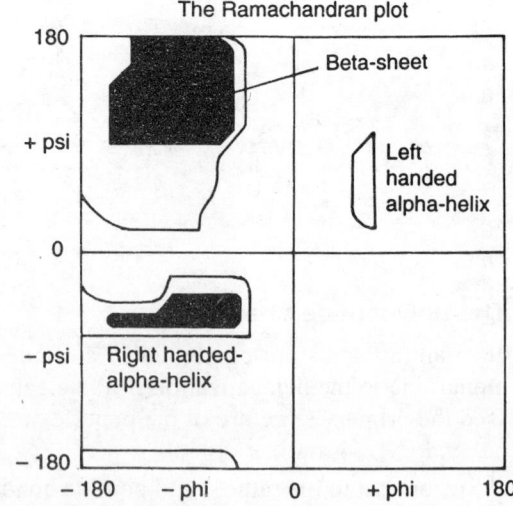

Fig. 4.4. Ramachandran plot.

The peptide bond has partial double bond character that forces the OCNH atoms of the polypeptide backbone to be planar. Thus, the only degrees of freedom for rotation in the polypeptide backbone are around the bonds to the Cα carbon - phi (φ) or psi (ψ). However, there are significant limitations as to which angles of φ and ψ can be used due to steric clashes between atoms. The Ramachandran plot shows those regions of φ and ψ where there are no steric conflicts.

Proteins are organized with the hydrophobic side-chains in the interior and the hydrophilic side chains on the surface. Because the main chain peptide bond elements, C=O and N-H, are polar, placing them in the hydrophobic interior of a protein could create a major problem. This problem is solved by the formation of hydrogen bonds between the amide protons and carbonyl oxygens of the peptide bonds in the main chain. These hydrogen bonds cause the main chain to adopt α-helix and β-sheet conformations.

In the α-helix, the protein twists to form a tightly wound spiral with the R groups facing out from the central axis. The helical structure is held together by extensive formation of hydrogen bonds that form between the carbonyl oxygens and amino hydrogens from residues four places further along the chain. In the β-conformation (or β-pleated sheet), the β-pleated sheet consists of peptide chains running side by side with hydrogen bonds holding the chains together. The sheet is most stable with the chains in an anti-parallel array; although a parallel arrangement may be seen as well. In the α-helix, intra-chain hydrogen bonds are formed between the peptide bond elements 4 residues apart in the primary sequence. The peptide bond has a dipole moment. Because the peptide bond has a dipole moment arising from the polarity of the NH and C=O groups, the helix itself has a dipole moment. (That runs the length of the helix with the amino terminal end of the helix carrying a partial positive charge and the carboxyl terminal a partial negative charge). The helix dipole moment plays an important role in binding charged ligands to proteins.

Loops and Turns

Most proteins contain combinations of α-helices and β-sheets, which are connected by loops. Loops have irregular lengths and shapes and are on the surface of the protein. The elements of the loop do not usually form hydrogen bonds to each other, but do form hydrogen bonds to water. Loop regions that connect two anti-parallel b-strands are called hairpin loops or turns. Turns are classified into Types I and II according to the (phi, psi) angles of the two central residues. Since a beta-turn has several unsaturated backbone hydrogen bond donors and acceptors, it is polar, and is usually found near the surface of the protein. Proline is very common in beta-turns, as it always has the correct phi angle (−60) and it has one less unsaturated hydrogen donor.

Folds and motifs of protein structure

The concept of a molecular motif is essentially the same as the literary one; a motif is a recurring thematic element, i.e. it is found in many molecules not uniquely in just one, and it is usually a dominant or central theme. Motifs can be seen in both molecular sequences and structures and provide a means to bridge these views of molecules. An example of a DNA motif is a repressor binding sequence - it occurs in many locations as part of its regulatory function, and it is centrally important because it mediates the interaction between the repressor molecule and the gene it regulates. Examples of protein motifs range from substructures such as the calcium binding EF-hand, to whole domains or "folds" such as the globin fold.

While the profile method can be used with either nucleic acids or proteins, the intimate coupling between sequence and structure in proteins makes the profile method especially well suited to describing protein motifs. When one looks at sequence alignments of protein families, a distinctive pattern of conserved (slowly evolving) regions and unconserved (rapidly evolving) regions can be easily seen.

This pattern arises because mutations in amino acid residues that lie in the tightly packed core of the structure are much more likely to disrupt the three-dimensional structure than are mutations in residues that lie on the surface.

Profiles provide a means to describe the sequence features that are important to a motif. This information is encoded in a two dimensional table in which the rows correspond to the positions in the motif, and the columns to all of the possible nucleotide bases or amino acid residues that could be found at each position. More simply, a profile is similar to a multiple sequence alignment where the rows are the aligned positions and the columns tabulate the frequencies of the residues or bases at each position.

Despite that there are about 100,000 different proteins expressed in eukaryotic systems, there are much fewer different structural motifs and folds, partly as a consequence of evolved pathways and mechanisms. Motif in this sense does refer to a small specific combination of secondary structure elements (such as helix-turn-helix), and not to the contents of the asymmetric unit cell as used as a crystallographic term. Fold refers to a global type of arrangement, like helix-bundle or β-barrel.

Motif example : EF hand

A typical small motif is the calcium binding EF-hand in calmodulin, a ubiquitions molecule undergoing Ca-dependent conformational changes. It contains 4 Ca^{++} ions which are coordinated in a typical fashion in a helix-turn-helix motif called the EF-hand.

The positively calcium atom Ca^{++} is coordinated through hydrogen bonds with acidic (negatively charged) aspartate and glutamate residues as well as with backbone oxygen atoms. Other typical motif in the alpha-domain structures is the 4-helix bundle. Ferritin, cytochrome b562 and apo-E are typical examples. The helices are amphipathic (hydrophobic residues on one side, charged ones on the other and pack antiparallel with the hydrophobic sides towards each other forming a hydrophobic core.

4.5. TERTIARY STRUCTURE

Most proteins are globular, essentially spherical. They posses both secondary structure and are folded into compact tertiary structures : every protein has a unique three dimensional structure made up of a variety of helices, beta-sheets and non-regular regions, which are folded in a specific manner.

Domains

Polypeptide chains of >200 amino acids that fold into two or more compact globular clusters are called domains. There are three main types of domains:

a) α domains are composed of α-helices.
b) β domains contain anti-parallel β sheets and usually contain two β sheets packed against each other.
c) α/β domains contain the β-α-β motif of parallel β sheets.

Adjacent domains are connected by one or two segments of the polypeptide chain.

Generalizations about Protein Structure

All globular proteins have a defined inside and outside. In the tertiary structure of proteins almost all the hydrophobic side-chains are found in the interior of the protein and almost all hydrophilic side-chains are found on the outside of the protein, interacting with water. Globular proteins are compact. There is no space inside, so water is effectively excluded from the hydrophobic interior. Nearly all buried hydrogen bond donors, e.g., Ser, form hydrogen bonds with hydrogen bond acceptors, e.g., Gln. In essence hydrogen bond formation neutralizes the polarity of the hydrogen bonding group. β-sheets are usually twisted or wrapped into *barrel* structures and *loops* and *turns* are on the outside of the protein.

Mutations, which place a hydrophobic side-chain on the surface, can cause significant changes in the folding of the protein.

4.6. QUATERNARY STRUCTURE

Many large proteins contain more than one polypeptide chain. The spatial arrangement of these sub-units is the quaternary structure of the protein (e.g. haemoglobin). The forces that hold subunits together are the same weak bonds as those that stabilize the tertiary structure of proteins - van der Waals and London Dispersion forces, salt bridges and hydrogen bonds. The contact region between sub-units resembles the interior of a protein. The sub-units may be identical or non-identical, but there is always a defined stoichiometery.

Several proteins function by forming transient complexes with other proteins. For example electron transfer from cytochrome *c* to cytochrome *c* peroxidase involves the formation of such a complex. Because such complexes are transient, the interactions are weaker than those that stabilize the quaternary structure of hemoglobin. In the cytochrome *c*-cytochrome *c* peroxidase complex there are specific electrostatic interactions that guide the two proteins together in the correct orientation.

4.7. PROTEIN FOLDING

The amino acid sequence of a protein contains all the information required for the protein to fold into the correct, biologically active, three-dimensional structure. One of the important unsolved problems in biochemistry is the "folding problem" by which we mean, "how do proteins fold?"

- The process most likely begins with the formation of secondary structural elements, which serve as nucleation foci around which the native structure of the protein can fold.
- It is likely that α-helices are the most important nucleation foci because they are formed from amino acids that are next to each other in the linear sequence, whereas β sheets are often formed by the interaction of strands that are far apart in the linear sequence.
- Nuclei with the proper native-like secondary structure probably interact with each until they form a native-like domain.
- Ultimately these secondary structural domains will come together to form a structure with extensive secondary structure, but disordered tertiary structure - the molten globule state.
- Finally, small rearrangement of the molten globule generates the native conformation.

While it is accepted that the amino acid sequence of a protein contains all the information necessary for the protein to adopt its correct three-dimensional structure, it is becoming clear that there are several accessory proteins that assist in the folding process. Among these are the molecular chaperones, multi-subunit proteins that utilize ATP to "guide" proteins along the correct folding pathway

Some proteins get misfolded. While most misfolded proteins are simply degraded in the cell, there are some situations in which the misfolded protein accumulates in the cell and leads to a pathological condition. What seems to happen is that the misfolded intermediate forms inappropriate aggregates leading to the formation of large polymers. Among the known examples of diseases caused by misfolded proteins are: cystic fibrosis, scurvy, and Alzheimer's disease.

4.8. PROTEIN FUNCTION

Many proteins function by interacting with other molecules. This often involves reversible binding. A molecule that binds reversibly with a protein is called a ligand. Just about any kind of molecule (or a single atom) can act as a ligand. A ligand binds to a protein at a part of the protein called the binding site, and this binding site is generally designed to bind very specifically to a particular ligand. Enzymes not only bind ligands, but they catalyze chemical reactions that transform the ligands. The ligand that is acted on by an enzyme is referred to as the enzyme's substrate, and the binding site of the enzyme is referred to as the active site.

Myoglobin and haemoglobin are globular proteins that reversibly bind oxygen. Note that these proteins are not enzymes, because they do not alter the ligand.

4.9. PROTEINS - PURIFICATION AND CHARACTERISATION

1. Source of Protein

- In order to purify a protein you need a source. It might be blood or some other biological fluid, but most often it is a cell, usually a specific type - liver, muscle, yeast, bacteria, etc.
- The cells must be broken open - homogenized - to release the protein in a soluble form.
- Homogenization conditions must be worked out that release the protein from the cell without damaging the protein.

2. Fractional Precipitation

- In concentrated salt solutions, usually ammonium sulfate is used, some proteins are more soluble than others. By varying the concentration of ammonium sulfate, one can achieve some limited purification of proteins. This technique is often used in the first step of protein purification.
- In general,
  1. Small proteins are more soluble than large proteins.
  2. The larger the number of charged side chains, the more soluble the protein.

3. Column Chromatography

- Column chromatography is the basis for the development of procedures for obtaining pure proteins. Studies on pure proteins are essential for understanding the structural and functional properties of proteins.
  a) In column chromatography an absorbent is placed in a glass tube.
  b) A protein mixture is passed into the column and binds to the absorbent.
  c) By proper choice of the eluting buffer, specific proteins can be eluted from the absorbent and separated from other proteins in the mixture.
  d) By repeating this procedure with several different absorbents, pure protein can be obtained.
- Because proteins are not very stable, low temperature (4° C) and neutral pH must often be employed.

4. Ion Exchange Chromatography

- Ion exchange resins have fixed charges - either positive or negative.
- Proteins bind to the resin via electrostatic interactions.
- The strength of these interactions depends on the net charge on the protein, which is a function of pH and the nature of the weak acid amino acid side chains, and the salt concentration of the buffer - high salt concentrations reduce the interaction.

5. Affinity Chromatography

- This is a more specific interaction in which a ligand specifically recognized by the protein of interest is attached to the column material.
- When a mixture of proteins is passed through the column, only those few that bind strongly to the ligand will stick, while the others will pass through the column.
- By changing the buffer one weakens the interaction between the protein and the ligand, which causes the protein to be eluted from the column.
- A variation is immunoaffinity chromatography, in which an antibody specific for a protein is immobilized on the column and used to affinity purify the specific protein.

6. Gel Filtration Chromatography

- The column consists of material that separates proteins based on their size and shape.
- Wide ranges of molecular exclusion limits are available for separating proteins of all sizes.
- For any particular column dimensions and material, the volume of buffer required to elute a specific protein depends on the molecular weight of the protein. Thus, one can separate proteins by size.
- If one calibrates the column by determining the elution volume of proteins with known molecular weights, then a calibration curve relating elution volume and molecular weight can be constructed.
- Such a calibration curve can then be used to estimate the molecular weight of an unknown protein.

7. Dialysis/Ultrafiltration

- Semipermeable membranes are available, which allow passage of small molecules but exclude the passage of proteins. Sacs made of such material allow the salt and buffer components of a protein solution to be changed to another buffer.

8. Electrophoresis : Protein Characterization

- In an electric field a protein or other charged macromolecule will move with a velocity that depends directly on the charge on the macromolecule and inversely on its size and shape.
- Gel electrophoresis is carried out in some supporting media, usually polyacrylamide or agarose, which has pores of sufficient size to allow passage of the macromolecule.
- The proteins in the gel are easily stained for detection purposes.
- Because the net charge on a protein and its molecular weight are characteristic properties of a protein, electrophoresis is a powerful method for characterizing the purity of a protein preparation
- *SDS-PAGE (sodium dodecyl sulfate-polyacrylamide gel electrophoresis)* is a variant of electrophoresis in which the buffers contain SDS, a detergent that binds to proteins. It is a very useful method for determining the molecular weight of a protein
- Most proteins bind SDS at a constant ratio, about 1 SDS for every 2 amino acids.
- The large negative charge resulting from the bound SDS masks the native charge on the protein, so that all proteins have essentially the same charge to mass ratio.
- This means that that the rate of movement in the electric field depends only on the molecular weight.

- In addition, the SDS causes all proteins to adopt a random-coil structure, which means that shape does not effect movement through the gel.
- *Western blotting* is a technique for detecting a specific protein in a mixture.

9. Isoelectric Focusing

- In this technique electrophoresis occurs through a stable pH gradient.
- Under these conditions the proteins will migrate in the electric field until they reach a point in the pH gradient where their net charge becomes 0 - the isoelectric point.
- The isoelectric point depends on the exact number and type of weak acid amino acid side chains present in the protein. Therefore, isoelectric focusing is a useful purification procedure.
- Often isoelectric focusing is combined with SDS PAGE in two-dimensional electrophoresis

10. Centrifugation : Molecular Weight Estimation.

- Estimates of molecular weight can be obtained using SDS-PAGE or gel filtration, as described above.
- One very useful technique for measuring molecular weight and shape is *centrifugation.*
- Ultracentrifugation is used in two ways to characterize proteins :
  a) In sedimentation equilibrium experiments, the centrifuge is operated at a relative low speed so that the forces of sedimentation and diffusion balance and the protein distributes in the centrifuge cell in a manner proportional to its molecular weight.
  b) In sedimentation velocity experiments, the centrifuge is operated at maximal speed, which causes the protein to sediment to the bottom of the tube. The rate at which the boundary moves gives S, which when combined with M gives f, a measure of the shape of the protein.

11. Mass Spectrometry

- Mass spectrometry has become an important technique in peptide/protein chemistry. Mass spectrometers consist of three basic parts :
  a) An ion source that creates charged molecules in the gas phase
  b) A mass analyzer that uses a physical property, e.g., time-of-flight (TOF), to separate ions
  c) A detector.
- Two important methods are used to create protein ions:
  a) In matrix-assisted laser desorption ionization (MALDI), using a laser to excite proteins in a crystalline matrix creates ions. MALDI is particularly suited for determining the molecular weight of proteins, often to accuracy of a few parts per million.
  b) In electrospray applying a potential to a flowing liquid creates ionization (ESI) ions. This causes the liquid to spray and protein ions to be created.

5

Using the Linux Operating System

5.1. INTRODUCTION TO LINUX

Linux has found its way onto the servers and desktops of major corporations as well as personal computers. It offers one of the most powerful and reliable systems available—and as an open source system, it can be altered to meet the needs of its users.

Linux is an operating system that can be downloaded free and "belongs" to an entire community of developers, not one corporate entity. That's why Linux is known as "open source" or "free software," because there is nothing secret about this system. This freedom also allows companies to sell and distribute Linux on CD-ROM or by other means, although those companies must keep their code open to the public.

With more and more people looking for an alternative to Windows, Linux has recently grown in popularity and is quickly becoming a favourite among major corporations and curious desktop users. Not only does it give users a choice of operating systems, it also proves itself valuable with its power, flexibility and reliability.

How did Linux get started?

The concept of open source programming has been around for many years—its roots stem from universities that needed to be able to share information as well as allow students and developers to adapt programs to meet their needs. In 1984, Richard Stallman, a researcher at the MIT AI Lab, started a project he called GNU to counter the fast-moving trend toward proprietary, fee-based software. Stallman, who remains an open advocate of open source, believes that making source code available to anyone who wants it is integral to furthering computer science and innovation.

This concept served as the basis of Linux development, the brainchild of Linus Torvalds. When Torvalds began developing Linux in 1991, he was a student at the University of Helsinki and originally targeted Linux at the Intel 386 (although it is now one of the most widely ported operating systems available for PCs).

What are the advantages and disadvantages of using Linux?

Linux is an extremely powerful and reliable operating system that gives users a certain flexibility not found within other systems. Aside from the fact that Linux can be downloaded and upgraded for free (and therefore becomes attractive to small businesses and individuals on a small budget), it can also be altered by the user to fix bugs or meet specific operating needs. The disadvantages to using Linux currently includes the simple fact that it can be tricky to install if there isn't support to help guide new users through the process. Likewise, users who are accustomed to using a Windows interface will have to adjust to a different system—although the adjustment generally isn't a complicated one.

What software is available for Linux users?

Almost all Linux software is available for free to users, and many people don't realize the variety of programs available.

Examples include :

Graphics programs like the GIMP (GNU Image Manipulation Program)

Development software like BASIC and Perl

Word processing programs like Word Perfect

Office suites like StarOffice and Applixware

Games like Civilization: Call to Power, Quake II, Flightgear and Majik 3D.

Speed

Linux machines are also known to be extremely fast, because the operating system is very efficient at managing resources such as memory, CPU power, and disk space. More of the Web than one might expect is actually powered by old 486 boxes running Linux and the Apache Web Server, while NASA, Sandia, Fermilabs and others have built very powerful yet inexpensive supercomputers by creating clusters of Linux boxes running in parallel.

5.2. THE BASICS OF LINUX SYSTEM

Linux operating system

Linux is a layered operating system. The innermost layer is the hardware that provides the services for the OS. The operating system, referred to in Linux/Unix as the kernel, interacts directly with the hardware and provides the services to the user programs. These user programs don't need to know anything about the hardware. They just need to know how to interact with the kernel and it's up to the kernel to provide the desired service. One of the big appeals of Linux to programmers has been that most well written user programs are independent of the underlying hardware, making them readily portable to new systems. User programs interact with the kernel through a set of standard system calls. These system calls request services to be provided by the kernel. Such services would include accessing a file: open close, read, write, link, or execute a file; starting or updating accounting records; changing ownership of a file or directory; changing to a new directory; creating, suspending, or killing a process; enabling access to hardware devices; and setting limits on system resources. Linux is a multi-user, multi-tasking operating system. You can have many users logged into a system simultaneously, each running many programs. It's the kernel's job to keep each process and user separate and to regulate access to system hardware, including CPU, memory, disk and other I/O devices.

Graphical Interface

As for an intuitive graphical interface, Linux has at least a dozen different, highly configurable graphical interfaces (known as window managers) which run on top of XFree86, a free implementation of the X

Window System. The most popular window managers at the moment are KDE (the K Desktop Environment) and GNOME (the GNU Network Object Model Environment). These offer the point-and-click, drag-and-drop functionality associated with other user-friendly environments (for example, Macintosh), but are extremely flexible and can take on a number of different looks and feels. If you want a Linux box running KDE to look just like a Mac, Windows, BeOS, or NextStep machine, you can do it with a few mouse clicks. Today, even complex tasks like system administration, package installation, upgrading, and network configuration can be done easily through graphical programs. Programs that work with one window manager nearly always work with all the others.

Networking

Networking comes naturally to Linux. After all, Linux is based on UNIX, where computer networking more or less developed. Probably all networking protocols in use on the Internet are native to UNIX and/or Linux, so one can expect that UNIX and Linux would network better than any other platforms. Setting up a network on a Linux machine is surprisingly simple, because Linux handles most of the work; you just have to give it the correct addresses. Linux is made for networking. A large part of the Web is running on Linux boxes.

Prompt

If you login as root (or the superuser), the prompt will be machinename:~# and if you login as user, the prompt will be machinename:~$. The tilde character (~) represents the home directory; appended to the end of a filename, it means a backup of a file that has been edited.

Shell Account

A good place to start is to find out what kind of shell you have. There are many shells (Bourne, C, Korn etc.), each of which has slightly different ways of working. To do this, at your prompt give the command "echo $SHELL."

    If you get the response: /bin/sh, that means you have the Bourne shell.

    If you get: /bin/bash, then you are in the Bourne Again (bash) shell.

    If you get: /bin/ksh, you have the Korn shell.

    If the "echo $SHELL" command doesn't work, try the command "echo $shell".This will likely get you the answer: /bin/csh. This means that you are in the C shell.

    Why is it important to know which shell you have? For right now, you'll want a shell that is easy to use. If you are a beginner, you will find bash to be the easiest shell to use. You may be able to get the bash shell by simply typing the word "bash" at the prompt. If this doesn't work, ask tech support at your ISP for a shell account set up to use bash.

Processes

A shell acts as the intermediary between the user and the operating system, interpreting your commands into a form that the operating system can understand. The shell has the capacity to run multiple commands at one time, and can run commands in the background using the ampersand (&) after the command.

    Multiple requests to the shell are called processes. As these requests are made, beginning with init during boot, the shell numbers them. These numbers are important if you want to stop a process: use the command ps to to see a list of current processes, then the command kill and the number of the process you want to stop.

Common Linux commands

Some of the commands most frequently used are :

1. man : This command brings up the online Unix manual.
2. ls : Lists files. Use "ls -alF|more" for listing. "|" is known as the pipe character. The "pipe" allows the output (file) of the command to be piped to the command "more" which lets you scroll through the list one page at a time.
3. pwd : Present working directory; shows what directory you are in.
4. cd : Change directory
5. more : This shows the contents of text files. You can also use "cat" which is for concatenation. (Linux, as discussed above treats the devices also as files. When you do a cat (concatenation of a file with the terminal screen, which is the other file), you can see the contents of the file on the screen.
6. whereis : Lets you find a file. Similar commands are "find" and "locate."
7. vi : Visual editor, an editing program.
8. grep : Extracts information from files, especially useful for seeing what's in syslog and shell log files. Similar commands are "egrep," "fgrep," and "look."
9. chmod : Change file permissions.
10. rm : Delete file.
11. cp : Copy file, and "mv" for move file.

LAN and Internet exploration tools

1. telnet : Telnet allows you to login remotely from a remote computer to a host server running any unix or unix clone system. Other variation is called RLOGIN/rlogin.
2. who : Shows you who else is currently logged in on your LAN. Other good commands to explore the other users on your LAN are "w," "rwho, " "users."
3. whois : Get information on Internet hosts outside you LAN.
4. ftp : File transfer protocol, use it to upload and download files to and from other computers.

5.3. USING LINUX FILE SYSTEM AND DIRECTORIES

File System

If one is comfortable with the DOS prompt, one can see a lot of similarities in Linux. However, if most of your experience has been in Windows or menu driven operating systems, the command line may seem a little awkward at first.

Linux has a hierarchical, unified filesystem (hierarchical means that there are directories within directories; and unified means that files, directories, and device drivers are treated as files). All command line entries are case sensitive.

Also note that Linux uses the slash (/) rather than the backslash (\) used in DOS (Fig. 5.1).

There is extensive online help available on any command on your system called the man pages (or manual pages). You can type in man CommandInQuestion to get a summary of what the command does and a brief summary of the options.

Linux, like all Unix, assumes you know what you're doing and that you do not make typographical errors. Linux, like all Unix, will execute whatever command you give it - all that matters is that it's a valid command. If it's not what you intended, that's your mistake.

There are four types of file:

> Ordinary files - text files (plain vanilla ASCII)
> Data files (contain special characters not contained in the ASCII set)
> Command text files (shell scripts)
> Executable files (binaries)

Files form directories and there can be many directories in a directory.

The main subdirectories ("/" is the root directory of the tree structured filesystem) are:

> /bin - binary files
> /boot - information need to boot the system
> /cdrom - CD-ROM drive
> /dos - DOS partition
> /dev - device drivers
> /etc - miscellaneous files (mostly system administration)
> /home - home directories for users
> /lib - programming libraries
> /tmp - temporary files
> /usr - commands
> /lost+found - recovered files

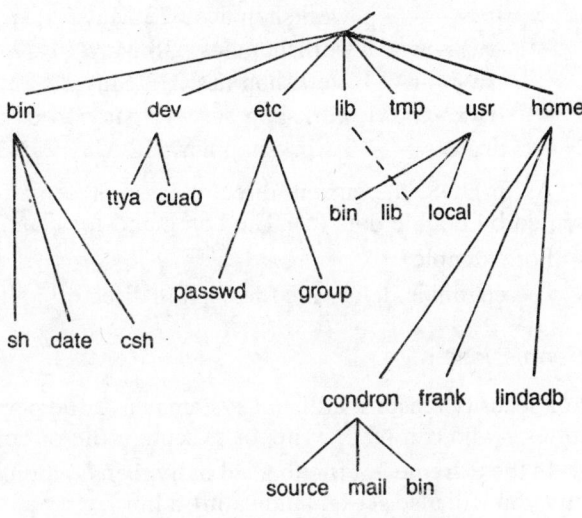

Fig. 5.1. Linux operating system.

Listing Directories

You can get a listing with dir, or ls (with any shell). The default is to list files in alphabetical order (capitals and numbers first).

Some of the most useful options with ls are:

> -a : lists all files, including hidden files
> -A : lists all files, except the current and parent directory
> -c : sorts file by time (oldest first)
> -d : lists only the name of a directory, not its contents
> -l : lists in long format (showing permissions and other details)
> -r : lists in reverse order
> -t : sorts files by time (newest first)
> -x : lists all files across the page instead of in columns.

Example

To get a long listing:

> % ls -al
> total 24
> drwxr-sr-x 5 workshop acs 512 Apr 7 11:12 .
> drwxr-xr-x 6 root sys 512 Mar 29 09:59 ..
> -rwxr-xr-x 1 workshop acs 532 May 20 15:31 .cshrc
> -rw------- 1 workshop acs 525 May 20 21:29 .emacs

```
-rw——— 1 workshop acs 622 May 24 12:13 .history
-rwxr-xr-x 1 workshop acs 238 May 14 09:44 .login
-rw-r—r— 1 workshop acs 273 May 22 23:53 .plan
-rwxr-xr-x 1 workshop acs 413 May 14 09:36 .profile
drwx——— 3 workshop acs 512 May 24 11:18 demofiles
```

As in DOS, the current directory is represented by a single dot (.); the parent directory is represented by double dots (..). The command for change directory is cd .

For example,

cd /bin ls -l, lists the files in /bin directory; all files here are binaries and end with an asterisk (*).

Permissions

For security reasons, all Unix systems have file permissions that allow you to control access to directories - who can read, write, or execute a file or command in a directory.

In the extreme left is either a d or hyphen (-) indicating whether this is a directory or a file (occasionally you will also see an l indicating a link).

Then you see three groups of the same three letters in the same order: r for read, w for write, x for execute, and the hyphen (-) for no permission given in that type. The first group of three letters is for the owner, the second group for the group, and the third the world. Whoever creates the file is the owner, and if more than one person is working on a project or needs access to this file they are given permission as a group, and finally how the file is open to anyone who has access to the system.

The command to change file permissions is chmod (change mode). There are two ways for doing this: the numeric system and the symbolic system.

The numeric system uses numbers to track permissions. Using the table below you add together the numeric equivalent for the permissions you want.

400 - owner has read permission 200 - owner has write permission 100 - owner has execute permission

040 - group has read permission 020 - group has write permission 010 - group has execute permission

004 - world has read permission 002 - world has write permission 001 - world has execute permission

Thus "chmod 764 TestFile", gives the owner permission to read, write, and execute "TestFile"; the group has permission to read and write; the world permission to read only.

The other method for changing modes is the symbolic method. With this method, you have to know the existing permissions because the commands are added or removed relative to how permissions are currently set. The plus sign (+) adds a permission, the minus sign (-) removes a permission.

u - user (owner) g - group o - other (world) a - everyone - user, group, and other

r - read permission w - write permission x - execute permission

Thus chmod g+x TestFile gives permission to the group to execute TestFile. You can also change the owner with the chown command, and change the group with chgrp.

Directory Navigation and Control

Command/Syntax	What it will do
cd [directory]	change directory
ls [options] [directory or file]	list directory contents or file permissions

mkdir [options] *directory*	make a *directory*
pwd	print working (current) directory
rmdir [options] *directory*	remove a *directory*
mkdir	· make a directory

You can extend your home hierarchy by making sub-directories below it. This is done with the *mkdir*, make directory, command.

Common Options

-p create the intermediate (parent) directories, as needed
-m mode access permissions (SVR4).

Examples

% mkdir /home/frank/data
or, if your present working directory is /home/frank the following would be equivalent:
% mkdir data
rmdir - remove directory

A directory needs to be empty before you can remove it. If it's not, you need to remove the files first. Also, you can't remove a directory if it is your present working directory; you must first come out of it.

Linking Files

Rather than having multiple copies of a file, Linux uses links to one file to save disk space and administrative headaches trying to keep multiple copies up to date and synchronized. Linux supports two types of links, hard links and symbolic links.

Hard links are set with the command :
        ln FileName /New Directory Location

The problem with hard links is that Linux treats all hard links equally, and before you can delete the original file, you have to remove all hard links. On the other hand, symbolic links don't need to be physically removed in order to delete the file.

Wildcards

Linux has three types of wildcards - the question mark (?), which is used to match a single character, the same as in DOS; the asterisk (*), which is much more expansive than anything in DOS because it can be used to return any number of letters at the beginning or end of an expression; and the final wildcard used to return specific characters as defined within brackets ([ ]).

A symbolic link is used to create a new path to another file or directory. If a group of users, for example, is accustomed to using a command called *chkmag*, but the command has been rewritten and is now called *chkit*, creating a symbolic link so the users will automatically execute *chkit* when they enter the command *chkmag* will ease transition to the new command.

A symbolic link would be done in the following way:
        % ln -s chkit chkmag
        The long listing for these two files is now as follows:
        16 -rwxr-x— 1 lindadb acs 15927 Apr 23 04:10 chkit

1 lrwxrwxrwx 1 lindadb acs 5 Apr 23 04:11 chkmag -> chkit

Note that while the permissions for *chkmag* are open to all, since it is linked to *chkit*, the permissions, group and owner characteristics for *chkit* will be enforced when *chkmag* is run. With a symbolic link, the link can exist without the file or directory it is linked to existing first.

A hard link can only be done to another file on the same file system, but not to a directory (except by the superuser). A hard link creates a new directory entry pointing to the same inode as the original file. The file linked to must exist before the hard link can be created. The file will not be deleted until all the hard links to it are removed. To link the two files above with a hard link to each other do:

% ln chkit chkmag

Then a long listing shows that the inode number (742) is the same for each:

% ls -il chkit chkmag

742 -rwxr-x— 2 lindadb acs 15927 Apr 23 04:10 chkit

742 -rwxr-x— 2 lindadb acs 15927 Apr 23 04:10 chkmag

Working With Files

This section describes a number of commands that you might find useful in examining and manipulating the contents of your files.

cmp [options] *file1 file2* compare two files and list where differences occur (text or binary files)

cut [options] [*file*(s)] cut specified field(s)/character(s) from lines in file(s)

diff [options] *file1 file2* compare the two files and display the differences (text files only)

file [options] *file* classify the file type

find directory [options] [actions] find files matching a type or pattern

ln [options] *source_file target* link the *source_file* to the *target*

paste [options] *file* paste field(s) onto the lines in *file*

sort [options] *file* sort the lines of the *file* according to the options chosen

strings [options] *file* report any sequence of 4 or more printable characters ending in <NL> or <NULL>. Usually used to search binary files for ASCII strings.

tee [options] *file* copy stdout to one or more files

touch [options] [date] *file* create an empty file, or update the access time of an existing file

tr [options] *string1 string2* translate the characters in string1 from stdin into those in string2 in stdout

uniq [options] *file* remove repeated lines in a file

wc [options] [*file*(s)] display word (or character or line) count for *file*(s)

cmp - compare file contents

The *cmp* command compares two files, and (without options) reports the location of the first difference between them. It can deal with both binary and ASCII file comparisons. It does a byte-by-byte comparison.

Syntax

cmp [options] file1 file2 [skip1] [skip2]

The skip numbers are the number of bytes to skip in each file before starting the comparison.

Common options

-l report on each difference

'   -s report exit status only, not byte differences

find - find files

The *find* command will recursively search the indicated directory tree to find files matching a type or pattern you specify. *find* can then list the files or execute arbitrary commands based on the results.

Syntax

find directory [search options] [actions]

Common Options

For the time search options the notation in days, n is:

+n more than n days

n exactly n days

-n less than n days

Some file characteristics that *find* can search for are:

time that the file was last accessed or changed

-atime n access time, true if accessed n days ago

-ctime n change time, true if the files status was changed n days ago

-mtime n modified time, true if the files data was modified n days ago

-newer filename true if newer than filename

-*type type of file, where type can be:*

b block special file

c character special file

d directory

l symbolic link

p named pipe (fifo)

f regular file

-fstype type of file system, where type can be any valid file system type, e.g.: ufs (Unix File System) and nfs (Network File System)

-user username true if the file belongs to the user username

-group groupname true if the file belongs to the group groupname

-perm [-]mode permissions on the file, where mode is the octal modes for the *chmod* command. When mode is precede by the minus sign only the bits that are set are compared.

-exec command execute command. The end of command is indicated by an escape and semicolon (\;). The command argument, {}, replaces the current path name.

-name filename true if the file is named filename. Wildcard pattern matches are allowed if the meta-character is escaped from the shell with a backslash (\).

-ls always true. It prints a long listing of the current pathname.

-print print the pathnames found

5.4 TEXT PROCESSING

Text Processing Commands

This section provides an introduction to the use of regular expressions and *grep*. The *grep* utility is used to search for generalized regular expressions occurring in Unix files. Regular expressions, such as those shown above, are best specified in apostrophes (or single quotes) when specified in the *grep* utility. The *egrep* utility provides searching capability using an extended set of meta-characters. The syntax of the *grep* utility, some of the available options, and a few examples are shown below.

Syntax

> *grep* [options] regexp [file[s]]

Common Options

-i ignore case

-c report only a count of the number of lines containing matches, not the matches themselves

-v invert the search, displaying only lines that do not match

-n display the line number along with the line on which a match was found

-s work silently, reporting only the final status:

0, for match(es) found

1, for no matches

2, for errors

-l list filenames, but not lines, in which matches were found

grep/egrep/fgrep [options] 'search string' *file* search the argument (in this case probably a file) for all occurrences of the search string, and list them.

sed [options] *file* stream editor for editing files from a script or from the command line

Example

Consider the following file:

{unix prompt 5} cat num.list

```
 1  15 fifteen
 2  14 fourteen
 3  13 thirteen
 4  12 twelve
 5  11 eleven
 6  10 ten
 7   9 nine
 8   8 eight
 9   7 seven
10   6 six
11   5 five
12   4 four
13   3 three
14   2 two
15   1 one
```

Here are some *grep* examples using this file.

(i) Search for the number 15:

```
    {unix prompt 6} grep '15' num.list
       1  15 fifteen
      15   1 one
```

(ii) Now we'll use the "-c" option to count the number of lines matching the search criterion:

{unix prompt 7} grep -c '15' num.list
2

(iii) Here we'll be a little more general in our search, selecting for all lines containing the character 1 followed by either of 1, 2 or 5:

{unix prompt 8} grep '1[125]' num.list
   1 15 fifteen
   4 12 twelve
   5 11 eleven
 11 5 five
 12 4 four
 15 1 one

(iv) Now we'll search for all lines that begin with a space:

{unix prompt 9} grep '^ ' num.list
 1 15 fifteen
 2 14 fourteen
 3 13 thirteen
 4 12 twelve
 5 11 eleven
 6 10 ten
 7 9 nine
 8 8 eight
 9 7 seven

(v) Search all lines that don't begin with a space:

{unix prompt 10} grep '^[^]' num.list
10 6 six
11 5 five
12 4 four
13 3 three
14 2 two
15 1 one

(vi) The latter could also be done by using the -v option with the original search string, e.g.:

{unix prompt 11} grep -v '^ ' num.list
10 6 six
11 5 five
12 4 four
13 3 three
14 2 two
15 1 one

(vii) Search for all lines that begin with the characters 1 through 9:

{unix prompt 12} grep '^[1-9]' num.list
10 6 six
11 5 five
12 4 four
13 3 three

14 2 two
15 1 one

(viii) Search for any instances of t followed by zero or more occurrences of e:
{unix prompt 13} grep 'te*' num.list

1 15 fifteen
2 14 fourteen
3 13 thirteen
4 12 twelve
6 10 ten
8 8 eight
13 3 three
14 2 two

(ix) Search for any instances of t followed by one or more occurrences of e:
{unix prompt 14} grep 'tee*' num.list

1 15 fifteen
2 14 fourteen
3 13 thirteen
6 10 ten

awk, nawk, gawk

awk is a pattern scanning and processing language. Its name comes from the last initials of the three authors: Alfred. V. Aho, Brian. W. Kernighan, and Peter. J. Weinberger. *nawk* is new *awk*, a newer version of the program, and *gawk* is gnu *awk*, from the Free Software Foundation. Each version is a little different. Here we'll confine ourselves to simple examples which should be the same for all versions. On some OSs *awk* is really *nawk*.

awk searches its input for patterns and performs the specified operation on each line, or fields of the line, that contain those patterns. You can specify the pattern matching statements for *awk* either on the command line, or by putting them in a file and using the -f program_file option.

Syntax

awk program [file]

where program is composed of one or more: pattern { action } fields. Each input line is checked for a pattern match with the indicated action being taken on a match. This continues through the full sequence of patterns, then the next line of input is checked. Input is divided into records and fields. The default record separator is <newline>, and the variable NR keeps the record count. The default field separator is whitespace, spaces and tabs, and the variable NF keeps the field count. Input field, FS, and record, RS, separators can be set at any time to match any single character. Output field, OFS, and record, ORS, separators can also be changed to any single character, as desired. $n, where n is an integer, is used to represent the nth field of the input record, while $0 represents the entire input record. BEGIN and END are special patterns matching the beginning of input, before the first field is read, and the end of input, after the last field is read, respectively. Printing is allowed through the *print*, and formatted print, *printf*, statements.

Patterns may be regular expressions, arithmetic relational expressions, string-valued expressions, and boolean combinations of any of these. For the latter the patterns can be combined with the boolean operators below, using parentheses to define the combination:

‖ or

&& and

! not

Comma separated patterns define the range for which the pattern is applicable, e.g.:

/first/,/last/

selects all lines starting with the one containing first, and continuing inclusively, through the one containing last.

To select lines 15 through 20 use the pattern range:

NR == 15, NR == 20

Regular expressions must be enclosed with slashes (/) and meta-characters can be escaped with the backslash (\). Regular expressions can be grouped with the operators:

| or, to separate alternatives

+ one or more

? zero or one

A regular expression match can be either of:

~ contains the expression

!~ does not contain the expression

So the program:

$1 ~ /[Ff]rank/

is true if the first field, $1, contains "Frank" or "frank" anywhere within the field. To match a field identical to "Frank" or "frank" use:

$1 ~ /^[Ff]rank$/

Relational expressions are allowed using the relational operators:

< less than

<= less than or equal to

== equal to

>= greater than or equal to

!= not equal to

> greater than

Off-hand you don't know if variables are strings or numbers. If neither operand is known to be numeric, than string comparisons are performed. Otherwise, a numeric comparison is done. In the absence of any information to the contrary, a string comparison is done, so that:

$1 > $2

will compare the string values. To ensure a numerical comparison, do something similar to:

($1 + 0) > $2

The mathematical functions: exp, log and sqrt are built-in. Some other built-in functions include:

index (s,t) returns the position of string s where t first occurs, or 0 if it doesn't

length (s) returns the length of string s

substr (s,m,n) returns the n-character substring of s, beginning at position m

Arrays are declared automatically when they are used, e.g.

arr[i] = $1

assigns the first field of the current input record to the ith element of the array.

Flow control statements using if-else, while, and for are allowed with C type syntax:

for (i=1; i <= NF; i++) {actions}
while (i<=NF) {actions}
if (i<NF) {actions}

5.5. WRITING SHELL PROGRAMS

You can write shell programs by creating scripts containing a series of shell commands. The first line of the script should start with #! which indicates to the kernel that the script is directly executable. You immediately follow this with the name of the shell, or program (spaces are allowed), to execute, using the full path name. Generally you can count on having up to 32 characters, possibly more on some systems, and can include one option. So to set up a Bourne shell script the first line would be:

#! /bin/sh

or for the C shell:

#! /bin/csh -f

where the "-f" option indicates that it should not read your .cshrc. Any blanks following the magic symbols, #!, are optional.

You also need to specify that the script is executable by setting the proper bits on the file with *chmod*, e.g.:

% chmod +x shell_script

Within the scripts # indicates a comment from that point until the end of the line, with #! being a special case if found as the first characters of the file.

Setting Parameter Values

Parameter values, e.g. param, are assigned as:

Bourne shell   C shell
param=value   set param = value

where value is any valid string, and can be enclosed within quotations, either single ('value) or double ("value"), to allow spaces within the string value. When enclosed with backquotes ('value') the string is first evaluated by the shell and the result is substituted. This is often used to run a command, substituting the command output for value, e.g. after the parameter values have been assigned, the current value of the parameter is accessed using the $param, or ${param}, notation.

Quoting

We quote strings to control the way the shell interprets any parameters or variables within the string. We can use single (') and double (") quotes around strings. Double quotes define the string, but allow variable substitution. Single quotes define the string and prevent variable substitution. A backslash (\) before a character is said to escape it, meaning that the system should take the character literally, without assigning any special meaning to it. These quoting techniques can be used to separate a variable from a fixed string. As an example lets use the variable, var, that has been assigned the value bar, and the constant string,man. If you want to combine these to get the result "varman", try:

$varman

but this doesn't work, because the shell will be trying to evaluate a variable called varman, which doesn't exist. To get the desired result we need to separate it by quoting, or by isolating the variable with curly braces ({}), as in:

"$var"man - quote the variable
$var""man - separate the parameters
$var"man" - quote the constant
$var"man - separate the parameters
$var'man' - quote the constant
$var\man - separate the parameters
${var}man - isolate the variable

These all work because ", ', \, {, and } are not valid characters in a variable name. We could not use either of

'$var'man
\$varman

because it would prevent the variable substitution from taking place.

When using the curly braces they should surround the variable only, and not include the $, otherwise, they will be included as part of the resulting string, e.g.:

% echo {$var}man
{var}man

Variables

There are a number of variables automatically set by the shell when it starts. These allow you to reference arguments on the command line. These shell variables are:

$#	number of arguments on the command line x
$-	options supplied to the shell x
$?	exit value of the last command executed x
$$	process number of the current process x x
$!	process number of the last command done in background x
$n	argument on the command line, where n is from 1 through 9, reading left to right x x
$0	the name of the current shell or program x x
$argv[n]	selects the nth word from the input list x
${argv[n]}	same as above x
$#argv	report the number of words in the input list x

Functions

The Bourne shell has functions, somewhat similar to aliases in the C shell, but allow more flexibility. A function has the form:

fcn () { command; }

where the space after {, and the semicolon (;) are both required; the latter can be dispensed with if a <newline> precedes the }. Additional spaces and <newline>'s are allowed. For example :

ls() { /bin/ls -sbF "$@";}
ll() { ls -al "$@";}

The first one redefines *ls* so that the options -sbF are always supplied to the standard */bin/ls* command, and acts on the supplied input, "$@". The second one takes the current value for *ls* (the previous function) and tacks on the -al options. Functions are very useful in shell scripts. The following is a simplified version of a function that automatically backup up system partitions to tape.

```sh
#!/bin/sh
# Cron script to do a complete backup of the system
HOST='/bin/uname -n'
admin=frank
Mt=/bin/mt
Dump=/usr/sbin/ufsdump
Mail=/bin/mailx
device=/dev/rmt/0n
Rewind="$Mt -f $device rewind"
Offline="$Mt -f $device rewoffl"
# Failure - exit
failure () {
$Mail -s "Backup Failure - $HOST" $admin << EOF_failure
$HOST
```

Cron backup script failed. Apparently there was no tape in the device.

```sh
EOF_failure
exit 1
}
# Dump failure - exit
dumpfail () {
$Mail -s "Backup Failure - $HOST" $admin << EOF_dumpfail
$HOST
```

Cron backup script failed. Initial tape access was okay, but dump failed.

```sh
EOF_dumpfail
exit 1
}
# Success
success () {
$Mail -s "Backup completed successfully - $HOST" $admin << EOF_success
$HOST
```

Cron backup script was apparently successful. The /etc/dumpdates file is:

```sh
'/bin/cat /etc/dumpdates'
EOF_success
}
# Confirm that the tape is in the device
$Rewind || failure
$Dump 0uf $device / || dumpfail
$Dump 0uf $device /usr || dumpfail
$Dump 0uf $device /home || dumpfail
$Dump 0uf $device /var || dumpfail
($Dump 0uf $device /var/spool/mail || dumpfail) && success
```

$Offline

This script illustrates a number of applications. It starts by setting various parameter values. HOST is set from the output of a command. Admin is the administrator of the system, Mt, Dump, and Mail are program names, device is the special device file used to access the tape drive, Rewind and Offline contain the commands to rewind and off-load the tape drive, respectively, using the previously referenced Mt and the necessary options. There are three functions defined: failure, dumpfail, and success. The functions in this script all use a here document to form the contents of the function. We also introduce the logical OR (||) and AND (&&) operators here; each is position between a pair of commands. For the OR operator, the second command will be run only if the first command does not complete successfully. For the AND operator, the second command will be run only if the first command does complete successfully.

The main purpose of the script is done with the Dump commands, i.e. backup the specified file systems. First an attempt is made to rewind the tape. Should this fail, || failure, the failure function is run and we exit the program. If it succeeds we proceed with the backup of each partition in turn, each time checking for successful completion (|| dumpfail). Should it not complete successfully we run the dumpfail subroutine and then exit. If the last backup succeeds we proceed with the success function ((...) && success). Lastly, we rewind the tape and take it offline so that no other user can accidentally write over our backup tape.

Control Commands

Conditional if

The conditional if statement is available in both shells, but has a different syntax in each.

Sh

> *if* condition1
> *then*
> command list if condition1 is true
> [*elif* condition2
> *then* command list if condition2 is true]
> [*else*   ·
> command list if condition1 is false]
> *fi*

The conditions to be tested for are usually done with the *test* command. The if and then must be separated, either with a <newline> or a semicolon (;).

```
#!/bin/sh
if [ $# -ge 2 ]
then
echo $2
elif [ $# -eq 1 ]; then
echo $1
else
echo No input
fi
```

while

The *while* commands let you loop as long as the condition is true.

Sh

> *while* condition
> do
> command list
> [*break*]
> [*continue*]
> done

A simple script to illustrate a while loop is:

> #!/bin/sh
> while [$# -gt 0]
> do
> echo $1
> shift
> done

This script takes the list of arguments, echoes the first one, then shifts the list to the left, losing the original first entry. It loops through until it has shifted all the arguments off the argument list.

test

Conditional statements are evaluated for true or false values. This is done with the *test* operators. It the condition evaluates to true, a zero (TRUE) exit status is set, otherwise a non-zero (FALSE) exit status is set. If there are no arguments a non-zero exit status is set. The operators used by the Bourne shell conditional statements are given below.

For filenames the options to *test* are given with the syntax:

> -option filename

The options available for the *test* operator for files include:

> -r true if it exists and is readable
> -w true if it exists and is writable
> -x true if it exists and is executable
> -f true if it exists and is a regular file (or for csh, exists and is not a directory)
> -d true if it exists and is a directory
> -h or -L true if it exists and is a symbolic link
> -c true if it exists and is a character special file (i.e. the special device is accessed one character at a time)
> -b true if it exists and is a block special file (i.e. the device is accessed in blocks of data)
> -p true if it exists and is a named pipe (fifo)
> -u true if it exists and is setuid (i.e. has the set-user-id bit set, s or S in the third bit)
> -g true if it exists and is setgid (i.e. has the set-group-id bit set, s or S in the sixth bit)
> -k true if it exists and the sticky bit is set (a t in bit 9)
> -s true if it exists and is greater than zero in size

There is a test for file descriptors:

> -t [file_descriptor] true if the open file descriptor (default is 1, stdin) is associated with a terminal

There are tests for strings:

> -z string true if the string length is zero

    -n string true if the string length is non-zero
    string1 = string2 true if string1 is identical to string2
    string1 != string2 true if string1 is non identical to string2
    string true if string is not NULL
There are integer comparisons:
    n1 -eq n2 true if integers n1 and n2 are equal
    n1 -ne n2 true if integers n1 and n2 are not equal
    n1 -gt n2 true if integer n1 is greater than integer n2
    n1 -ge n2 true if integer n1 is greater than or equal to integer n2
    n1 -lt n2 true if integer n1 is less than integer n2
    n1 -le n2 true if integer n1 is less than or equal to integer n2

The following logical operators are also available:
    ! negation (unary)
    -a and (binary)
    -o or (binary)
    () expressions within the () are grouped together. You may need to quote the () to prevent the shell from interpreting them.

6

Programming with Perl

6.1 INTRODUCTION TO PERL

What is Perl?

Perl is a *"Practical Extraction and Report Language"* freely available for Unix, MVS, VMS, MS/DOS, Macintosh, OS/2, Amiga, and other operating systems. Perl has powerful text-manipulation functions. It eclectically combines features and purposes of many command languages. Perl has enjoyed recent popularity for programming World Wide Web electronic forms and generally as glue and gateway between systems, databases, and users.

Why Perl?

Perl is a preferred language in bioinformatics, because of the following reasons:
1. Perl is excellent for processing text (sequence analysis, database management)
2. Perl is excellent for CGI-programming (used extensively on the web for programming)
3. Perl is easy to learn

How Perl functions?

When you run the program on the command line, the whole program is compiled into an internal format and then immediately executed. With few exceptions, Perl scripts are interpreted, not compiled. "Interpretation" is kind of "compilation" done on the fly. Interpretation is not as fast during run-time, but allows for fast program execution. There's no "binary" copy of program left behind (only the source script).

6.2. PROGRAMMING IN PERL

Basic format

```
#!/usr/bin/perl –w
print "all Perl statements end in semicolons";
```

74

```
# comments in Perl
# are written like this with
# signs in front of every comment line
print "spaces do not matter "; print "to Perl ";
print "sometimes there is an error"
print "and you forget one...the program will fail";
```

Program execution begins at the top and steps line-by-line to the bottom until the file ends or an "exit;" is called.

Example

Each statement ends with a semicolon (;). $a, $b and $result in this example are variables. A variable is a name for a container that holds one or more values. 2 and 5 in this example are values (or "literals"). The = sign indicates an assignment. Values are assigned to $a and $b. The sum of $a and $b is assigned to $result.

```
#!/usr/bin/perl
$a =2;
$b =5;
$result = $a + $b; #calculate sum
print "Result is: $result\n"; #print it
```

Name Conventions

Scalar variables start with '$', even when referring to an array element. The variable name reference for a whole list starts with '@', and the variable name reference for a whole associative array starts with '%'.

Lists are indexed with square brackets enclosing a number, normally starting with [0]. In Perl 5, negative subscripts count from the end. Thus, $things[5] is the 6th element of array @things, and ('Sun','Mon','Tue','Wed','Thu','Fri','Sat')[1] equals 'Mon'.

Associative arrays are indexed with curly brackets enclosing a string. $whatever, @whatever, and %whatever are three different variables.

```
@days = (31,28,31,30,31,30,31,31,30,31,30,31);     # A list with 12 elements.
$#days       # Last index of @days; 11 for above list
$#days = 7; # shortens or lengthens list @days to 8 elements
@days  # ($days[0], $days[1],... )
@days[3,4,5]   # = (30,31,30)
@days{'a','c'} # same as ($days{'a'},$days{'c'})
%days  # (key1, value1, key2, value2, ...)
```

Case *is* significant: "$FOO", "$Foo" and "$foo" are all different variables. If a letter or underscore is the first character after the $, @, or %, the rest of the name may also contain digits and underscores. If this character is a digit, the rest must be digits. Perl has several dozen special variables whose second character is non-alphanumeric. For example, $/ is the input record separator, newline "\n" by default. An uninitialized variable has a special "undefined" value which can be detected by the function defined(). Undefined values convert depending on context to 0, null, or false.

The variable "$_" Perl presumes when needed variables are not specified. Thus:

```
<STDIN>; assigns 1 record from filehandle STDIN to $_
print; prints the curent value of $_
```

chop; *removes the last character from $_*

@things = split; *parses $_ into white-space delimited words, which become successive elements of list @things.*

, Subroutines and functions are referenced with an initial '&', which is optional if reference is obviously a subroutine or function such as following the sub, do, and sort directives:

sub square { return $_[0] ** 2; }

print "5 squared is ", &square(5);

Filehandles don't start with a special character, and so as to not conflict with reserved words are most reliably specified as uppercase names: INPUT, OUTPUT, STDIN, STDOUT, STDERR, etc.

Printing Strings

The print construct:

- The string to print is enclosed by double quotes (").
- On output, all variable are replaced by their values - i.e $result is displayed as 7.
- \n denotes a newline.

Variables

Perl provides three kinds of variables: *scalars*, *arrays*, and *associative arrays*. The initial character of the name identifies the particular type of variable and, hence, its functionality.

scalar variable: either a number or string; Perl does not differentiate between the two, nor does it differentiate between integers and reals.

$aVar = 4;

$bVar = "a string of words";

$cVar = 4.5; # a decimal number

$dVar = 3.14e10; # a floatingpoint number

@name()

array : a one-dimensional list of scalars. Perl uses the "at" symbol and parentheses with respect to the name of an array as a whole, whereas individual elements within an array are referred to as scalars and the index is placed in square brackets.

@aList = (2, 4, 6, 8);

@bList = @aList; # creates new array and gives it values of @aList

$aList[0] = 1; # changes the value of first item from 2 to 1

%name{}

associative array : a special, 2-dimensional array, ideal for handling attribute/value pairs. The first element in each row is a key and the second element is a value associated with that key. Perl uses the "percent" symbol and curly braces with respect to the name of an associative array as a whole, whereas individual elements within an array are referred to as scalars, although the index is still placed in curly braces (unlike the shift in nomenclature used for arrays). Instead of using numbers to index an associative array, key values, such as $name{"QUERY_STRING"}, are used to reference the value associated with that particular key, i.e., QUERY_STRING. Since the associated value is a scalar, the variable has a $ prefix.

$aAA{"A"} = 1; # creates first row of assoc. array

$aAA{"B"} = 2; # creates second row of assoc. array

%bAA = %aAA; # creates new assoc. array and gives it values of %aAA

$aAA{"A"} = 3; # changes the value of first item from 1 to 3

%aAA = ("A", 1, "B", 2); # same as first two stmts., above

Example : *Program strings.pl*

Here the scalar variables $lecturer and $course contain strings. Therefore, the values assigned to them are enclosed by quotes.

```
#!/usr/bin/perl -w
$school = "University";
$course = "Bioinformatics Core";
print "We are enrolled in $course at $school\n";
```

When strings are enclosed by double quotes, several things happen:

1. The combination of a backslash and certain character(s) has special meaning (backslash escape). Examples:
   \n newline
   \t tab

2. Variable names names inside the string are replaced by their current values
   $name ="Fred";
   print "My name is $name";

3. If you wish to have a literal double quote inside your string, precede it with a backslash (\").
   Same thing if you want to have a literal backslash (\\).

Operators

If variables are the *nouns* Perl provides, *operators* are the *verbs*. Operators access and change the values of variables. Some, such as assignment, apply to all three kinds of variables, discussed above; however, most are specialized with respect to a particular type. Consequently, operators will be discussed with respect to the three basic types of variables.

(i) Scalar Operators

assignment

```
hex and octal assignment
$aVar1 = 0xff; # hex assign. for 255 decimal
$aVar2 = 0377; # octal assign. for same thing
single and double quote strings
$aVar1 = 0xff; # set $aVar1 = 255 decimal
$aVar2 = 'aVar2 = $aVar1'; # set $aVar2 = literal string
$aVar3 = "aVar3 = $aVar1"; # set $aVar3 = variable interpolated string, with $aVar1 replaced by
255
$aVar4 = 'only single quote interpolated characters are \' and \\'
double quote interpolated characters include:
  \n newline
  \a bell
  \\ backslash
  \" double quote
  \l lowercase next letter
  \u uppercase next letter
  \L lowercase letters follow
  \U uppercase letters follow
  \E terminate \L or \E
```

operators for numbers

+ plus
- minus
* multiply
/ divide
** exponentiation
% modulus # e.g., 7 % 3 = 1
== equal
!= not equal
< less than
> greater than
<= less than or equal to
>= greater than or equal to
+= binary assignment # e.g., $A += 1;
-= same, subtraction
*= same, multiplication
++ autoincrement # e.g., ++$A; also, $A++
— autodecrement

operators for strings

. concatenate
x n repetition # e.g., "A" x 3 => "AAA"
eq equal
ne not equal
lt less than
gt grater than
le less than or equal to
ge greater than or equal to
chop() # remove last character in string
index ($string, $substring) # position of substring in string, zero-based; -1 if not found
index ($string, $substring, $skip) # skip number of chars
substr($string, $start, $length) # substring
substr($string, -$start, $length) # defined from end
substr($string, $start) # rest of string

conversion between numbers and strings

Automatic, determined by the operator, if reasonable (e.g., "1.23" as string converts to 1.23 as number). If unreasonable, string converts to zero (0) as number (e.g., "not_a_number" converts to 0).

conversion between packed and unpacked forms

It is often necessary to convert from a character or scalar form to a packed binary representation, and back. A common example is building an IP address data structure. The two operators for doing this are *pack* and *unpack*. Pack takes a format specification and a list of values and packs them into a character string; conversely, unpack takes a format and a character string and breaks the string apart, according to the format, and assigns the parts to a list of variables.

Form:

pack("format", $value1, $value2, . . .);

unpack ("format", character_string);

Example:

$IP = pack("CCCC", 152, 2, 128, 184); # create IP address

($var1, $var2, $var3, $var4) = unpack("CCCC", $IP); # inverse of the above

Format specifications can be given in context (in quotes) or they can be assigned to a string variable. There are a number of options available. See a standard text or the Perl man page for a complete list. In the example above, the "C" stands for an unsigned character value. One useful format to know is the following, which can be used to construct the address structure needed to bind a socket to a remote host:

$socket_addr_ptrn = 'S n a4 x8';

The "S" denotes a "short" unsigned integer. The "n" is a short integer in network order. The "a4" is an unpadded ASCII string, four bytes long. And, the "x8" is eight bytes of padding.

    <STDIN> as scalar

Designates the next line of text from *standard input*.

(ii) Array Operators

assignment

@aList = (2, 4, 6, 8); # explicit values

@aList = (1..4); # range of values

@aList = (1, "two", 3, "four"); # mixed values

@aList = (); # empty list

@bList = @aList;

access

Individual items in array accessed as scalars.

$aList[0] # first item in @aList

$aList[0,1] # *slice*, first two items in @aList

$aList[$too_big] # access beyond array bounds returns *undef*, i.e., 0 or ''

additional operators

$#aList # index of last item

push (@aList, $aNewItem); # @aList = @aList, $aNewItem

$LastItem = pop (@aList); # inverse of push

unshift (@aList, $aNewItem); # @aList = $aNewItem, @aList

$FirstItem = shift (@aList); # inverse of unshift

@aList = reverse (@aList); # reverse items

@aList = sort (@aList); # sort items, *alphabetically*

chop (@aList); # remove last character from each item

@aList = <STDIN>; # one line of input per item

(iii) Associative Array Operators

assignment

> $aAA{"A"} = 1; # creates first row of assoc. array
> $aAA{"B"} = 2; # creates second row of assoc. array
> %aAA = ("A", 1, "B", 2); # same as first two stmts., above
> %bAA = %aAA; # creates new assoc. array and gives it values of %aAA
> $aAA{"A"} = 3; # changes the value of first item from 1 to 3

additional operators

> keys (%aAA) # list of keys for %aAA
> values (%aAA) # list of values for %aAA
> each (%aAA) # next key/value pair, as list
> delete $aAA{"A"}; # deletes key/value pair referenced

Functions

Functions are a fundamental part of most programming languages. They often behave like an operator, producing a change in the value of some variable or returning a value that can be assigned to a variable. They also control the flow of execution, transferring control from the point of invocation to the function definition block and back. Thus, they combine properties of the two preceding discussions. The discussion will cover both the *designation* of functions and their *invocation* and use.

invocation

The function is invoked within the context of some expression. It is recognized in context by the form of its name: an ampersand is placed before the name when the function is called. If the function takes arguments, they are placed within parentheses following the name of the function.

> Form:
> &name()
> Example :
> &aFunction()
> *definition*

The function definition is marked by the keyword, sub; followed by the name of the function, without the ampersand prefix. It is followed by the block of code that is executed when the function is called, enclosed within curly braces.

> Example:
> sub aFunction {
>   stmt_1;
>   stmt_2;
>   stmt_3;
> }

To use functions effectively, we need three additional concepts: *return values*, *arguments*, and *local variables*.

return values

The value returned by a Perl function is the value of the last expression evaluated in the function.

Example:

```
sub aFunction {
    stmt_1;
    stmt_2;
    $a = $b + $c;
}
```

In this example, the function will return the value of $a at the time when the function ends. Note: operators, such as print return values of 0 or 1, indicating failure or success. Thus, print ($a); as the last statement in a function would result in a return of 0 or 1 for the function, not the value of $a.

arguments

Arguments are enclosed in parenthses following the name of the function during invocation; thus, they constitute a *list*. They are available within the function definition block through the predefined (list) variable, @_.

Example:

```
&aFunction ($a, "Literal_string", $b);
sub aFunction {
    foreach $temp(@_) {
        print "$temp \n";
    }
}
```

local variables

Any variables defined within the body of a Perl program are available inside a Perl function as global variables. Consequently, Perl provides an explicit *local* operator that can be used to limit the scope of variables. Thus, one can define variables that are local to a function so that their use will not produce inadvertent side effects with any global variables that may have the same names. By the same token, they will not be visible outside of the function.

Local variables are, by convention, defined at the top of a Perl function. They are defined by the keyword, local, followed by a list of variable names, within parentheses.

Example:

```
&aFunction ($a, $b);
sub aFunction {
    local ($aLocal, $bLocal);
    $aLocal = $_[0];
    $bLocal = $_[1];
}
```

$aLocal and $bLocal will have the same values inside the function as $a and $b have at the time the function was invoked. Changes to either local variable inside the function, however, will not affect the values of $a or $b.

The sort function

The sort function receives a list of variables (or an array) and returns the sorted list.

Example:

```
#!/usr/bin/perl -w
@countries = ("Israel", "Norway", "France", "Argentina");
@sorted_countries = sort ( @countries);
print "ORIG: @countries\n",
"SORTED: @sorted_countries\n";
Output:
ORIG: Israel Norway France Argentina
SORTED: Argentina France Israel Norway
```

The push and shift functions

The push function adds a variable or a list of variables to the end of a given array.

```
$a = 5;
$b = 7;
@array = ("David", "John", "Gadi");
push (@array, $a, $b);
# @array is now ("David", "John", "Gadi", 5, 7)
```
The shift function removes the first element of a given array and returns this element.
```
@array = ("David", "John", "Gadi");
$k = shift (@array);
# @array is now ("John", "Gadi");
#$kisnow"David"
```

Control Structures

Perl is an *iterative language* in which control flows from the first statement in the program to the last statement unless something interrupts. Some of the things that can interrupt this linear flow are conditional branches and loop structures. Perl offers approximately a dozen such constructs.

statement block

Statement blocks provide a mechanism for grouping statements that are to be executed as a result some expression being evaluated. They are used in all of the control structures discussed below. Statement blocks are designated by pairs of curly braces.

Form: BLOCK

Example:

```
{
    stmt_1;
    stmt_2;
    stmt_3;
}
```

if statement

   Form: if (EXPR) BLOCK
   Example:
```
  if (expression) {
      true_stmt_1;
      true_stmt_2;
      true_stmt_3;
  }
```

if/else statement

Form: if (EXPR) BLOCK else BLOCK
   Example:
```
  if (expression) {
      true_stmt_1;
      true_stmt_2;
      true_stmt_3;
  } else {
      false_stmt_1;
      false_stmt_2;
      false_stmt_3;
  }
```

if/elseif/else statement

Form: if (EXPR) BLOCK elseif (EXPR) BLOCK . . . else BLOCK
   Example:
```
  if (expression_A) {
      A_true_stmt_1;
      A_true_stmt_2;
      A_true_stmt_3;
  } elseif (expression_B) {
      B_true_stmt_1;
      B_true_stmt_2;
      B_true_stmt_3;
  } else {
      false_stmt_1;
      false_stmt_2;
      false_stmt_3;
  }
```

while statement

Form: LABEL: while (EXPR) BLOCK
   The LABEL in this and the following control structures is optional. In addition to description, it also provides function in the quasi-goto statements: last, next, and redo. Perl conventional practice calls for labels to be expressed in uppercase to avoid confusion with variables or key words.

Example:
```
ALABEL: while (expression) {
    stmt_1;
    stmt_2;
    stmt_3;
}
```

until statement

Form: LABEL: until (EXPR) BLOCK

Example:
```
ALABEL: until (expression) { # while not
    stmt_1;
    stmt_2;
    stmt_3;
}
```

for statement

Form: LABEL: for (EXPR; EXPR; EXPR) BLOCK

Example:
```
ALABEL: for (initial exp; test exp; increment exp) { # e.g., ($i=1; $i<5; $i++)
    stmt_1;
    stmt_2;
    stmt_3;
}
```

foreach statement

Form: LABEL: foreach VAR (EXPR) BLOCK

Example:
```
ALABEL: foreach $i (@aList) {
    stmt_1;
    stmt_2;
    stmt_3;
}
```

last operator

The last operator, as well as the next and redo operators that follow, apply only to loop control structures. They cause execution to jump from where they occur to some other position, defined with respect to the block structure of the encompassing control structure. Thus, they function as limited forms of *goto* statements.

Last causes control to jump from where it occurs to the first statement following the enclosing block.

Example:
```
ALABEL: while (expression) {
    stmt_1;
```

```
        stmt_2;
        last;
        stmt_3;
    }
    # last jumps to here
```

If last occurs within nested control structures, the jump can be made to the end of an outer loop by adding a label to that loop and specifying the label in the last statement.

Example:

```
    ALABEL: while (expression) {
        stmt_1;
        stmt_2;
        BLABEL: while (expression) {
            stmt_a;
            stmt_b;
            last ALABEL;
            stmt_c;
        }
        stmt_3;
    }
    # last jumps to here
```

next operator

The next operator is similar to last except that execution jumps to the end of the block, but remains *inside* the block, rather than exiting the block. Thus, iteration continues normally.

Example:

```
    ALABEL: while (expression) {
        stmt_1;
        stmt_2;
        next;
        stmt_3;
    # next jumps to here
    }
```

As with last, next can be used with a label to jump to an outer designated loop.

redo operator

The redo operator is similar to next except that execution jumps to the top of the block without re-evaluating the control expression.

Example:

```
    ALABEL: while (expression) {
    # redo jumps to here
        stmt_1;
        stmt_2;
        redo;
        stmt_3;
    }
```

As with last, next can be used with a label to jump to an outer designated loop.

6.3 ILLUSTRATIONS OF PRORAMMING IN PERL

Example 1 :

```perl
#!/usr/bin/perl -w
# receive a number from user
print "enter number: ";
my $n = <>;
chomp ($n);
# make a decision and act accordingly
if ($n > 10) {
print "large number\n";
}else {
print "small number\n";
```

Example 2 :

```perl
#!/usr/bin/perl -w
my ($grade, $evaluation);
# receive a grade from user
print "enter student grade (between 0 - 100): ";
$grade = <>;
chomp ($grade);
# decide what will the evaluation be
if ($grade >=0 and $grade <= 40) {
$evaluation = "failed";
} elsif ($grade > 40 and $grade <= 60) {
$evaluation = "bad";
} elsif ($grade > 60 and $grade <= 80) {
$evaluation = "good";
} elsif ($grade > 80 and $grade <= 100) {
$evaluation = "very good";
}else{
$evaluation = "invalid input - grade should be between 0 and 100";
}
print "Evaluation: $evaluation\n"; # print out the evaluation
```

Exampe 3 :

```perl
#!/usr/bin/perl -w
my $n = "protein"; # a string
if ($n) {
print "OK\n";
}else{
print "NO\n";
}
```

Example 4 :

```perl
#!/usr/bin/perl -w
my $k = 53 - 53; # the number 0
```

```perl
if ($k) {
print "OK\n";
}else{
print "NO\n";
}
```

Examples 5 :

```perl
#!/usr/bin/perl -w
my @a = (3, 6, 9, 12); # an array
if (@a) {
print "OK\n";
}else{
print "NO\n";
}
```

Example 6 : count from a given number up to 10

```perl
#!/usr/bin/perl -w
# receive a number from user
print "enter an integer: ";
my $n = <>;
chomp ($n);
#count up to 10
while ($n <= 10) {
print "$n\n";
$n++; # same as $n +=1;
};
print "DONE\n";
```

Note that if the entered number is greater than 10, the while loop will never be executed.

Example 7 : same program, but using until loop

```perl
#!/usr/bin/perl -w
# receive a number from user
print "enter an integer: ";
my $n = <>;
chomp ($n);
#count up to 10
until ($n > 10) {
print "$n\n";
$n++; #same as $n +=1;
};
print "DONE\n";
```

Example 8 :

```perl
#!/usr/bin/perl -w
my ($nuc, $aa);
do {
print "please enter no. of translated nucleotides: ";
```

```
$nuc = <>;
chomp ($nuc);
} until ($nuc > 0 and $nuc % 3 == 0);
$aa = $nuc / 3;
print "no. of amino acids: $aa\n";
```

Example 9 :

```
#!/usr/bin/perl -w
@genes=("POLR2A","RCV1","TP53","TRK1");
# print genes and their indexes
foreach $i (0 .. $#genes) {
print "$i. $genes[$i]\n";
}
```

Output:

```
0. POLR2A
1. RCV1
2. TP53
3. TRK1
```

Example 10 : print all even numbers between 4 and 12:

```
for ($i = 4; $i <= 12; $i += 2) {
 print "$i\n";
}
```

Same as:

```
$i = 4; # set initial state of $i
while ($i <= 12) { # condition to test $i
print "$i\n";
$i += 2 # modify $i
```

6.4 OPERATIONS WITH ASSOCIATIVE ARRAYS (HASHES)

Examples:

%student = ("name" $\Rightarrow$ "Shirley","department" $\Rightarrow$ "Brain Research","degree" $\Rightarrow$ "MSc","phone" $\Rightarrow$ "3579","email" $\Rightarrow$ "brshir\@weizmann.weizmann.ac.il");

%prices = ("shirt" $\Rightarrow$ 45,"pullover" $\Rightarrow$ 90,"trousers" $\Rightarrow$ 120,"socks" $\Rightarrow$ 15);

%genetic_code = ("TGT"$\Rightarrow$"Cys", # partial list"TGC"$\Rightarrow$"Cys","GAT"$\Rightarrow$"Asp","GAC"$\Rightarrow$"Asp", "GAA" $\Rightarrow$ "Glu","GAG" $\Rightarrow$ "Glu","TTT" $\Rightarrow$ "Phe");

You may use scalar variables instead of literal strings. e.g.

%gene = ("name" $\Rightarrow$ $gene_name,"description" $\Rightarrow$ $gene_desc,"cDNA sequence" $\Rightarrow$ $cDNA_seq, "genomic sequence" => $genomic_seq);

Assignment into a hash variable

To create a hash with all of its key-value pairs, you can use one of several equivalent ways:

%hash = ("key1" => "val1","key2" => "val2","key3" => "val3");

%hash = ("key1" => "val1", "key2" => "val2", "key3" => "val3");

%hash = ("key1", "val1", "key2", "val2", "key3", "val3");

Actually, the => operator is just a synonym for a comma. Its sole role here is to increase readability.

Therefore, in all the above examples, we write data to be assigned to the hash variable as a list. Each pair of elements in the list (which should always have an even number of elements) defines a key and its corresponding value. Hashes are internally stored in a way that will optimize retrieval of values by their keys. Therefore, the order in which the elements were assigned to the hash is irrelevant.

For example, if you assign a hash variable back to an array variable, the order of the key value pairs might be different than the one used while defining the hash:

```
#!/usr/bin/perl
my%hash=("a","b","x","y","m","n");
my @list = %hash;
print "@list\n";
```
This would result in:
```
x ya bmn
```

Creating an empty hash

To create an empty hash, assign an empty list into it, e.g.:
```
%empt = ();7
```

Accessing individual hash elements

Whereas array elements are accessed by their (numerical) index, their keys access hash elements (values).

Syntax : Assuming that @arr is some array and %assoc is some hash:
```
Array       Hash
$arr[2]     $assoc{"some_key"}
$arr[$n]    $assoc{$k}
```

Example:
```
#!/usr/bin/perl -w
%prices = ("shirt" => 45,"pullover" => 90,"trousers" => 120,"socks" => 15);
$s = $prices{"shirt"};
$t = $prices{"trousers"};
print "EXAMPLE PRICES:\n";
print "SHIRT: $s DOLLARS, TROUSERS: $t DOLLARS\n";
Result:
EXAMPLE PRICES:
SHIRT: 45 DOLLARS, TROUSERS: 120 DOLLARS
```

Adding an element to a hash

Simply assign a value to a hash individual element, e.g.:
```
$prices{"coat"} = 250;
# coat, 250 will be added to the %prices hash
```

Deleting an element from a hash

Use the delete function, e.g.:
```
delete $prices{"coat"};
```

Checking whether a hash is empty

```
if (%hash_name) { # will be false if hash is empty
.......;
}
```

The keys function

The keys function yields a list of all the current keys in a given hash.

Example:
```
#!/usr/bin/perl -w
my %prices = ("shirt" => 45,"pullover" => 90,"trousers" => 120,"socks" => 15);
my @items = keys (%prices);
print "ITEMS: @items\n";
Result:
ITEMS: pullover shirt socks trousers
```

Iterating over all hash elements using the keys function

Example - printing all keys and values of the %prices hash:
```
my @items_list = keys (%prices);
foreach $item (@items_list) {
print "$item : $prices{$item} DOLLARS\n";
}
or, shorter:
foreach $item (keys (%prices)) {
print "$item : $prices{$item} DOLLARS\n";
}
Result:
pullover : 90 DOLLARS
shirt : 45 DOLLARS
socks : 15 DOLLARS
trousers : 120 DOLLARS
```

The values function

The values function yields a list of all the current values in a given hash.

Example:
```
#!/usr/bin/perl -w
my %prices = ("shirt" => 45,"pullover" => 90,"trousers" => 120,"socks" => 15);
my @dollars = values (%prices);
print "PRICES: @dollars\n";
Result:
PRICES: 90 45 15 120
```

Iterating over all elements of a hash using the each function

Example - demonstrating how the each function works:
```
%prices = ("shirt" => 45,"pullover" => 90,"trousers" => 120,"socks" => 15);
```

@a = each (%prices); # @a is now (pullover, 90)
@b = each (%prices); # @b is now (shirt, 45)
@c = each (%prices); # @c is now (socks, 15)
@d = each (%prices); # @d is now (trousers, 120)
@e = each (%prices); # @e is now *null*;
@f = each (%prices); # @f is now (shirt, 45)
@g = each ... etc.

Instead of
@a = each (%prices);
you may write:
($item, $dollars) = each (%prices);
and then $item will be "pullover" and $dollars will be 90.
Example - printing all keys and values of the %prices hash:
%prices = ("shirt" => 45,"pullover" => 90,"trousers" => 120,"socks" => 15);
while (($item, $dollars) = each (%prices)) {
print "$item : $dollars DOLLARS\n";
}
Result:
pullover : 90 DOLLARS
shirt : 45 DOLLARS
socks : 15 DOLLARS
trousers : 120 DOLLARS

The each function returns a key-value pair as a two-element list. On each evaluation of this function for the same hash, the next successive key-value pair is returned until all the elements have been accessed. When there are no more pairs, each returns an empty list.

6.5. FILE INPUT AND OUTPUT

standard files

Perl provides access to the standard files: STDIN, STDOUT, and STDERR.

STDIN is accessed through the angle brackets (<>) operator. When placed in a scalar context, the operator returns the next line; when place in an array context, it returns the entire file, one line per item in the array.

Examples:
$a = <STDIN>;# returns next line in file
@a = <STDIN>; # returns entire file
STDOUT is the default file accessed through a print statement.
STDERR is the file used by the system to which it writes error messages; it is usually mapped to the terminal display.

open file

Files are accessed within a Perl program through *filehandles* which are bound to *filenames* within the UNIX file system through an open statement. By convention, Perl filehandle names are written in all uppercase, to differentiate them from keywords and function names.

Form:

  open (FILEHANDLE, "filename");

Example:

  open (INPUT, "index.html");

In the above, the file is opened for read access. It may also be opened for write access and for update. The difference between the two is that write replaces the file contents, whereas update appends new data to the end of the current contents. These two options are indicated by appending either a single or a double greater than (>) symbol to the file name as a prefix:

Form:

  open (FILEHANDLE, ">filename"); # write access
  open (FILEHANDLE, ">>filename"); # update

Examples:

  open (INPUT, ">index.html");
  open (INPUT, ">>index.html");

Since Perl will continue operating regardless of whether the open was successful or not, you need to test the open statement. Like other Perl constructs, the open statement returns a true or false value, indicating success or failure. One convenient construct in which this value can be tested and appropriate response taken is with the logical or and die operators. die can be used to deliver a message to STDERR and terminate the Perl program. The following construct can be paraphrased: "open or die."

Form:

  open (FILEHANDLE, "filename") || die "Message written to STDERR";

Example:

  open (INPUT, "index.html") || die "Error opening file index.html ";

close file

Files are closed implicitly when another open is encountered. they may also be closed explicitly.

Form:

  close (FILEHANDLE);

Example:

  close (INPUT);

read file

The file, once opened and associated with a filehandle, can be read with the angle brackets operator (<>), which can be used in a variety of constructs.

Form:

  <FILEHANDLE>

Example:

  while (<INPUT>) { # read one line at a time until EOF
      chop; # remove newline
      print line = $_ \n"; # print line read using default scalar variable
  }

write file

Once a file has been opened for either *write* or *update* access, data can be sent to that file through the print operator.

Form:

   print FILEHANDLE (content);

Example:

print OUTPUT "$next \n"; # outputs contents of $next followed by newline char.

file tests

There are a number of circumstances where the actions taken by the Perl program should take into account attributes of the file, such as whether or not the file currently exists, whether or not it has content, etc. A number of tests can be performed on files through the dash (-) operator.

Form:

   -SYMBOL # where SYMBOL is a single character designator

Examples :

   -r # readable
   -w # writeable
   -x # executable
   -o # owned by user
   -e # exists
   -z # zero content
   -s # nonzero content (size)
   -f # plain file
   -d # directory
   -l # symbolic link
   -T # text file
   -B # binary file
   -M # modification age
   -A # access age

Redirection of standard output to a file

The print command we been using sends its argument (the string in parentheses) to standard output, which is normally the terminal.A simple way to send program output to a file (instead of printing it on the screen) is to use the Unix redirection sign ">".

Example :

   To print the results of the protocol.pl program to a file named my_protocol, use the following Unix command:

   ./protocol.pl > my_protocol

Example :

   # open a filehandle for appending:
   open (LOGFILE, ">>filename";
   # open a filehandle for both reading and writing:
   open (IN_OUT_FILE, "+>filename"); # or
   open (IN_OUT_FILE, "+<filename");

Example :
```
    my $in_file = "filename1";
    open (SOURCE_FILE, "$in_file");
    my $out_file = "filename2";
    open (RESULT_FILE, ">$out_file");10
```

6.6 PERL APPLICATIONS FOR BIOINFORMATICS

Processing Text

Text processing applications involve :

- Extract relevant information from text files written in a certain format.
- Analyze / modify the extracted information.
- Store information.
- Allow user to query for information.

Text processing functions

The substr function

The substr function extracts a substring out of a string and returns it. The function receives 3 arguments: a string value, a position on the string (starting to count from 0) and a length.

Example:
```
    $a = "university";
    $k =substr ($a,3,5);
    $k is now "versi"
    $a remains unchanged.
```

If length is omitted, everything to the end of the string is returned.

Text Processing (fixed-length)

The *substr* function example: a Swiss-Prot entry
```
    ID ACM1_HUMAN STANDARD; PRT; 460 AA.
    AC P11229;
    012345678..... ....n
```
To extract the field names and values it is enough to specify their positions on the line.
Field: start at position 0 and count 2 characters.
Value: start at position 5 and continue to end of line. (Notice that we count from 0).

```
    #!/usr/bin/perl -w
    my $sp_file;
    my $id, $ac;
    $sp_file = "sp_entry";
    open (SP, "<$sp_file") || die "Cannot open \"$sp_file\".\n Bye!";
    while (my $line = <SP>)
    {
    chomp ($line);
    my $field = substr ($line, 0, 2);
```

```
my $value = substr ($line, 5);
if( $field eq "ID")
{
$id = $value;
}
if( $field eq "AC")
{
$ac = $value;
}
}
print "Identification: $id\n";
print "Accession No. : $ac\n";
```

ID ACM1_HUMAN STANDARD; PRT; 460 AA.
AC P11229;
012345678..... .....n

To extract the field names and values it is enough to specify their positions on the line.
Field: start at position 0 and count 2 characters.
Value: start at position 5 and continue to end of line.Notice that we count from 0.

Identification: ACM1_HUMAN STANDARD; PRT; 460 AA.
Accession No. : P11229;
Output
Acetylcholine (muscarinic) receptors
==
ACM1_HUMAN (P11229) MUSCARINIC ACETYLCHOLINE M1 [CHRM1] - HUMAN
ACM1_MOUSE (P12657) MUSCARINIC ACETYLCHOLINE M1 [CHRM1] - MOUSE
ACM1_PIG (P04761) MUSCARINIC ACETYLCHOLINE M1 (BRAIN) [CHRM1] - PIG
ACM1_RAT (P08482) MUSCARINIC ACETYLCHOLINE M1 [CHRM1] - RAT
ACM2_BOVIN (P41985) MUSCARINIC ACETYLCHOLINE M2 [CHRM2] - BOVINE
ACM2_CHICK (P30372) MUSCARINIC ACETYLCHOLINE M2 [CM2] - CHICKEN
ACM2_HUMAN (P08172) MUSCARINIC ACETYLCHOLINE M2 [CHRM2] - HUMAN
ACM2_PIG (P06199) MUSCARINIC ACETYLCHOLINE M2 (CARDIAC) [CHRM2] - PIG
ACM2_RAT (P10980) MUSCARINIC ACETYLCHOLINE M2 [CHRM2] - RAT
ACM3_BOVIN (P41984) MUSCARINIC ACETYLCHOLINE M3 [CHRM3] - BOVINE
ACM3_HUMAN (P20309) MUSCARINIC ACETYLCHOLINE M3 [CHRM3] - HUMAN
ACM3_PIG (P11483) MUSCARINIC ACETYLCHOLINE M3 [CHRM3] - PIG
ACM3_RAT (P08483) MUSCARINIC ACETYLCHOLINE M3 [CHRM3] - RAT
ACM3_CHICK (P49578) MUSCARINIC ACETYLCHOLINE M3 - CHICKEN
ACM4_BOVIN (P41986) MUSCARINIC ACETYLCHOLINE M4 [CHRM4] - BOVINE
ACM4_CHICK (P17200) MUSCARINIC ACETYLCHOLINE M4 - CHICKEN
ACM4_HUMAN (P08173) MUSCARINIC ACETYLCHOLINE M4 [CHRM4] - HUMAN
ACM4_MOUSE (P32211) MUSCARINIC ACETYLCHOLINE M4 [CHRM4] - MOUSE
ACM4_RAT (P08485) MUSCARINIC ACETYLCHOLINE M4 [CHRM4] - RAT
ACM4_XENLA (P30544) MUSCARINIC ACETYLCHOLINE M4 - XENOPUS LAEVIS
ACM5_HUMAN (P08912) MUSCARINIC ACETYLCHOLINE M5 [CHRM5] - HUMAN
ACM5_RAT (P08911) MUSCARINIC ACETYLCHOLINE M5 [CHRM5] - RAT
ACM1_DROME (P16395) MUSCARINIC ACETYLCHOLINE DM1 [ACRC] - DROSOPHILA

Example : extract all accession numbers from a Swiss-Prot list of muscarinic acetylcholine receptors.

```perl
#!/usr/bin/perl -w
my $sp_list_file = "sp_list";
open (SP, $sp_list_file) || die "cannot open \"$sp_list\": $!";
foreach (1 .. 3) { #skip title lines
<SP>;
}
my @acc_nos = ();
while (my $line = <SP>) {
chop ($line);
my $n = substr ($line, 12, 6);
push (@acc_nos, $n);
}
print "@acc_nos\n";
```

Output:
P11229 P12657 P04761 P08482 P41985 P30372 P08172 P06199
P10980 P41984 P20309 P11483 P08483 P49578 P41986 P17200
P08173 P32211 P08485 P30544 P08912 P08911 P16395

The split function

The split function splits a string to a list of substrings according to the positions of a given delimiter. The delimiter is written as a pattern enclosed by slashes:

/PATTERN/.

Examples:
```perl
$string = "perl::programming::for::bioinformatics";
@list = split (/::/, $string);
# @list is now ("perl", "programming", "for", "bioinformatics")
# $string remains unchanged.
$string = "protein kinase C\t450 Kilodaltons\t120 Kilobases";
@list = split (/\t/, $string); #\t indicates tab
# @list is now ("protein kinase C", "450 Kilodaltons", "120 Kilobases")
```

Parsing a tab-delimited file using split

You can assign the result of the split function to an array containing a list of scalar variable names.

Example:
```perl
$string = "protein kinase C\t450 Kilodaltons\t120 Kilobases";
($name, $mol_weight, $seq_length) = split (/\t/, $string);
# Now $name contains "protein kinase C"
# $mol_weight contains "450 Kilodaltons" and
# $seq_length contains "120 Kilobases".
CHRM1 GDB:125213 cholinergic receptor, muscarinic 1
CHRM2 GDB:125214 cholinergic receptor, muscarinic 2
```

CHRM3 GDB:125215 cholinergic receptor, muscarinic 3
CHRM4 GDB:125216 cholinergic receptor, muscarinic 4
CHRM5 GDB:125217 cholinergic receptor, muscarinic 54

```perl
#!/usr/bin/perl -w
my $gdb_list_file = "gdb_list";
open (GDB, $gdb_list_file) || die "cannot open \"$gdb_list_file\": $!";
my @acc_nos = ();
while (my $line = <GDB>) {
chop ($line);
my ($gene_symbol, $acc_no, $gene_name) = split (/\t/, $line);
push (@acc_nos, $acc_no);
}
print "@acc_nos\n";
output:
GDB:125213 GDB:125214 GDB:125215 GDB:125216 GDB:125217
```

The join function

The join function does the opposite of split. It receives a delimiter and a list of strings, and joins the strings into a single string, such that they are separated by the delimiter.

Note that the delimiter is written inside quotes.

Examples:

```perl
@list = ("perl", "programming", "for", "bioinformatics");
$string = join ("::", @list);
# $string is now "perl::programming::for::bioinformatics"
$name = "protein kinase C";
$mol_weight = "450 Kilodaltons";
$seq_length = "120 Kilobases";
$string = join ("\t", $name, $mol_weight, $seq_length);
#$stringisnow:
# "protein kinase C\t450 Kilodaltons\t120 Kilobases"
```

In hashes, keys point to only one value. However, we can use the split and join functions to store many fields in each value.

```perl
#!/usr/bin/perl -w
my (%refs);
%refs = ("ref1" => "Cohen et al.|Nature|123|45-49|1998",
"ref2" => "Zilman|Cell|54|127-130|1997",
"ref3" => "Grinberg et al.|PNAS|1142|345|1997");
while (($key, $value) = each (%refs)) {
($author, $journal, $volume, $pages, $year) = split (/\|/, $value);
print "$key: $author ($year) $journal $volume: $pages.\n";
}
Output:
ref3: Grinberg et al. (1997) PNAS 1142: 345.
ref2: Zilman (1997) Cell 54: 127-130.
ref1: Cohen et al. (1998) Nature 123: 45-49.
```

Using split and join in hashes

The index function allows you to find a substring within a larger string, returning the integer location of the larger string (starting at 0). If it isn't found, index returns -1.

Examples:

```
$where = index("hello", "e"); # $where = 1;
$person = "geddy";
$where = index("neil alex geddy", $person); # $where = 10
@rush = ("alex", "neil", "geddy");
$where = index(join(" ", @rush), $person); # $where = 10
```

The index function

- The default iterator variable in a foreach loop if no other variable is supplied.
- The various list functions like print and chomp.
- The default place to put an input record when a <FILEHANDLE> operation's result is tested by itself as the sole criterion of a while test.
- The pattern matching operations m//, s///, and tr/// when used with an =~operator.
- The implicit iterator variable in the grep function.

The $_ variable (a Global Special Variable). The $_ variable is the default input and pattern matching space. Perl assumes it in the following contexts:

Preface/Review

```
In a foreach:
@a = (1, 2, 3, 4, 5);
foreach $b (reverse @a) {
print $b;
}
The following code is equivalent:
@a = (1, 2, 3, 4, 5);
foreach (reverse @a) { # perl pretends you've specified $_
print;
Input from STDIN in a list context.
@a = <STDIN>;
Read all lines one at a time, processing each line:
while (defined($line = <STDIN>)) {
chomp($line);
# other line processing statements here
}
The following is equivalent:
while (<STDIN>) { # like "while (defined($_ = <STDIN>)) {"
chomp; # like "chomp($_);
#otheroperationswith $_here
}
```

Processing Regular Expressions

Regular expressions are strings that can be recognized by a regular grammar, a restricted type of context-free grammar. Basically, they are strings that can be parsed left to right, without backtracking, and requiring only exact symbol matching, matching of a symbol by a category of symbols, or matching of a symbol by a specified number of sequential occurrences of a symbol or category.

Perl includes an evaluation component that, given a pattern and a string in which to search for that pattern, determines whether — and if so, where — the pattern occurs. These patterns are referred to as *regular expressions*.

Perl provides a general mechanism for specifying regular expressions. By default, regular expressions are strings that are bounded or *delimited* by slashes, e.g., /cat/. By default, the string that will be searched is $_. However, the delimiter can be changed to virtually any nonalphanumeric character by preceding the first occurrence of the new delimiter with an m, e.g., m#cat#. In this example, the pound sign (#) becomes the delimiter. And, of course, one can apply the expression to strings other than those contained in the default variable, $_, as will be explained below. In addition to providing a general mechanism for evaluating regular expressions, Perl provides several operators that perform various manipulations on strings based upon the results of the evaluation.

(i) Patterns

literals

The simples form of pattern is a *literal string*. Thus, one can search for /cat/, as discussed in the introduction to this section. Normally, such an expression would appear in some conditional context, such as an if statement.

Example:

```
if (/cat/) {
print "cat found in $_\n";
}
```

single-character patterns

In addition to including literal characters, expressions can contain categories of characters. The period (.) stands for any single character.

Example:

```
/.at/ # matches "cat," "bat", but not "at"
```

An explicit *category* or *class* of characters can be specified by placing the characters in square brackets.

Example:

```
/[0123456789]/
```

Ranges of characters can also be specified:

Examples:

```
/[0-9]/
/[a-z]/
/[A-Z]/
/[0-9a-zA-Z]/
```

Several predefined categories are available. These include:

\d # digits
\w # words
\s # space
\D # not digits
\W # not words
\S # not space

Any character or range can be turned into a *not* condition by placing a carat (^) in front of it.
Example:

/[^0-9]/ # not a digit

sequences

In addition to the literals and single category instances discussed above, patterns can include sequences in which a given symbol or category can occur a variable, but specified, number of times. An Asterisk (*) indicates any number of occurrences of any character that occurs in the position where the asterisk occurs in the pattern. A plus sign (+) indicates one or more of the preceding character. The question mark (?) indicates zero or one of the preceding character. The concept of *multiplier* implied by these facilities can be generalized by placing curly braces around a minimum and a maximum number of occurrences of the preceding character. Specialized forms of the general multiplier exist, as shown in the examples that follow.

Examples :

/a*t/ # any number of a's followed by t
/a+t/ # one or more a's followed by t
/a?t/ # zero or one a followed by t
/a{2,4}t/ # between 2 and 4 a's followed by t
/a{2,}t/ # 2 or more a's followed by t
/a{2}t/ # exactly 2 a's followed by t

Pattern matching is *greedy*, meaning that if a pattern can be found at more than one place in the string but one instance is longer than the others, the longest match will be identified, thereby affecting patterned-based operators such as *substitution*, discussed below.

memory

The portion of the string that matches a pattern can be assigned to a variable for use later in the statement or in subsequent statements. This is done by placing the portion to be *remembered* in parentheses (()). Within the same statement, the matched segment will be available in the variable, \1. Multiple segments, specified by multiple occurrences of parentheses through the pattern, are available in variables, \1, \2, \3, etc. in the order corresponding to the different parenthesized components. Beyond the scope of the statement, these stored segments are available in the variables, $1, $2, $3, etc.

Other information available in variables include $&, the sequence that matched; $', everything in the string up to the match; and $', everything in the string beyond the match.

Examples:

/c(.*)t/ # in caaat, \1 is "aaa"; $1 has the same value
$& is "aaa"
$' is "c"
$' is "t"

anchors

The pattern that is searched for in the string can be restricted to several specified locations, such as the beginnings and endings of words or the beginnings and endings of the string. \b indicates a word boundary. \B indicates any place but a word boundary. Carat (^) restricts the pattern to the beginning of the string. Dollar sign ($) specifies the end of the string. If a literal dollars sign occurs in the pattern, mark it with the backslash.

Example:

/\bat/ # matches "at" and "attention", but not "bat"

/at\b/ # matches "at" and "bat", but not "attention"

/at\B/ # matches "attention" but not "at" and "bat"

/^at/ # matches "at $5.00, it is a bargain" but not "where you are at"

/at$/ # matches "where you are at" but not "at $5.00, it is a bargain"

/\$/ # matches "at $5.00, it is a bargain"

variable interpolation

Variables are interpolated. Since the dollar sign is used to mark ends of strings, as explained above, it should not conflict with interpolation of scalar variables that begin with a dollar sign.

Example:

$word = "cat;

/$word/ # matches strings that contain "cat"

precedence

Know that it exists. Look it up in a text on Perl, if you like. Use parentheses!

explicit target string

The (=~) operator takes two arguments: a string on the left and a regular expression pattern on the right. Instead of searching in the string contained in the default variable, $_, the search is performed in the string specified on the left.

Example:

$a =~ /cat/ # does the content of $a contain "cat"?

<STDIN> =~ /cat/ # does the next line of input contain "cat"?

case

Case can be ignored in the search by placing an (i) immediately after the last delimiter.

Example:

/cat/i # matches "cat", "CAT", "Cat", etc.

(ii) Regular expression operators

Regular expression operators include a regular expression as an argument but instead of just looking for the pattern and returning a truth value. They perform some action on the string, such as replacing the matched portion with a specified substring, like the well-known "search and replace" commands in word processing programs.

substitution

Looks for the specified pattern and replaces it with the specified string. By default, it does this for only the first occurrence found in the string. Appending a (g) to the end of the expression tells the operator to make the substitution for all occurrences.

Form:

s/pattern/replacement/

s/pattern/replacement/gi

$var =~ s/pattern/replacement/

In the second version, (g) and (i) indicate that the replacement should be made for all occurrences and that the match should ignore case. In the third version, the action is performed on the variable indicated — $var — instead of on the default variable, $_. Thus, the operator behaves somewhat like the assignment operator; hence its form that includes an "equal" symbol as part of it.

Examples:

s/cat/dog/ # replaces "cat" with "dog" in $_

s/cat/dog/gi # same thing, but applies to "CAT", "Cat" wherever they appear

$a =~ s/cat/dog/ # applies the operation to $a

split( )

Split searchers for a pattern in a specified string and, if it finds it, throws away the portion that matched and returns the "before" and "after" substrings, as a list.

Form:

@var = split(/pattern/, string);

@var = split(/pattern/)

If no string is specified, the operator is applied to $_.

Examples:

@a = split(/cat/, $aString);

@a = split(/cat/);

In the first example, the contents of $aString are split on "cat" and the two parts assigned to the array, @a. In the second, the operator is applied to the contents of $_.

join( )

Approximately the opposite of split. Takes a list of values, concatenates them, and returns the resulting string.

Form:

$var = join("item_1", $item2, . . .);

Example:

$a = join('cat", "dog", "bird"); # returns "catdogbird"

$a = join($b, $c);

Applications

1. Determine whether the string contains the pattern, and return "true" or "false"
   if ($string =~ /PATTERN/) {
   ....
   }

2. Extract from the string a substring that matches the pattern.
   $string =~ /PATTERN1(PATTERN2)PATTERN3(PATTERN4)/;
   # The patterns inside parentheses will be "remembered" and assigned to
   # the special variables $1 and $2
   ($name1, $name2) = $string =~
   /PATTERN1(PATTERN2)PATTERN3(PATTERN4)/;
   # The patterns inside parentheses will be assigned
   # into the variables $name1 and $name2

3. Look for the pattern in the string and replace it with something else.
   $string =~ s/PATTERN/SOMETHING_ELSE/;

4. Look for all appearances of the pattern in the string and extract the parts of the string that are not
   matching the pattern.
   @array = split (/PATTERN/, $string); 6
   Acetylcholine (muscarinic) receptors
   ==
   ACM1_HUMAN (P11229) MUSCARINIC ACETYLCHOLINE M1 [CHRM1] - HUMAN
   ACM1_MOUSE (P12657) MUSCARINIC ACETYLCHOLINE M1 [CHRM1] - MOUSE
   ACM1_PIG (P04761) MUSCARINIC ACETYLCHOLINE M1 (BRAIN) [CHRM1] - PIG
   ACM1_RAT (P08482) MUSCARINIC ACETYLCHOLINE M1 [CHRM1] - RAT
   ACM2_BOVIN (P41985) MUSCARINIC ACETYLCHOLINE M2 [CHRM2] - BOVINE
   ACM2_CHICK (P30372) MUSCARINIC ACETYLCHOLINE M2 [CM2] - CHICKEN
   ACM2_HUMAN (P08172) MUSCARINIC ACETYLCHOLINE M2 [CHRM2] - HUMAN
   ACM2_PIG (P06199) MUSCARINIC ACETYLCHOLINE M2 (CARDIAC) [CHRM2] - PIG
   ACM2_RAT (P10980) MUSCARINIC ACETYLCHOLINE M2 [CHRM2] - RAT
   ACM3_BOVIN (P41984) MUSCARINIC ACETYLCHOLINE M3 [CHRM3] - BOVINE
   ACM3_HUMAN (P20309) MUSCARINIC ACETYLCHOLINE M3 [CHRM3] - HUMAN
   ACM3_PIG (P11483) MUSCARINIC ACETYLCHOLINE M3 [CHRM3] - PIG
   ACM3_RAT (P08483) MUSCARINIC ACETYLCHOLINE M3 [CHRM3] - RAT
   ACM3_CHICK (P49578) MUSCARINIC ACETYLCHOLINE M3 - CHICKEN
   ACM4_BOVIN (P41986) MUSCARINIC ACETYLCHOLINE M4 [CHRM4] - BOVINE
   ACM4_CHICK (P17200) MUSCARINIC ACETYLCHOLINE M4 - CHICKEN
   ACM4_HUMAN (P08173) MUSCARINIC ACETYLCHOLINE M4 [CHRM4] - HUMAN
   ACM4_MOUSE (P32211) MUSCARINIC ACETYLCHOLINE M4 [CHRM4] - MOUSE
   ACM4_RAT (P08485) MUSCARINIC ACETYLCHOLINE M4 [CHRM4] - RAT
   ACM4_XENLA (P30544) MUSCARINIC ACETYLCHOLINE M4 - XENOPUS LAEVIS
   ACM5_HUMAN (P08912) MUSCARINIC ACETYLCHOLINE M5 [CHRM5] - HUMAN
   ACM5_RAT (P08911) MUSCARINIC ACETYLCHOLINE M5 [CHRM5] - RAT
   ACM1_DROME (P16395) MUSCARINIC ACETYLCHOLINE DM1 [ACRC] - DROSOPHILA

Example: Match to a sequence of characters

```
#!/usr/bin/perl -w
$sp_list_file = "sp_list";
open (SP, $sp_list_file) || die "cannot open \"$sp_list_file\": $!";
while ($line = <SP>) {
if ($line =~ /HUMAN/) { # match line against "HUMAN"
print $line; # print line if matches
}
}
```

Output:

```
ACM1_HUMAN (P11229) MUSCARINIC ACETYLCHOLINE M1 [CHRM1] - HUMAN
ACM2_HUMAN (P08172) MUSCARINIC ACETYLCHOLINE M2 [CHRM2] - HUMAN
ACM3_HUMAN (P20309) MUSCARINIC ACETYLCHOLINE M3 [CHRM3] - HUMAN
ACM4_HUMAN (P08173) MUSCARINIC ACETYLCHOLINE M4 [CHRM4] - HUMAN
ACM5_HUMAN (P08912) MUSCARINIC ACETYLCHOLINE M5 [CHRM5] - HUMAN
```

Example: Matching to a sequence of characters

The EcoRI restriction enzyme cuts at the consensus sequence GAATTC.

To find out whether a sequence contains a restriction site for EcoR1, write;

```
$sequence =~ /GAATTC/;
```

Example: Match to a character class

The BstYI restriction enzyme cuts at the consensus sequence rGATCy, namely A or G in the first position, then GATC, and then T or C in the sixth position. To find out whether a sequence contains a restriction site for BstYI, write;

```
$sequence =~ /[AG]GATC[TC]/;
# This will match all of AGATCT, GGATCT, AGATCC, GGATCC.
```

Usage of Regular Expressions

- When a list of characters is enclosed in square brackets [ ], one and only one of these characters must be present at the corresponding position of the string in order for the pattern to match.
- You may specify a range of characters using a hyphen -.
- A caret ^ at the front of the list negates the character class.

Examples

```
$string =~ /[AGTC]/; # matches any nucleotide
$string =~ /[a-z]/; # matches any lowercase letter
$string =~ /chromosome[1-6]/; # matches chromosome1, chromosome2 ...
# chromosome6
$string =~ /[^xyzXYZ]/; # matches any character except x, X, y, Y, z, Z
```

Quantifiers

Quantifiers affect the character before them in the regular expression, and determine how many times this character must or may occur. If you want the quantifier to affect a sequence of characters, enclose those characters in parentheses.

The quantifiers are:

{n} Must occur exactly n times

{n,m} Must occur at least n times but no more than m times

{n,} Must occur at least n times
* 0 or more times (same as {0,})
+ 1 or more times (same as {1,})
? 0 or 1 time (same as {0,1})

Example :

We would like to find out whether the consensus sequence is contained (somewhere) in a given sequence $a.

Without quantifiers:

$a =~ /ACCCC[AG][AG][AG]GTGT/;

With quantifiers:

$a =~ /AC{4}[AG]{3}(GT){2}/;

To check whether a given sequence contains 2 or more repeats of the GATA tetranucleotide write:

if ($seq =~ /(GATA){2,}/) { }

note that we enclosed the sequence to be repeated in parentheses

The Genome Database accession IDs are composed of the characters GDB,followed by several digits. To check whether a Genome Database accession ID is entered correctly, use the following conditional:

if ($entry =~ /GDB:\d+/) { }

i.e. "GDB:" followed by one or more digits

Alternation

Alternation allows matching any one of several subexpressions. The alternative subexpressions are separated by vertical bar(s) |.

Example:

Recall the example we used for extracting all lines about human proteins from the Swiss-Prot list of muscarinic acetylcholine receptors.

Let us now change it to extract all lines including either human, rat or mouse proteins:

if ($line =~ /HUMAN|RAT|MOUSE/) { }

match line against either HUMAN, RAT or MOUSE

Example:

In the same file, let us now restrict our search only for the ACM1 receptors in either human, rat or mouse.

if ($line =~ /ACM1_(HUMAN|RAT|MOUSE)/) { }

We enclosed the alternative expressions in parentheses (HUMAN|RAT|MOUSE)

and added the receptor name prefix ACM1_ before them.

Anchoring a pattern to the beginning or end of a string

Example:

To print the "description" line from a SwissProt entry, which starts with DE:

```
#!/usr/bin/perl -w
$sp_file = "sp_entry";
open (SP, $sp_file) || die "cannot open \"$sp_file\": $!";
while ($line = <SP>) {
if ($line =~ /^DE/) {
```

```
print $line;
}
}
```
Result:

DE MUSCARINIC ACETYLCHOLINE RECEPTOR M1.
Regular Expressions

6.7 PERL APPLICATION FOR BIOINFORMATICS - BIOPERL

Bioperl is a collection of perl modules that facilitate the development of perl scripts for bioinformatics applications. As such, it does not include ready to use programs in the sense that may commercial packages and free web-based interfaces (e.g Entrez, SRS) do. On the other hand, bioperl does provide reusable perl modules that facilitate writing perl scripts for sequence manipulation, accessing of data-bases using a range of data formats and execution and parsing of the results of various molecular biology programs including Blast, clustalw, TCoffee, genscan, ESTscan and HMMER. Consequently, bioperl enables developing scripts that can analyze large quantities of sequence data in ways that are typically difficult or impossible with web based systems.

Sequence objects: Seq, PrimarySeq, LocatableSeq, LiveSeq, LargeSeq, SeqI

Seq is the central sequence object in bioperl. When in doubt this is probably the object that you want to use to describe a dna, rna or protein sequence in bioperl. Most common sequence manipulations can be performed with Seq.

Seq objects can be created explicitly.However usually Seq objects will be created for you automatically when you read in a file containing sequence data using the SeqIO object.In addition to storing its identification labels and the sequence itself, a Seq object can store multiple annotations and associated "sequence features". This capability can be very useful - especially in development of automated genome annotation systems.

On the other hand, if you need a script capable of simultaneously handling many (hundreds or thousands) sequences at a time, then the overhead of adding annotations to each sequence can be significant. For such applications, you will want to use the PrimarySeq object. PrimarySeq is basically a "stripped down" version of Seq. It contains just the sequence data itself and a few identifying labels (id, accession number, molecule type = dna, rna, or protein). For applications with hundreds or thousands or sequences, using PrimarySeq objects can significantly speed up program execution and decrease the amount of RAM the program requires.

The LocatableSeq object is just a Seq object which has "start" and "end" positions associated with it. It is used by the alignment object SimpleAlign and other modules that use SimpleAlign objects (eg AlignIO, pSW). In general you don't have to worry about creating LocatableSeq objects because they will be made for you automatically when you create an alignment (using pSW, Clustalw, Tcoffee or bl2seq) or when input an alignment data file using AlignIO. However if you need to input a sequence alignment by hand (ieg to build a SimpleAlign object), you will need to input the sequences as LocatableSeqs.

A LargeSeq object is a special type of Seq object used for handling very long (eg >100 MB) sequences.

A LiveSeq object is another specialized object for storing sequence data. LiveSeq addresses the problem of features whose location on a sequence changes over time. This can happen, for example, when sequence feature objects are used to store gene locations on newly sequenced genomes - locations which can change as higher quality sequencing data becomes available. Although a LiveSeq object is not implemented in the same way as a Seq object, LargeSeq does implement the SeqI interface. Consequently, most methods available for Seq objects will work fine with LiveSeq objects.

SeqI objects are Seq "interface objects". They are used to ensure bioperl's compatibility with other software packages. SeqI and other interface objects are not likely to be relevant to the casual bioperl user.

Alignment objects : SimpleAlign, UnivAln

There are two "alignment objects" in bioperl: SimpleAlign and UnivAln. Both store an array of sequences as an alignment. However their internal data structures are quite different and converting between them - though certainly possible - is rather awkward. In contrast to the sequence objects - where there are good reasons for having 6 different classes of objects, the presence of two alignment objects is just an unfortunate relic of the two systems having been designed independently at different times.

Since each object has some capabilities that the other lacks it has not yet been feasible to unify bioperl's sequence alignment methods into a single object. However, recent development in bioperl involving alignments has been focused on using SimpleAlign and the new user should generally use SimpleAlign where possible.

Using bioperl

Bioperl provides software modules for many of the typical tasks of bioinformatics programming. These include:
- Accessing sequence data from local and remote databases
- Transforming formats of database/ file records
- Manipulating individual sequences
- Searching for "similar" sequences
- Creating and manipulating sequence alignments
- Searching for genes and other structures on genomic DNA
- Developing machine readable sequence annotations

Illustration of Bioperl application : Parsing BLAST

No matter how Blast searches are run, they return large quantities of data that are tedious to sift through. Bioperl offers different objects for this purpose - Blast.pm and BPlite.pm (along with its minor modifications, BPpsilite and BPbl2seq) for parsing Blast reports.

The parser contained within the Blast.pm module is the original Blast parser developed for Bioperl. It is very full featured and has a large array of options and output formats. BPlite is less complex and easier to maintain than Blast.pm. Although it has fewer options and display modes than Blast.pm, it contains the functionality that is usually need.

The syntax for using BPlite is as follows where the method for retrieving hits is now called "nextSbjct" (for "subject"), while the method for retrieving high-scoring-pairs is called "nextHSP":

```
use Bio::Tools::BPlite;
$report = new BPlite(-fh=>\*STDIN);
$report->query;
while(my $sbjct = $report->nextSbjct) {
    $sbjct->name;
    while (my $hsp = $sbjct->nextHSP) { $hsp->score; }
}
```

Illustration of Bioperl application : Aligning 2 sequences with Blast using bl2seq and AlignIO

Two sequences çan also be aligned in Bioperl using the bl2seq option of Blast within the StandAloneBlast object. To get an alignment - in the form of a SimpleAlign object - using bl2seq, it is needed to parse the bl2seq report with the AlignIO file format reader as follows:

```
$factory = Bio::Tools::StandAloneBlast->new('outfile' => 'bl2seq.out');
$bl2seq_report = $factory->bl2seq($seq1, $seq2);
# Use AlignIO.pm to create a SimpleAlign object from the bl2seq report
$str = Bio::AlignIO->new('-file '=>' bl2seq.out','-format' => 'bl2seq');
$aln = $str->next_aln();
```

7

Relational Databases for Biological Information

7.1 INTRODUCTION

This chapter discusses types of databases and using relational databases for storing biological information. Creating and managing the biological databases is one of the key tasks for bioinformatics. Deciding the structure of a database is a technical decision and has to be done after due consideration to the database strategy. The database strategy includes evolving the norms like: limited versus unlimited access to the database, curated versus non-curated databases, frequency of updation, mirroring of the database etc. While these are "strategy" guidelines, one also needs to decide the structure of the database. The identification of key fields (fields that can be used as identifiers of the data-set) is an important consideration and should be done in consultation with the users (molecular biologists).

It is important to understand the basic underlying principles to appreciate the considerations in decisions related to the databases. The understanding of the databasing principles would also help in their better use.

All databases perform the following four tasks :

1. To collect and preserve data
2. To make data easy to find and search
3. To standardize data representation
4. To organize data into knowledge

Biological databases are crucial from the following points of view :

1. They provide a record of scientific work
2. They can be used to share data on the web (as a close proxy to publication)
3. They can be used to add-on visualisation functions (maps, 3D structures, pathways, trees, morphology, taxonomy etc.)
4. Several biological databases provide support for data analysis and tools that were hitherto not available to biologists. They are exceptionally useful for making high throughput technologies being available on the scientists desktops.

7.2 TYPES OF DATABASES

There are three basic types of databases : flat files, relational databases and object oriented databases. Object oriented databases would be discussed in a later chapter.

Flat file databases

The flat file database consists of a collection of records, each containing several data fields. It is a rudimentary database - an ordered collection of similar files following the same standard format. For example, three records in a database of cell stocks might look like this:

```
Cell_Stock : "SK11.pEA215.3"
Species  "Escherichia coli"
Plasmid  "pEA215.3"
Experiment      "SK11"-+
Freezer "AG334 -80C"
Box      "Pisum ESTs II"
Gridded  "Rack(BF7) Box(Pisum ESTs II)"

Cell_Stock : "SK11.pI206KS"
Species  "Escherichia coli"
Plasmid  "pI206KS"
Experiment      "SK11"
Freezer "AG334 -80C"
Box      "Pisum ESTs II"
Gridded  "Rack(BF7) Box(Pisum ESTs II)"

Cell_Stock : "SK11.pEA46.2"
Species  "Escherichia coli"
Plasmid  "pEA46.2"
Experiment      "SK11"
Freezer "AG334 -80C"
Box      "Pisum ESTs II"
Gridded  "Rack(BF7) Box(Pisum ESTs II)"
```

In this example, the data in the Species, Freezer, Box and Gridded fields are identical. This implies that the flat file databases are highly redundant. Not only does this redundancy waste space, it means that if a field has to change, it must be changed in all records. For example, if the box were moved to a different freezer, all Freezer fields would have to be changed. For large data storage requirements, working with flat files becomes very inefficient.

All transactions that change, add or delete records require rewriting the database. To add a record, the database is written to the point at which the record is to be added, the new record is written, and then the rest of the records are written. Similarly, changing and deleting records also requires that all records be rewritten.

Searching a flat file database implies that the entire text of the database be searched. Indexing can be used to make the searches faster; however indexing increases the size of the database. Another disadvantage of flat file databases is that the records must be organized by one of the fields.

GenBank entries retrieved by Entrez are flat file representations of data that are centered around

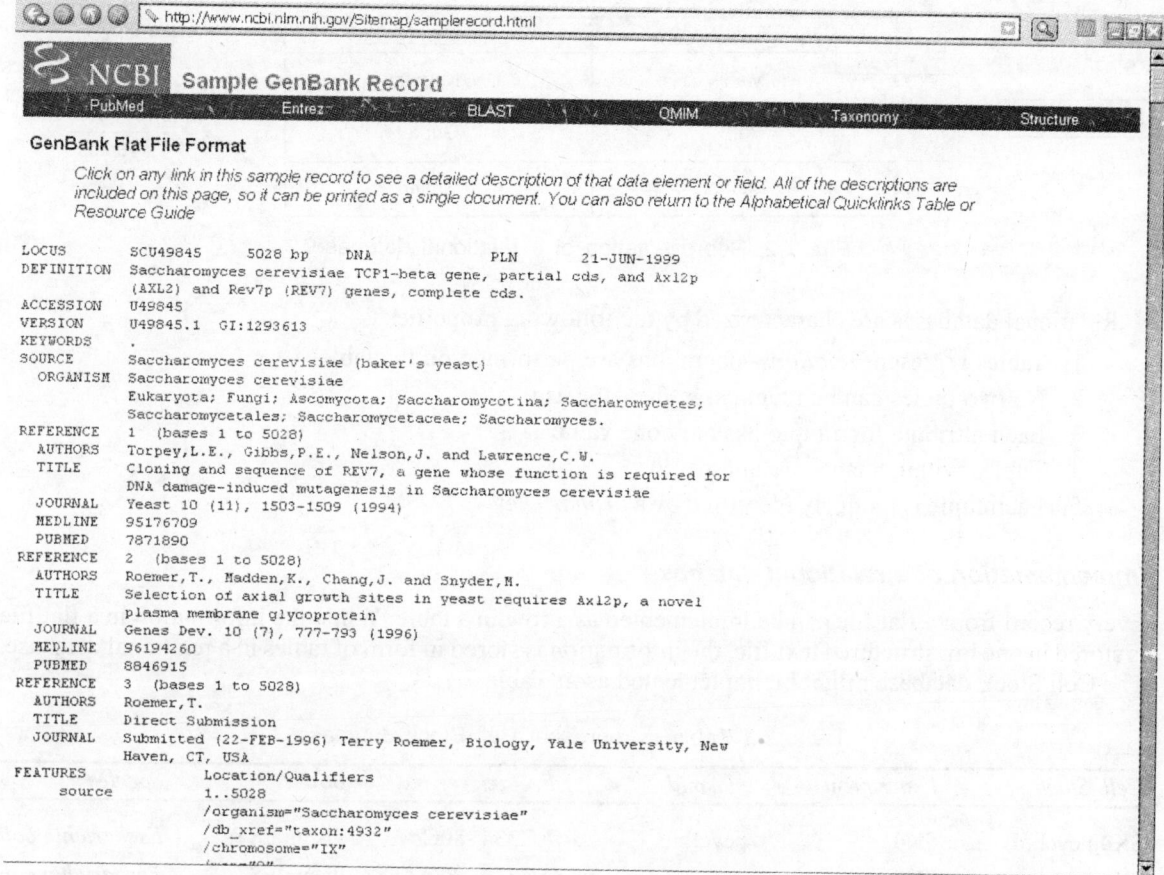

Fig. 7.1. GenBank flat file illustration.

DNA sequences. In a GenBank entry, every field appears to belong to a particular sequence (http://www.ncbi.nlm.nih.gov/Sitemap/samplerecord.html) (Fig. 7.1).

Most of the NCBI databases are flat files with indexes, based on ASN1 format (abstract syntax notation, which is semi-structured format) and some relational parts. These databases provide output in XML, FASTA and other formats.

PDB, the protein database started out as a flat file structure and was then restructured as an object oriented database.

2. Relational databases

Introduction

Relational databases can be thought of as comprehensive tables of data. A relational database is a collection of tables, each of which is assigned a unique name. Each table consists of a set of *attributes* and stores a set of records or *tuples*. Each record (tuple) in a relational table represents an *object* identified by a unique key and described by a set of *attribute values*. An *entity*-relationship model is usually used to model the relational databases (Fig. 7.2).

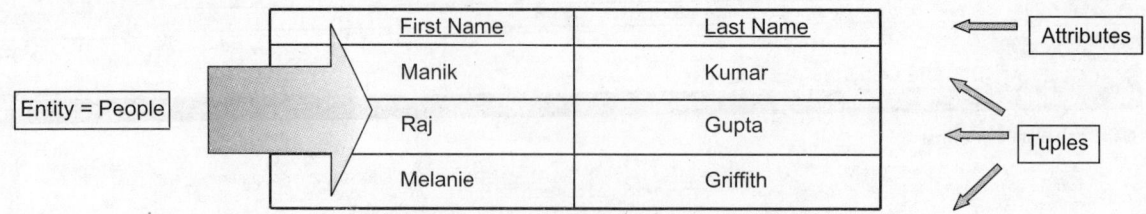

Fig. 7.2. Representation of a relational database.

Relational databases are characterized by the following properties :

1. Tables represent *relations*- operations are performed on the tables
2. No two tuples can be identical in the database
3. Each attribute for a tuple has only one value
4. Tuples within a table are unordered
5. Each tuple is uniquely identified by a *primary key*

Implementation of a relational database

Every record from a flat file can be implemented as a row in a table. While the information in a flat file is stored in one big structured text file, the information is stored in form of tables in a relational database. The Cell Stock database might be implemented as in Table 7.1.

Table 7.1 Table to represent Cell Stock database

Cell_Stock	Experiment	plasmid	Freezer	Box	Species
SK4.pcyclinB	SK4	pcyclinB	AG334 -80C	Pisum ESTs	*Escherichia coli*
SK4.pcyclinD	SK4	pcyclinD	AG334 -80C	Pisum ESTs	*Escherichia coli*
SK4.pNDK-P1	SK4	pNDK-P1	AG334 -80C	Pisum ESTs	*Escherichia coli*

From a relational database, many views of the data are possible as shown in Tables 7.2 (a) and (b).

Table 7.2 (a) Plasmid View

Plasmid	Species	Cell Stock
pEA25	*Escherichia coli*	SK10.2.pEA25
pEA46.2	*Escherichia coli*	SK11.pEA46.2
pEA207.2	*Escherichia coli*	SK11.pEA207.2

Table 7.2 (b). Experiment View

Experiment	Cell	Stock	Box Freezer
SK4	SK4.pPS-IAA4-5	PisumESTs I	AG334-80C
SK4	SK4.pPS-IAA6	PisumESTs I	AG334-80C
SK4	SK4.pTic110	PisumESTs I	AG334-80C

Relational databases can be organized across many files as illustrated below.

PLASMID	VECTOR	Insert	DNA_SAMPLE

DNA_SAMPLE	VECTOR	PLASMID	Exp#	Conc.	LOCATION

VECTOR	ACCESSION	DNA_SAMPLE

LOCATION	Freezer	Box#

Although a relational database can be implemented in a single large table or "relation", it is often advantageous to split the database up into multiple tables.

Four tables are shown in the above schema : PLASMID, DNA_SAMPLE, VECTOR and LOCA-TION. Fields in lowercase contain text or other data. Fields in uppercase contain names of items in other tables. Relational data can be accessed using database queries written in a query language like SQL. A given query is transformed into a set of relational operations like selection, join, projection etc.

Design of relational databases

Using Entity Relationship Diagrams

The design of relational databases is based on the use of *entity-relationship diagrams (ERDs)*. We first need to conceptualise the data elements in form of entities and then we identify the relationship in the data to create the ERD. An ERD can have three elements : entities, attributes and relationships.

For example, consider the ERD given in the Fig. 7.3, where people have addresses and phone numbers and phone numbers are part of the address. Entities, relationships and attributes are identified in this ERD.

This ERD can be converted into tables for a RDBMS as given in the Fig. 7.4.

Relationships can be of fours types : 1-to1, 1-to-many, many-to-1 and many-to-many (Fig. 7.5). Many-to-many relationships need to be converted to the first three types to clarify the relationships for a good design.

Consider the GenBank structure (Fig. 7.1) as discussed earlier. The attributes identified are as follows :

Locus, Definition, Accession, Version, Source Organism

Authors, Title, Journal, Medline Id, PubMed Id

Protein Name, Protein Description, Protein Id, Protein Translation, Locus Id, GI

A count, C count, G count, T count, Sequence

Grouping can be done to identify the entities as follows :

Gene

    – Locus, Definition, Accession, Version, Source Organism

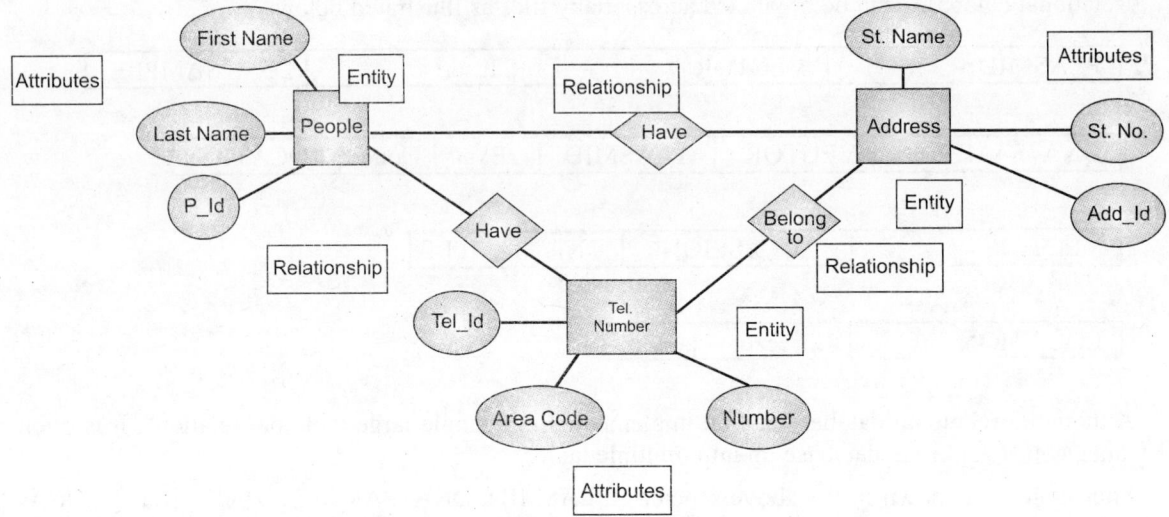

Fig. 7.3. An example of an ERD.

References
— Authors, Title, Journal, Medline Id, PubMed Id
Features
— Protein Name, Protein Description, Protein Id, Protein Translation, Locus Id, GI
Sequence Information
— A count, C count, G count, T count, Sequence

These entities can be conceptualized and the relationships are shown in Fig. 7.6.

The finalized ERD is shown in Fig. 7.7 ERD which shows various relationships and references.

Normalizing the database

Normalization is another step in design of the databases. Normalisation is done to avoid redundancy and make data manipulation "atomic". The method used is to identify functional dependencies, and group them together such that no two determinants (candidate keys) exist in the same tuple. The database is said to be well normalized when a tuple consists of a primary key to provide identification and zero or more mutually independent attributes that describe the entity in some way.

Popular biological databases like PIR, SwissProt, EMBL, GenBank etc. are now implemented as relational databases.

Using Relational Databases

We can perform several operations on the relational databases. The commonly used operations performed on relational databases are discussed here. The operations are as follows :

Restrict: remove tuples (rows) that don't satisfy some criteria.

Project: remove specified attributes (columns, fields)

Product: merge tuple pairs from two relations in all possible ways; both degree and cardinality increase

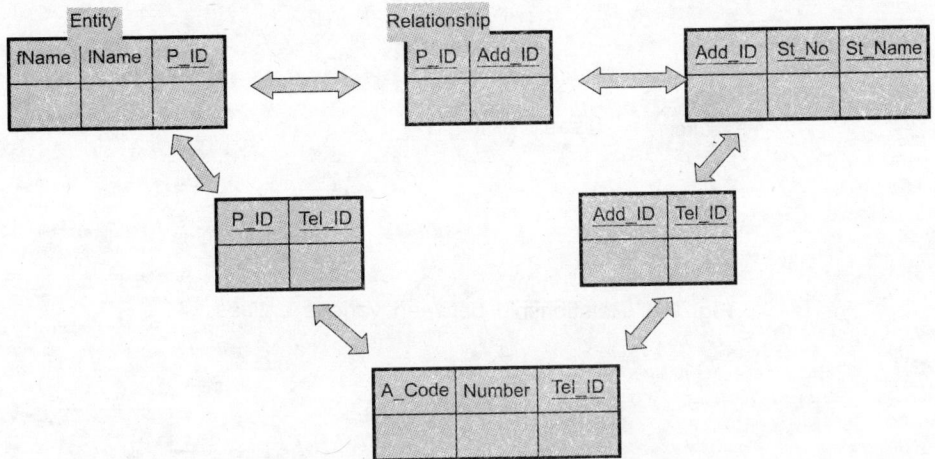

Fig. 7.4. ERD converted to a RDBMS.

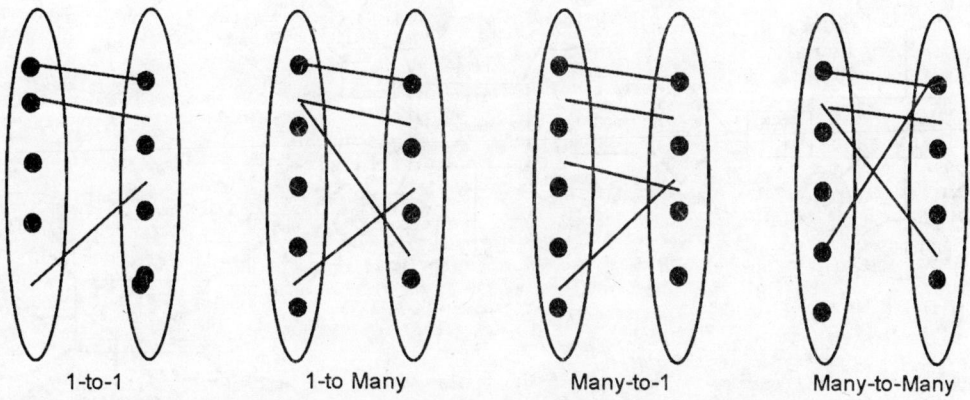

1-to-1   1-to Many   Many-to-1   Many-to-Many

Fig. 7.5. Illustration of various possible relationships between entities.

Join: Like "Product", but merged tuple pairs must satisfy some criteria for joining, otherwise the pair is removed

Union: concatenation of all tuples from two relations; degree remains the same, cardinality increases

Intersection: remove tuples that are not shared by both relations

Difference: remove tuples that are not shared by one of the relations

For example, consider the Table 7.3.

restrict on (species_id = 1) operation would result in the Table 7.4.

SQL (Structured Query Language) is a popular language used to perform such operations of relational databases. SQL is a non-procedural language.

Consider the Table 7.5 as part of a relational database.

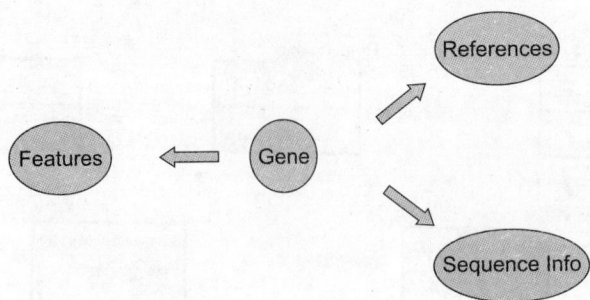

Fig. 7.6. Relationship between various entities.

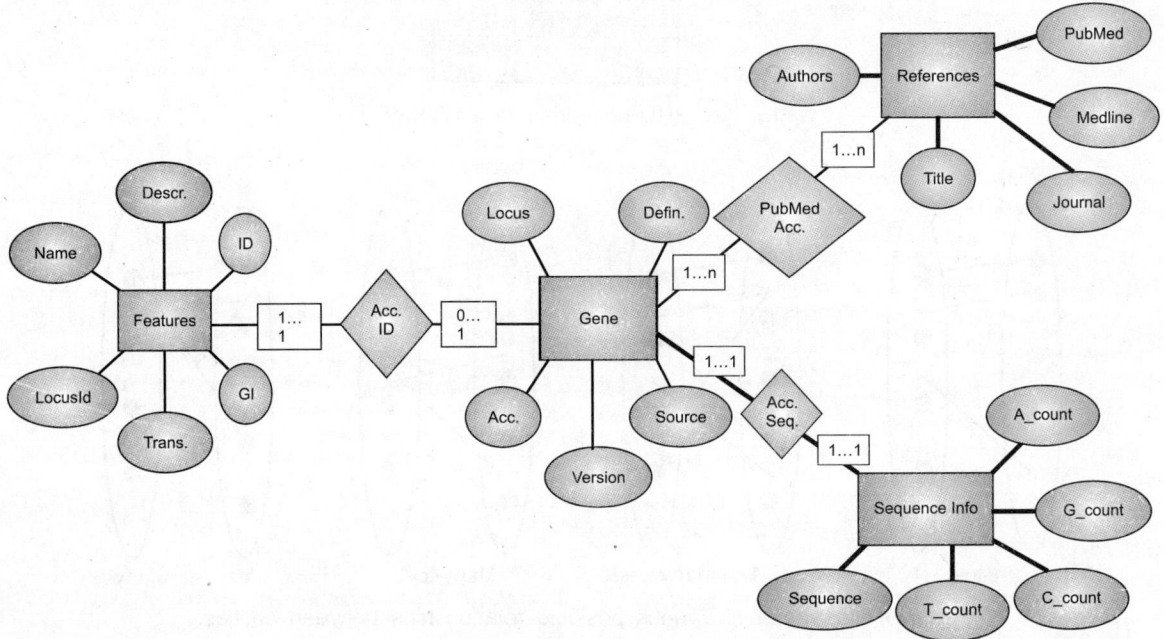

Fig. 7.7. ERD for GenBank.

Table 7.3 Sample database

protein_id	name	sequence	species_id
1	GTM1_HUMAN	MGTSHSMT...	1
2	GTM1_RAT	MGYTVSIT...	3
3	GTM1_MOUSE	MGSTKMLT...	2
4	GTM2_HUMAN	MGTSHSMT...	1

Table 7.4 Result of restrict operation

protein_id	name	sequence	species_id
1	GTM1 HUMAN	MGTSHSMT...	1
4	GTM2 HUMAN	MGTSHSMT...	1

Table 7.5 Sample tables from a relational database

protein relation (table)   *degree = 4*

prot_id	name	seq	species_id
1	GTM1_HUMAN	MGTSHSMT...	1
2	GTM1_RAT	MGYTVSIT...	3
3	GTM1_MOUSE	MGSTKMLT...	2
4	GTM2_HUMAN	MGTSHSMT...	1

tuples (rows)   *cardinality = 4*

species relation (table)

species_id	name	scientific_name
1	human	Homo sapiens
2	mouse	Mus musculus
2	house mouse	Mus musculus
3	rat	Rattus rattus

There are two types of operations that can be performed on such a relational database. The two types of operations are : Data Definition Language (DDL) and Data Manipulation Language (DML). The typical DDL and DML statements are as follows :

DDL

– CREATE DATABASE seqdb

   – CREATE TABLE protein (

     id INT PRIMARY KEY AUTOINCREMENT

     seq TEXT

     len INT)

– ALTER TABLE protein

– DROP TABLE protein, DROP DATABASE seqdb

DML

– SELECT : calculate new relations via Restrict, Project and Join operations

– UPDATE : make changes to existing tuples

– INSERT : add new tuples to a relation

– DELETE : remove tuples from a relation

Select is widely used DML operation and has the syntax as follows :

SELECT [attribute list]
FROM [relation]

For example, for the above sample database:

SELECT prot_id, protein.description,species.name
FROM [relation]

If you want to return attributes from tuples with conditions, you can use statements like this :

SELECT name FROM protein
WHERE name LIKE "glutathione %"

You can also extract data using join :

SELECT protein.*, species.*
FROM protein
JOIN species

This operation on the Table 7.6

Table 7.6 Sample table

protein id	name	sequence	species id
1	GTM1_HUMAN	MGTSHSMT...	1
2	GTM1_RAT	MGYTVSIT...	3
3	GTM1_MOUSE	MGSTKMLT...	2
4	GTM2_HUMAN	MGTSHSMT...	1

species id	name	scientific name
1	human	Homo sapiens
2	mouse	Mus musculus
3	rat	Rattus rattus

would result in the Table 7.7.

Table 7.7. Output table of the join operation

protein id	name	sequence	p.sid	s.sid	name
1	GTM1_HUMAN	MGTSHSMT...	1	1	human
2	GTM1_RAT	MGYTVSIT...	3	1	human
3	GTM1_MOUSE	MGSTKMLT...	2	1	human
4	GTM2_HUMAN	MGTSHSMT...	1	1	human
1	GTM1_HUMAN	MGTSHSMT...	1	2	mouse
2	GTM1_RAT	MGYTVSIT...	3	2	mouse
3	GTM1_MOUSE	MGSTKMLT...	2	2	mouse
4	GTM2_HUMAN	MGTSHSMT...	1	2	mouse
1	GTM1_HUMAN	MGTSHSMT...	1	3	rat
2	GTM1_RAT	MGYTVSIT...	3	3	rat
3	GTM1_MOUSE	MGSTKMLT...	2	3	rat
4	GTM2_HUMAN	MGTSHSMT...	1	3	rat

MySQL

MySQL is a relational database management system and is based on a client/server model. This implies that there is the MySQL server at the back-end and your interface to it is the MySQL client program. Data is organized as a relational database.

MySQL commands can be entered into the MySQL client command line. MySQL supports multi-line commands and uses a semicolon to designate the end of the command.

Creating a Database

The CREATE statement is used to create a database. The CREATE DATABASE <tablename>; syntax is very simple.

    CREATE DATABASE database1;
    Creates a database named database1.

Creating tables

There are many different data types to format the storage of data. There are storage types for text, numeric values, date and time, etc. Also there are optional settings you can apply to fields such as default settings, allow NULL fields and auto_increment value are some common ones.

```
CREATE TABLE table1 (
    id INT NOT NULL auto_increment,
    firstname varchar(20) NOT NULL,
    lastname varchar(25) NOT NULL,
    address1 varchar(40) NOT NULL,
    address2 varchar(40),
    city varchar(20) NOT NULL,
    state varchar(2) NOT NULL,
    zipcode varchar(10) NOT NULL,
    email text NOT NULL,
    primary key (id)
);
```

Here we created a table named table1 with nine fields. The id field is an integer. There are two modifiers to the id, NOT NULL and auto_increment. NOT NULL means that the value of that field cannot be left empty, while auto_increment means that every row the value of the field will be one higher.

Firstname, lastname, address1, address2, city, state, and zipcode are all of varchar type. The numbers in parentheses represent the length of the field. The email field is text type. The primary key is a field that is unique to each row. An ID field is the perfect column to set as a primary key because no two columns should have the same ID.

```
CREATE TABLE table2 (
    id INT NOT NULL auto_increment,
    login varchar(20) NOT NULL,
    password text NOT NULL,
    lastlogin datetime NOT NULL DEFAULT '0000-00-00 00:00:00',
    primary key (id)
);
```

In this CREATE TABLE statement we created table2. This table is similar to the first but we introduce the datetime field type and the DEFAULT statement. The datetime field type stores the time and date in YYYY-MM-DD HH:MM:SS format. By using the DEFAULT statement you can set the default value.

Inserting data

```
INSERT INTO users (name, number)
    values ('John', 21);
CREATE TABLE users
(
    ...
    password varchar(16) NOT NULL,
    ...
);
```

The *not null* means you need to have some value for the column.

Consider the line from the create table table2 command above :

```
CREATE TABLE users
(
    id INT NOT NULL auto_increment,
    ...
);
```

In the case of the id column, we have specified auto_increment and MySQL creates the value by adding 1 to the greatest value it finds in that column.

Displaying and updating data

SELECT command is used to display data from a table.

SELECT * FROM person;

The SELECT command here is used to visualize the columns of a table. SELECT * FROM person displays every column of the table person.

The general syntax is:

SELECT (column1, column2,...) FROM nameofTable;

The SELECT command can be combined with the WHERE option in order to refine a search. In the Table 7.8 "person" as follows :

Table 7.8 Table "person"

name	birth	nmbKids
Roger	1953-05-19	0
Luke	1963-09-27	2

The command :

SELECT * FROM person WHERE name = 'Luke' ;

displays the entries of the table 'person' where the name equals 'Luke' as in Table 7.9

Table 7.9 Result of the where operation

name	birth	nmbKids
Luke	1963-09-27	2

The WHERE option can be applied to any column in order to search a specific entry. The command:

SELECT * FROM person WHERE nmbKids = '2' ;

also works.

It is possible to update a table entry with the command UPDATE :

UPDATE nameofTable SET attribute = 'X' WHERE attribute = 'Y' ;

Example:

UPDATE person SET nmbKids = '0' WHERE name = 'Luke';

MySQL types and primary key

Primary key directive in the create table command is an important option.

CREATE TABLE users

(

   ...

   PRIMARY KEY (user_id),

   ...

)

This is a command to file things by using user_id field as the primary key. The constraint imposed on a primary key is that each row must have a unique value for the key. MySQL creates a B-tree to make lookup of a specific row by user_id fast. The command :

SELECT * from users WHERE user_id = 2;

is executed faster than

SELECT * from users WHERE favorite_number = 945;

Using Perl DBI to interface to MySQL

DBI stands for database interface. The Perl DBI module provides a generic interface for database access. You can write a DBI script that works with many different database engines without change. To use DBI, you must install the DBI module, as well as a DataBase Driver (DBD) module for each type of server you want to access. For MySQL, this driver is the DBD::mysql module.

To use DBI, first you need to load the DBI module:

use DBI;

Once you have the DBI and DBD::mysql modules installed, you can get information about them at the command line with the perldoc command:

perldoc DBI
perldoc DBI::FAQ
perldoc DBD::mysql

Then you need to "connect" to your data source and get a handle for that connection:

connect:
$dbh = DBI->connect($data_source, $user, $password)
or die $DBI::errstr;

The connect string above takes three arguments: a data source name, a username, and a password. The data source name is in the form dbi:DriverName:instance. "Connect" will return a true value on success, untrue otherwise. Also, DBI will place an error message in the package variable $DBI::errstr.

DBI allows an application to "prepare" statements for later execution. A statement handle held in a Perl variable identifies a prepared statement. The variable is $sth in the example. The typical sequence of calls for a SELECT statement is:

prepare, execute, fetch, fetch, ...

For example :

$sth = $dbh->prepare(q{SELECT term_id, term_synonym
        FROM term_synonym
        WHERE term_id<100 })
    or die "Can't prepare statement: $DBI::errstr";

Prepares a statement for later execution and returns a statement handle. q{ }puts the correct quotes around the string.

Sending the statement to the DBMS is done by using "execute".

$rc = $sth->execute or die $DBI::errstr;

A successful execute always returns true. It is always important to check the return status of execute. For SELECT statements, execute returns a true value. For non-SELECT statements (insert, update, delete), execute returns the number of rows affected, if known. If no rows were affected, then execute returns "0E0", which Perl will treat as 0 but will regard as true.

Data from a select is typically a sequence of rows. Use fetchrow_array to get one row at a time.

@ary = $sth->fetchrow_array;

It fetches the next row of data and returns it as a list containing the field values. Null fields are returned as undef values in the list. If there are no more rows or if an error occurs, then fetchrow_array returns an empty list. You should check $sth->err afterwards to discover if the empty list returned was due to an error.

When you have finished working with the data source, you should "disconnect" from it:

$dbh->disconnect;

8

Object Oriented Databases

8.1 INTRODUCTION

Object-oriented database management systems (OODBMSs) were developed in the 1980s. At that time, there were a few Object-Oriented Programming (OOP) languages, such as Smalltalk and C^{++}. Object oriented languages have some advantages over conventional languages for many programming applications :

1. *Strong encapsulation*, which makes it easier to program large applications.
2. *Inheritance,* which fosters code reuse.
3. *Persistence of objects*, which means that object lifetimes can extend beyond the single execution of a program.

Some of the important terms in OOP are as follows :

Object identity : Even if two objects have the same internal value, they are still different objects. Similarly, two variables are different even if temporarily they have the same value, because they have different locations, and hence in the future they can be updated differently. Object identity is connected to an "object-centric" view of programming: every operation is about some primary object.

Encapsulation : The state of an object is private to the object: the only way the state can be changed or observed is by calling one of the object's methods.

Overloading: Two objects of different classes can have a method with the same name. If these methods perform conceptually similar operations, the caller of the method does not need to know the exact class of the called object. Overloading is particularly important with inheritance.

An Object-Oriented Database Management System (OODBMS) can be seen as trying "to add DBMS capabilities to an OOP language", and in effect making it a *persistent* O-O language. Consequently application programmers who use OODBMSs typically write programs in a native O-O language such as Java or C^{++}, and the language has some kind of Persistent class, Database class, Database Interface, or Database API that provides DBMS functionality as, effectively, an extension of the O-O language. There are several OODBMS vendors, but persistent versions of O-O languages currently have limited popularity.

Object-Relational Database Management System (ORDBMS) as a system that "extends a relational database with O-O features". In particular ORDBMSs offer

1. A rich (abstract) type system
2. Inheritance mechanisms
3. OOP extensions to SQL

Object-oriented databases provide more powerful capabilities than relational databases. Following are important attributes of OOD :

1. Allow for the definition of data types
2. Define methods for those data types
3. Allow for manipulation of the data types within the queries of the database
4. Allow for inheritance of sub-data types from super-data types
5. Provide for object identity
6. Allow for abstract data types and encapsulation

8.2 OBJECT ORIENTED DATABASES

Object-oriented databases solve many of the problems that are inherent in relational databases to provide more powerful capabilities. The fundamental unit of Object-oriented databases (OODB) is the Class, which may have many attributes and methods as defined below.

Attributes

Attributes hold the information that is intrinsic to the class. Data items are usually simple types of data, such as text or numbers. Attributes can also be pointers to other classes. There may be either one or many data items or classes of each type.

Methods

Methods are procedures or tasks that an object can carry out. A method may contain its own data fields, and may point to other classes.

The representation of Class is given below :

> **Class**
>> **Attributes**
>>> **Data items**
>>> **Classes** →
>> **Methods**
>>> **Data items**
>>> **Classes** →

A class can be thought of as a formula for an object. An object is an instance of a class. Hence the representation of Object is given below :

> **OBJECT**
>> **Attributes**
>>> **Data items**
>>> **Objects** →
>> **Methods**
>>> **Data items**
>>> **Objects** →

Objects correspond to individual records in a relational database. There can be several objects of a given class. A class is an abstraction; while an object is a tangible thing. For example, pFF100 is an instance of the class PLASMID. The class definition allows it to point to two other classes, VECTOR and DNA_SAMPLE. DNA_SAMPLE might look like this:

CLASS	OBJECT
DNA_SAMPLE	SK99.pFF100
VECTOR | PLASMID	pFF100
EXPERIMENT	SK99
concentration [μg/μl]	0.5
BOX	Pisum ESTs I

In the DNA_SAMPLE class, the first field points to either a VECTOR or a PLASMID. In this example, the corresponding field in SK99.pFF100 points to PLASMID pFF100. The EXPERIMENT field points to an object of the type EXPERIMENT. The concentration field contains a floating point number whose units are μg/ μl. The BOX field points to an object of the type BOX, called "Pisum ESTs I".

Methods

The implementation of methods is highly dependent on the specific database software being used. In some cases, macros, that is, sets of database commands might be run. In other cases, an external program might be called. For example, the PLASMID class could have a method called MAP_VIEWER:

CLASS	OBJECT
PLASMID	pFF100
VECTOR	pBluescriptIISK+
insert	2500bp BamHI frag. from GB::X6638
MAP_VIEWER *filename*	xv pFF100.gif
DNA_SAMPLE	SK99.pFF100

The MAP_VIEWER and filename fields could be a template for a command that would launch a viewing program with a specific file. In the pFF100 object, the actual command that would be run is 'xv pFF100.gif'. This command would be passed to Linux, launching the xv image viewer with the GIF file pFF100.gif.

One-to-one versus one-to-many

One-to-one and one-to-many relationships have been discussed earlier in the section on entities for relational databases. The structure of relational databases makes implementation of one-to-many relationships difficult. In OODBs, it is very easy to modify a class to allow many fields of the same type.

AceDB is one of the oldest database schemas implemented for biological databases. The data modeling for AceDB is shown below :

In databases like ACeDB, all fields may be present in arbitrary numbers unless specifically implemented as UNIQUE fields (Genetic, Cytogenetic and Physical as above). For DNA_SAMPLE example,

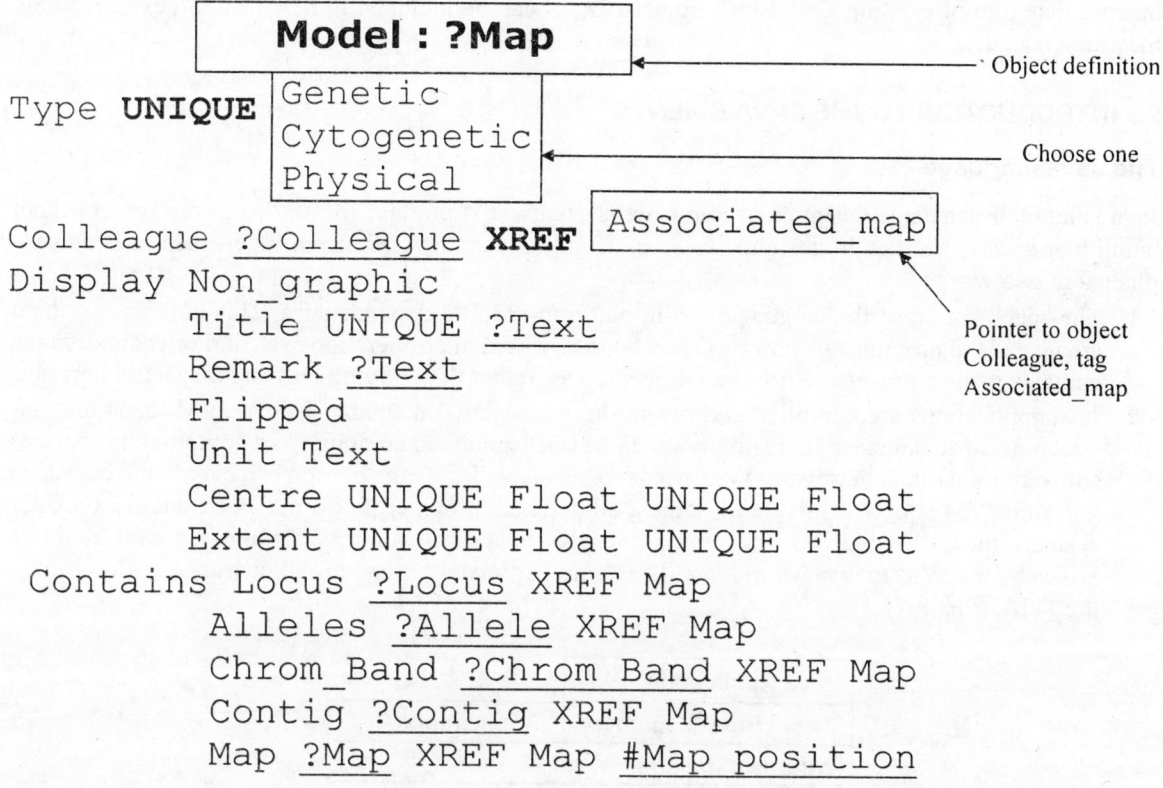

the Class and Object representation is as given below. Here, four plasmid constructs were made using the pBluescriptKSm13+ vector, and three DNA_SAMPLEs of this vector (not the plasmids) are listed.

CLASS	OBJECT
VECTOR	pBluescriptKSm13+
PLASMID	pI206KS
	pI49KS
	pI236KS
	pI230KS
ACCESSION	X52331
DNA_SAMPLE	AN29.pBluescriptKSm13+
	GK302.pBluescriptKSm13+
	FJ120.pBluescript.KSm13+

Many changes in classes have no effect on other classes. In particular, any number of attributes can be added, without changing objects that link to a class. When a class is changed, not all objects in that class need to be modified. OODBs, and to some extent other types of databases, do not require that all objects contain data for all possible attributes defined in the class. This allows a 'grandfathering' of preexisting objects. For example, if the class Cell_Stock was modified by the addition of an attribute called 'Date', listing the date on which the stock was made, it would not be necessary to go back and insert a date into of existing Cell_Stock objects. Dates can be included in new Cell_Stock objects, as they are created.

8.3 INTRODUCTION TO THE JAVA CLIENTS

The Java language

Java is an OOP language designed at Sun Microsystems. It is popular for many reasons, one of them being that it was specifically designed to be platform-independent. Platform independence is accomplished in two ways :

1. The specification of the language has no platform-specific dependencies. This implies that there are no calls to programs or libraries specific to any particular operating system. For example, Java contains its own procedures for drawing windows, rather than relying on system-specific libraries.

2. Java applications are compiled and run in the Java Virtual machine (JVM). JVM maps Java instructions to actual machine instructions. JVM is a "simulated computer" - a computer that runs as software rather than hardware. JVM needs to be adapted for each computer system on which Java will run. JVM is now available for almost all popular computer platforms. For example, on Unix systems, the CDE window manager might display Java applications, and some X11 calls might be issued by the JVM to create windows. The kernel, ultimately, executes all instructions emulated in the JVM. (Fig. 8.1).

Java Application	
Java Virtual Machines	Applications
Windows Manager	
Applications program interface	
Kernel	
Hardware	

Fig. 8.1. Java Virtual Machine Architecture.

Java is particularly well suited for network applications, because network capabilities are built into the Java language. The standard Java language includes libraries that implement network interfaces. In particular, a comprehensive set of network classes is found in the java.net libraries, which are standard with Java. The existence of network classes in Java saves the programmer from having to reinvent the wheel, when writing network-specific code.

Java applets (Fig. 8.2)

The major Web browsers include a JVM that allows them to run Java "applets". Applets are Java applications that are downloaded from a server at runtime, but run in a local JVM, by the Web browser. As a security measure, the JVM is implemented as a "sandbox", that is, a virtual machine that cannot read or write anywhere except in a protected area of memory. No disk files can be read or written, and no instructions can be executed outside of the sandbox. In contrast, normal Java applications, run from a user's account, can execute with the same read and write capabilities of any other program.

Java applets are implemented for the following reasons :

1. Java applets run as independent windows, or within the browser. Web browsers tend to move

from one page to another, defeating the purpose of having multiple windows. Applets can run in multiple windows for different types of data, or different procedures.

2. Java applets can implement more sophisticated user interfaces than are possible through HTML. HTML as a stand-alone has limited capabilities for user input and display of data. Applets can work on the data locally, in real time, with any type of control desired e.g. sliders, scroll bars.

3. Java applets are platform independent. For most purposes, the applet cannot run, regardless of the computer system at the client end. Only one version needs to be written, rather than many different versions for different platform.

4. Java applets are not permanently installed at client end. Since the Java applet is downloaded at runtime, the applet running at the server end would always be the latest.

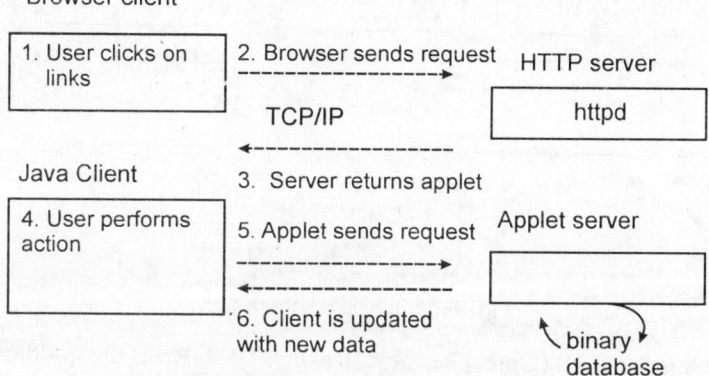

Fig. 8.2. Applet architecture overview.

Query mechanisms for Biological Databases

In order to support querying and data exploration, biological databases need to offer facilities for easy formulation of queries and interpretation of query results as well as support for easy manipulation of application-specific data. Most of the biological databases provide query interfaces. Existing public query interfaces for biological databases are usually either form-based or textual query language-based. Form-based query interfaces usually have a fixed structure involving a predetermined set of components and provide a limited number of options. Such interfaces provide a single fixed view of the database and do not reflect the structure of the underlying database, since the list of attributes or fields retrieved by the query may involve only a subset of the attributes and fields in the underlying database, and the classes or tables accessed may be only a subset of those in the underlying database.

One advanced object-oriented technique to provide a robust query mechanism for biological databases is *Object Protocol Model (OPM)*. OPM query tools are generic. They are driven by the metadata associated with the underlying database and allow ad-hoc queries to be constructed Query construction follows a two-stage approach:

(i) A query tree is constructed by browsing the object schema of the underlying database and iteratively selecting classes and attributes of interest.

(ii) A Web form is generated automatically from the query tree, which can be used for further specifying conditions or can be saved and customized.

The query tools generate queries in an object-oriented query language, OPM-QL, which are then processed using OPM query translators.

8.4 COMMON OBJECT REQUEST BROKER ARCHITECTURE (CORBA)

One of the primary motivations behind object-oriented programming is that objects can be reused and extended, and that objects can inherit attributes and methods from other objects on which they are based. CORBA is a set of protocols and standards for how objects are defined, and how objects on networks can communicate with each other. As communication protocols are standardized, new objects can be written to communicate with existing objects. The knowledge of how the existing objects are written is not required. You only needed is a definition of the interface for the object that you wish to communicate with. CORBA is illustrated in Fig. 8.3.

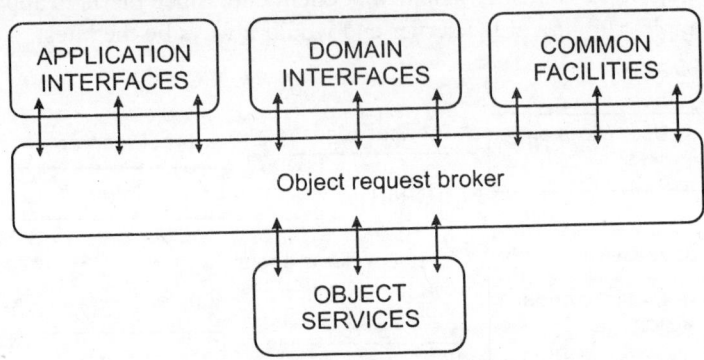

Fig. 8.3. CORBA schematic.

The key to CORBA is the ORB (Object Request Broker). The ORB is the middleware that establishes client-server relationships between objects. For example, an application program can ask for an object from the ORB, and the ORB locates the object and invokes its methods. The client does not need to know the location of the object, the computing platform, or the language in which the object is written. For example, if CORBA interfaces existed for important databases, anyone could write clients that can obtain and work with those objects in very different ways.

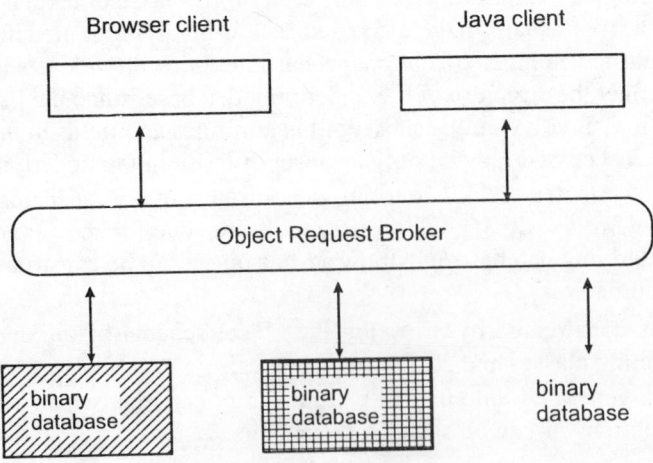

Fig. 8.4. CORBA Interfacing.

In the Fig. 8.4, three different databases are shown with CORBA interfaces. In one case, a web client has been written to obtain request data from the databases, and then translate the objects that are returned into HTML for display in the browser. On the right, a Java client obtains data from the same databases, to be displayed and manipulated in a Java client. In this example, data might be drawn from more than one database. In essence, combining objects from different real databases could create virtual databases.

8.5 SOME PROJECTS

Biocorba

Interface objects have facilitated interoperability between bioperl and other perl packages such as Ensembl and the Annotation Workbench. However, interoperability between bioperl and packages written in other languages requires additional support software. CORBA is a framework for interlanguage support.

The biocorba project (http://biocorba.org/) is currently implementing a CORBA interface for bioperl. With biocorba, objects written within bioperl would be able to communicate with objects written in biopython and biojava (Fig. 8.5).

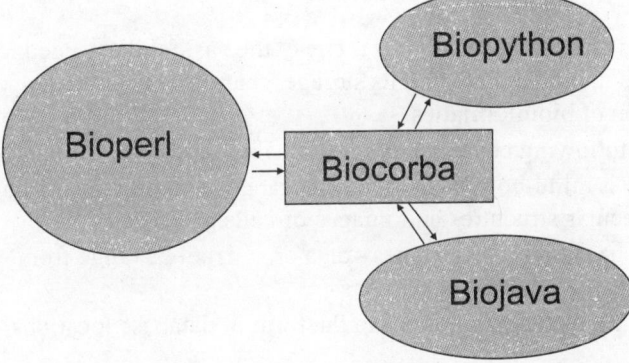

Fig. 8.5. Biocorba relationship with other modules.

Ensembl

Ensembl (http://www.ensembl.org/.) is an automated-genome-annotation project at EBI. Much of Ensembl's code is written in bioperl. Ensembl developers have contributed the bioperl code for automated sequence annotation.

Bioperl-db

Bioperl-db http://cvs.bioperl.org/cgi-bin/viewcvs/viewcvs.cgi/bioperl-db/?cvsroot=bioperl) is a project intended to transfer some of Ensembl's capability of integrating bioperl syntax with a standalone Mysql database to the bioperl code-base.

Biopython and biojava

Biopython (http://biopython.org/) and biojava (biojava http://biojava.org/) are open source projects. Their code is implemented in python and java, respectively. With the development of interface objects and biocorba, it is possible to write java or python objects which can be accessed by a bioperl script, or to call bioperl objects from java or python code.

9

Managing Biological Databanks

9.1 INTRODUCTION

Implementing and managing biological databases is one of the basic skills needed for a bioinformatician. While the data is generated in the laboratories, its storage, sharing and performing various operations is the fundamental application of bioinformatics.

Biological data has the following characteristics that makes it complex to handle :

Diversity : The diversity is mind-boggling - data types range from protein and nucleic acid sequences, texts, 3- dimensional molecular structures and images of cells and tissues.

Hierarchical : The data has several hierarchies - data organizations range from molecules, biochemical pathways, cells, tissues, organisms, populations.

Heterogeneity : Data is highly heterogenous – in the form of database locations, storage formats, and access methods.

Dynamic : Data is extremely dynamic - data contents and database schema are constantly changing.

This chapter discusses some of the issues related to implementation of databases for biological information.

9.2 SUBMISSION OF DATA

The biologist (researcher) needs to submit the data to the database. The generalized procedure for submission to a typical database is as follows :

1. Definition of who can submit data. Can the data be submitted directly or it has to be routed through a "data coordinator" or the "reporting laboratory"?
2. Data submissions normally receive an "accession" number that tracks the progress of the submission.
3. Data submissions typically need to be provided in a particular format. There are certain fields in the format that are mandatory.
4. There can be a policy of data restriction and that needs to be defined by the database when making the submission.

5. Usually the data so submitted is screened and sometimes curated before being uploaded on the database.

6. Most of the databases have user-friendly utilities that can be used for submission of data.

For example, consider EMBL (http://www.ebi.ac.uk/embl/). Webin is EBI's preferred submission medium. Webin guides the user through a sequence of screens (forms) in an interactive mode. All the information required to create a database entry is collected during this process:

1. Submitter Information

2. Release Date Information

3. Sequence Data, Description and Source Information

4. Reference Citation Information

5. Feature Information (e.g. coding regions, regulatory signals etc.)

Sequin is a multi-platform stand-alone software tool developed by the NCBI for submitting entries to the EMBL, GenBank, or DDBJ sequence databases. The Sequin program, along with detailed downloading and installation instructions plus general information are available from the EBI (Fig. 9.1).

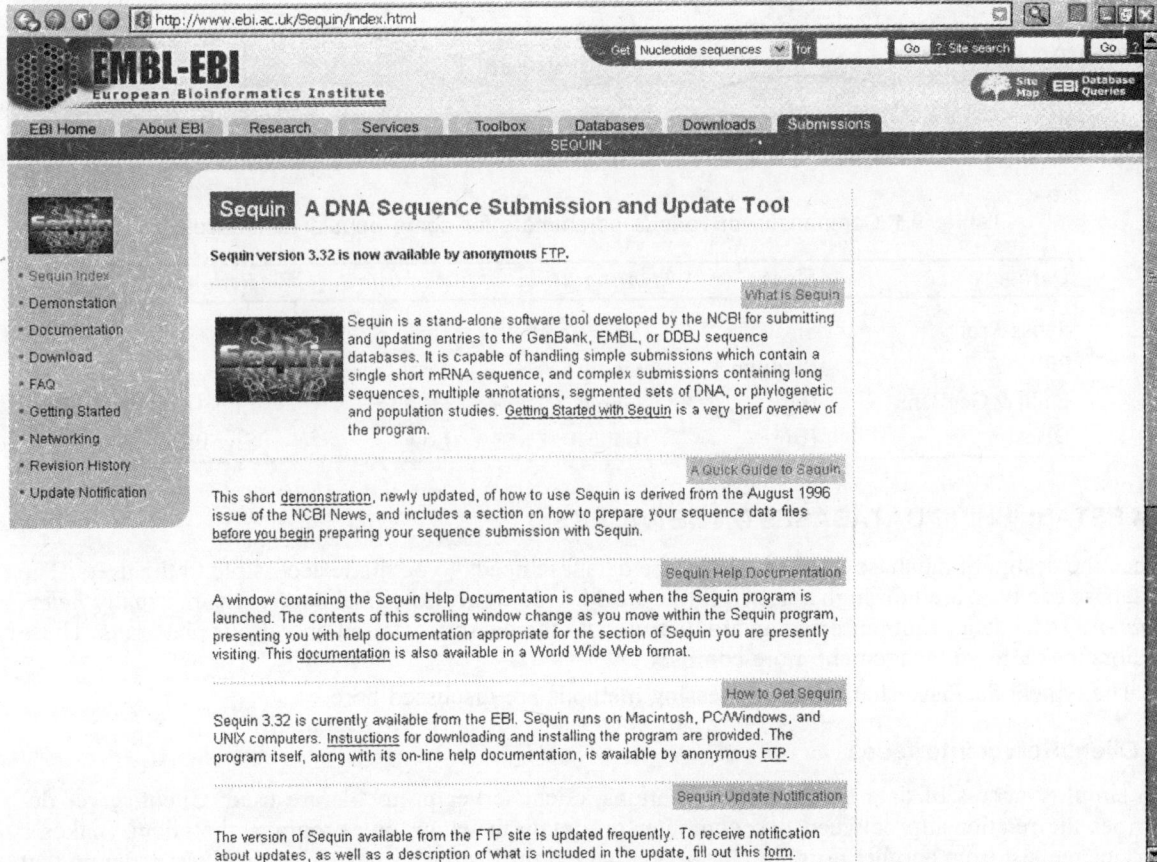

Fig. 9.1. Screen shot for Sequin.

9.3 CURATION OF DATABASES

Database curation involves modifying records, adding or deleting parts of the record; merging database records to produce nonredundant data sources; and deleting records that are judged to be false or inaccurate. The curator does curation. A Curator reviews, verifies and edits data in a database in order to improve the quality of the information that is made available to data consumers.

This process is shown in the Fig 9.2. The curated data is kept in the database. The quality of curation defines database qualities like annotation, accuracy and redundancy. A comparison of various parameters for some of the popular databases is shown in Table 9.1.

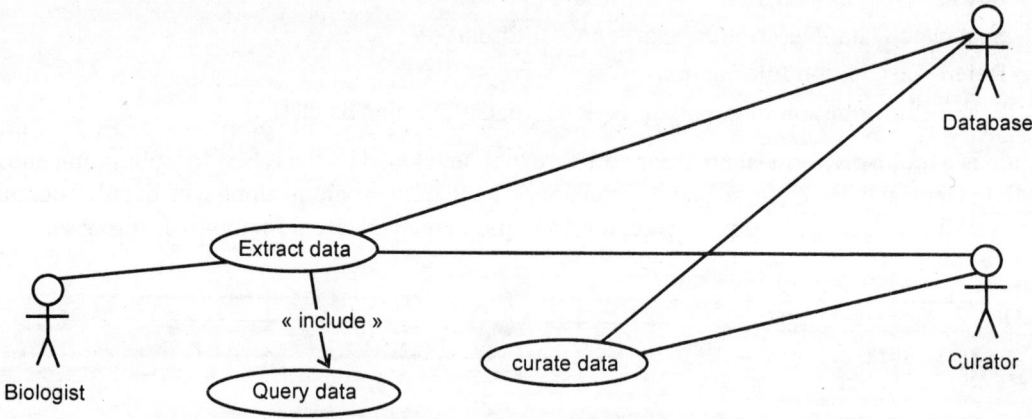

Fig. 9.2. Process of curation.

Table. 9.1 Comparison of various parameters for some popular databases

Database	Size	Annotation	Accuracy	Redundancy
Swiss-Prot	Small	Very good	Best	None
PIR	Medium	Good	Very Good	Low
Embl & GenBank	Big	Good	Good	Little
DBest	Huge	Little	Low	Significant

9.4 ESTABLISHING DATABASES ON NETWORKS

Once the design of database has been done, the database needs to be made accessible to the users. The database can be shared through a network like world wide web. Biological databases are usually *heterogenous* – the data is not uniform and are *distributed* - the data is scattered on various platforms. These factors make their management more complex.

The typical database sharing and accessing methods are discussed here.

1. Client/Server interfaces

To simplify access of data from remote locations, client/server protocols are used. Client/server describes the relationship between two computer programs in which one program, the client, makes a service request from another program, the server, which fulfills the request. The client is a program that runs on a local machine, processing user requests. The client "talks to" the server program across the

Internet, sending instructions for a transaction, and retrieving the results of that transaction. These results are then displayed locally. The server program retrieves the requested data from a database, and sends them back to the client.

File Transfer Protocol

File Transfer Protocol (FTP) is a standard Internet protocol. It is the simplest way to exchange files between computers on the Internet. Like the Hypertext Transfer Protocol (HTTP), which transfers displayable Web pages and related files, FTP is an application protocol that uses the Internet's TCP/IP protocols (Fig. 9.3). FTP is commonly used to transfer Web page files from their creator to the computer that acts as their server for everyone on the Internet. FTP is also used to download programs and other files to your computer from other servers. The ability to download databases across a network is important because it is often more useful to have locally-installed copies of databases. Local copies are useful for projects in which rapid retrieval of large numbers of sequences are important, such as creating database subsets. Every Linux shell has the FTP program. Remote databases are typically managed through a single database management system, whose files are unreadable by other programs.

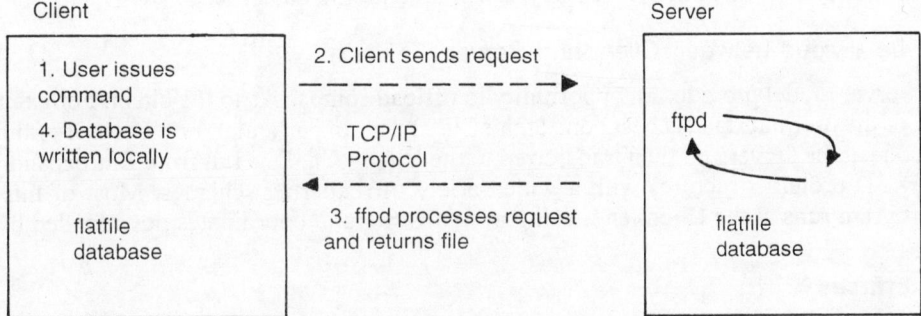

Fig. 9.3. Client/server architecture.

FINDKEY, FETCH and FEATURES can work directly with flat files. Automated retrieval of sequence and/or annotation data can be done in batches of hundreds of entries at a time. FASTA or BLAST programs can read the same flat-file database (Fig. 9.4). Finally, users can write scripts using Unix commands such as grep, awk, tr, sort etc. to search and process text lines from flat-file databases.

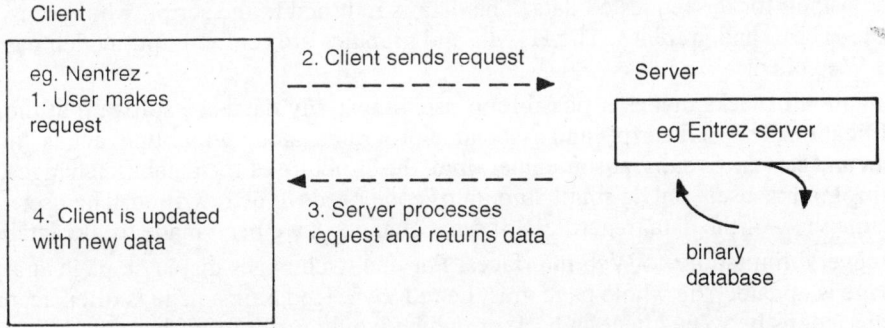

Fig. 9.4. Retrieval of data from a flat file database.

Interactive client/server programs

FTP is one special case of the more general client/server model. A more typical case is the NCBI program ENTREZ.

A client/server version of Entrez, called Network Entrez, provides remote Internet access to the Entrez database residing at the NCBI. To use the networked version, direct TCP/IP access to the Internet is a mandatory requirement.

Typically, a small number of database entries are requested at a time.

At the server end, the Entrez server finds and retrieves data from a binary version of the chosen database, converts the data into a human-readable form, and sends the data back to the client. Transactions between client and server are carried out using the common internet protocol TCP/IP.

Transactions can only occur through remote server

In the client/server model the only way to send of receive data to or from the database is with clients specifically written for the particular server program that talks to the database. This is good, in terms of system reliability, because potentially, databases that are updated by user transactions could conflict, which might result in a corrupt database. On the other hand, the requirement for going through a specific server program may limit the kind of things you can do with the database.

Tasks can be divided between Client and Server

The Client/Server model provides an opportunity to offload some tasks to the client. For example, most of the work of the user interface is best done at the Client end. In particular, rendering of graphics would be slow if done at the server and then transferred to the Client. Cn3D is run from Entrez, and allows the user to view 3D protein structures with a wide variety of rendering schemes. Most of this graphics-intensive program runs at the Client end, using protein structural coordinates downloaded by Entrez.

2. Web interfaces

Web interfaces to remote databases are often easy to implement, and are easy to use. They are easy to implement because no software development needs to be done at the client end. The client is simply the Web browser. All the work is done at the server end. The trick is to get HTTP requests translated into a form the database software can understand, and to convert output from the database program into HTML and graphics.

The Fig. 9.5 (web interfaces to database) shows that as with all Web pages, the HTTP daemon httpd receives an HTTP request, which is processed by a CGI script. A CGI script contains instructions for running programs at the server end. In this case, the CGI script would run programs that call the database software, asking for the requested data. The data is returned to the script, which runs further programs to create HTML and graphics. The HTML and graphics are sent to httpd, which passes them on to the remote Web client.

The organization of tasks makes it possible to use almost any database software at the server end, without modification. The CGI scripts and associated programs, along with httpd, act as "middleware", between client and server. Even if, at some later time, the structure of the database changes, or a different database program is used, only a small amount of code needs to be rewritten. The user can be given exactly the same view of the data, regardless of what changes have been made to the database itself.

There are several limitations to Web interfaces. For one, web pages display a page at a time. Every time a web page is updated, the whole page must be redrawn. Updating a page is often accompanied by additional transactions between client and server, which would result in further delays.

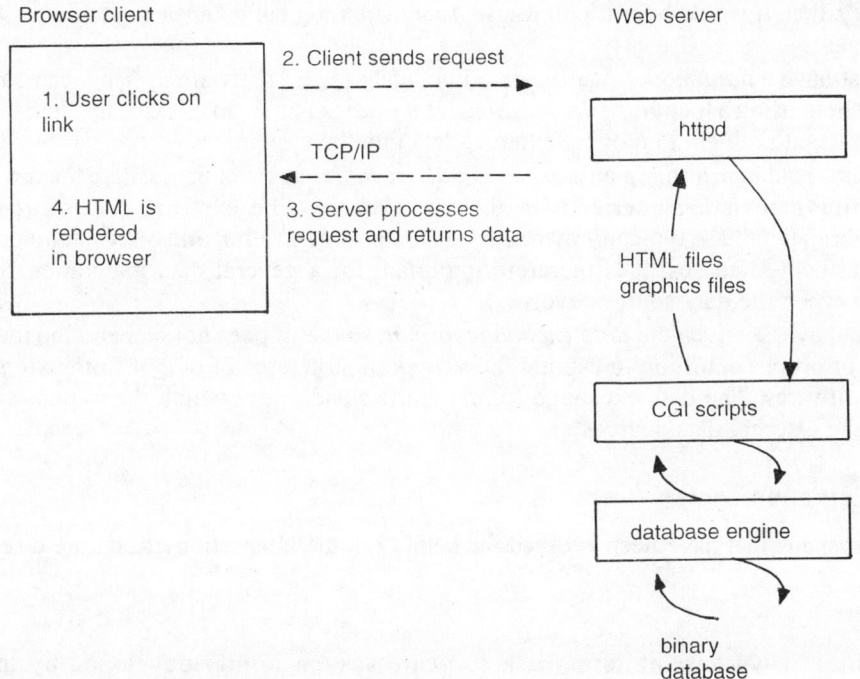

Fig 9.5. Web interfacing to databases.

9.5 INTEGRATION OF DATABASES

Introduction

Integration of diverse biological databases is one of the most important challenges for the bioinformatician. Integration helps in forming a unified view of the data and helps the scientist in making new discoveries.

The process of building a new database relevant to some field of study in bioinformatics involves transforming, integrating, and cleansing multiple data sources, as well as adding new material and annotations. In a dynamic heterogeneous environment such as that of bioinformatics, many different databases and software systems are used. A large proportion of these databases were designed and built by biologists. There are several databases that are several years old - when these databases were created, the amount of data was small and it was important that the database entries were human readable. Hence several older databases were created as flat files. As new types of data were captured, new databases were created using a variety of flat file formats. This resulted in a large number of different databases in different formats, using non-standard query software, and only accessible to bioinformatics experts. These databases and systems often do not have an explicit database schema. Further compounding the problem is that research biologists demand flexible access and queries in ad-hoc combinations. Simple retrieval of data is not sufficient for modern bioinformatics. The challenge is how to manipulate the retrieved data derived from various databases and re-structure the data.

A system that aims to be a general integration mechanism in the bioinformatics environment needs to satisfy the following four conditions:

1. It must not be dependent on the *availability of schemas*. It should be able to compile any query submitted based solely on the structure of that query. If it needs a schema before it can compile

a query, then it would be difficult to use, as most biological databases often do not have usable schemas.

2. It must have a *data model* that the external database and software systems can easily translate to, without using a lot of *type declarations*. If it does not have this flexibility, then there would be a significant problem in moving external data into the system.

3. An extra field appearing in an *external database table* must not necessitate the recompilation or rewriting of existing queries over that data source. The external data sources used by a bioinformatician are typically owned by different organizations that have autonomous right to evolve their databases. It is therefore important for a general data integration solution to be robust when the data sources evolve.

4. It must have a convenient *data exchange format*, so that it does not demand too much programming effort or contortion to capture the variety of structures of output from external databases and softwares. The data exchange format is the standard by which the system exchange data with the external data sources.

Database Integration Tools

Some of the systems that have been evolved for helping in the integration efforts are discussed below.

EnsEMBL

EnsEMBL (http://www.ensembl.org/) is a software system jointly developed by the European Bioinformatics Institute and the Sanger Institute. It provides an easy access to eukaryotic genomic sequence data. It also performs automatic prediction of genes in these sequence data and assembles supporting annotations for these predictions.

Enseml organizes raw sequence data from public databases into its internal database. It then assembles these sequences into their proper place in the genome. After that, it runs GenScan to predict the location of genes and applies various analysis programs to annotate these predicted genes. Finally, the results are presented for public access.

The main "entry points" to these results on the EnsEMBL Genome Browser are as follows :

1. Searching by sequence similarity via the built-in BLAST component of the EnsEMBL Genome Browser

2. Browsing from the chromosome level all the way down to the DNA sequence level searching using special EnsEMBL identifiers

3. Free-text matching using annotation of databases linked to EnsEMBL, including OMIM, SWISS-PROT, and InterPro.

EnsMart data retrieval tool can also be used to access these results. EnsMart has a good query builder interface that allows a user to conveniently specify certain types of genomic regions and filters on these results. EnsEMBL also provides a Perl-based interface for the access to its stored results.

EnsEMBL's strengths lie in its highly tailored functionalities for genome browsing. Once the sequences are imported into the system, assembly and annotation are automatically performed; the results are automatically prepared for browsing in a graphical user interface. However, it is not possible to use EnsEMBL to perform an ad hoc query in general, unless that particular type of query has been anticipated by the designer of the

EnsEMBL and its associated access tools. EnsEMBL also does not have a flexible data model nor exchange format, other than the structure of its highly specialized internal database.

GenoMax

GenoMax (http://register.informaxinc.com/support/genomax.html) is an enterprise-level integration of bioinformatics tools and data sources developed by InforMax.

GenoMax includes a sequence analysis module and a gene expression module, developed on top of a data warehouse of fixed design. The warehouse is an Oracle database designed to hold sequence data, gene expression data, 3D protein structures, and protein-protein interaction information.

Load routines are built in for standard data sources such as GenBank and SWISS-PROT. The modules provide capabilities of performing BLAST and GenScan. A special scripting language of limited expressive power is also supported for building analytical pipelines.

Its strengths are twofold. First, each of GenoMax's component point-solution modules is a very well designed application for a specific purpose. For example, its gene expression module provides self-organizing map clustering, principal component analysis, and so forth on microarray data via simple-to-use graphical user interfaces. Second, these components are integrated in a tight way via the specially designed data warehouse. Its weakness is its tight point-solution-like application integration.

SRS

SRS (http://srs.embl-heidelberg.de:8000/srs5/) is one of the most widely used database query and navigation system for biological databases. It provides easy-to-use graphical user interface access to a broad range of scientific databases, including biological sequences, metabolic pathways, and literature abstracts. SRS provides functionality to search across heterogenous databases.

In order to add a new data source into SRS, you need to have the data source available as a flat file and a description of the schema or structure of the data source must be available as an Icarus script, which is the special built-in wrapper programming language of SRS. The notable exception to this flat file requirement on the data source is when the data source is a relational database. SRS then indexes this data source on various fields parsed and described by the Icarus script. A biologist then accesses the data by supplying some keywords and constraints on them in the SRS Query Language. Then all records matching those keywords and constraints are returned.

The SRS Query language is primarily a navigational language. This query language has limited data joining capabilities based on indexed fields and has limited data restructuring capabilities. The results are returned as an aggregation of records that matched the search constraints. Hence, SRS is essentially an information retrieval system. It brings back records matching specified keywords and constraints. These records can contain embedded links that a user can follow individually to obtain deeper information. However, it does not offer much help in organizing or transforming the retrieved results in a way that might be needed for setting up an analytical pipeline. There is also a browser-based interface for formulating SRS queries and viewing results. Biologists often use this interface of SRS as a unified front end to independently access multiple data sources.

DiscoveryLink

DiscoveryLink (http://www-1.ibm.com/industries/healthcare/doc/content/solution/939513105.html) goes one step beyond SRS as a general data integration system for biological data. DiscoveryLink, when compared to SRS, EnsEMBL, and GenoMax has a distinct feature – it has an explicit data model. This data model dictates the way a DiscoveryLink user views the underlying data, the way she views results, as well as the way she queries the data. The data model is the relational data model. As a result, DiscoveryLink comes with SQL, which makes it a very powerful and convenient tool.

This however implies that it is not simple to add new data sources or analysis tools into the system.

For example, to put the SWISS-PROT database into a relational database in the third normal form would require us to break every SWISS-PROT record into nearly 30 pieces in a normalization process.

Object Protocol Management (OPM)

OPM is a general data integration system. It goes one step beyond DiscoveryLink in the sense that it has a more powerful data model, which is an enriched form of the ERD model. This data model can deal with the deeply nested structure of biological data in a natural way. An SQL-like query language that allows data to be seen in terms of entities and relationships also supports this data model. Queries across multiple data sources, as well as transformation of results, can be easily and naturally expressed in this query language. Queries are also optimized. Furthermore, OPM comes with a number of data management tools that are useful for designing an integrated data warehouse on top of OPM.

However, OPM has several weaknesses. First, OPM requires the use of a global integrated schema. It requires significant skill and effort to design a global integrated schema well. If a new data source needs to be added, the effort needed to re-design the global integrated schema potentially goes up significantly. OPM stores entities and relationships internally using a relational database management system. It achieves this by automatically converting the entities and relationships into a set of relational tables in the third normal form. This conversion process leads to an entity being broken up into many pieces when stored. This process is transparent to the OPM user.

Kleisli (discoveryHub)

Kleisli (http://www.geneticxchange.com) is one of the earliest systems that have been successfully applied to some of the earliest data integration problem in the human genome project. Kleisli is positioned as a mediator system encompassing a nested relational data model, a high-level query language, and a powerful query optimizer. It runs on top of a large number of light-weight wrappers for accessing various data sources.

The Kleisli system is highly extensible. It can be used to support several different high-level query languages by replacing its high-level query language module. Currently, Kleisli supports a "comprehension syntax"-based language called CPL and a "nested relationalized" version of SQL called sSQL. The Kleisli system can also be used to support many different types of external data sources by adding new wrappers, which forward Kleisli's requests to these sources and translate their replies into Kleisli's exchange format. (Wrappers are software interfaces to data sources and can be written to any data source and in any language). These wrappers are lightweight and new wrappers are generally easy to develop and insert into the Kleisli system. The optimizer of the Kleisli system can also be customized by different rules and strategies.

Kleisli does not have its own native database management system and has the ability to turn many kinds of database systems into an updatable store conforming to its nested relational data model. In particular, Kleisli can use relational database management systems such as Sybase, Oracle, MySQL, etc. to be its updatable store. It can even use all of these systems simultaneously. Kleisli stores nested relations into flat relational database management systems using an encoding scheme that does not require these nested relations to be fragmented over several tables.

Strategies for Integration

Integrating two databases fundamentally identifying information that is implicitly or explicitly shared, and can be used to create new relationships.

There are two generalized approaches in integration of databases : *consolidation* and *federation*.

Consolidation is used to create single homogenous large database. The pre-condition for consolidation is that the databases involved use same tables and concepts. The incompatible parts of the databases are "scrubbed out". Consolidation has limited applications, except for the legacy databases.

Federation involves incorporation of links from and between databases. Federation uses a common query language and data warehousing.

To link two databases, we need to have the following considerations:
1. Identify the critical shared data elements that allow relationships to be combined.
2. Need to be sure that semantics of the shared data is similar.
3. Need to create thesaurus for corresponding concepts.

For example, the inter-links between five databases could be of the type given in Fig. 9.6.

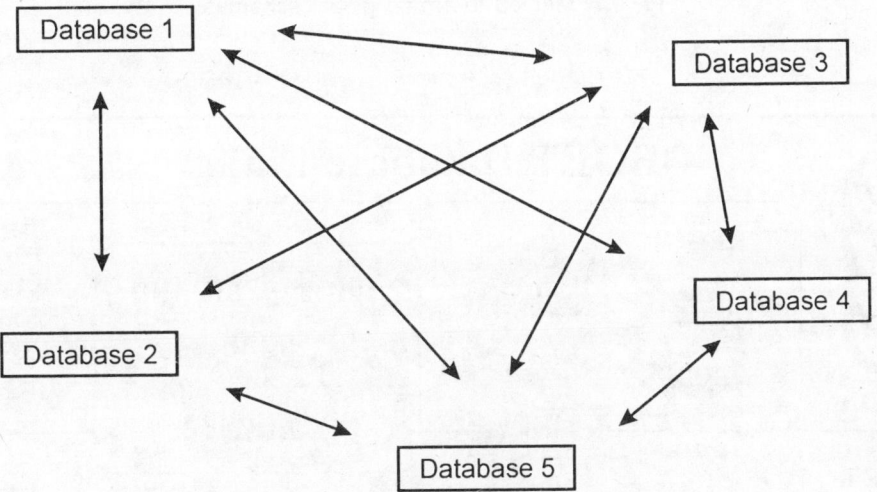

Fig. 9.6. Inter-links between databases.

The solution to avoid this cumbersome method of linking is to develop *global schemas* (Fig. 9.7). Global schemas are difficult to create, since they must be general enough to handle any type of data in the contributing databases. There has to be a global query model – where it is possible to write queries in local language, but then combine queries as needed at the global level. This is implemented in Kleisli model as discussed above.

Global data model and query model involves writing queries in global language – knowledge of local structure is less required. This is implemented in OPM-based models.

One of the methods of federation is to incorporate links within databases to one another. This is often implemented by providing hypertext links from item in database A to item in database B. Traversing the hypertext links accesses data. This method is prone to missing or inconsistent links and there is a difficulty in maintenance for rapidly growing databases, which is usually the case. Also, there is no general-purpose query facility to retrieve multiple records that satisfy some set of conditions. This technique is used in DBGET (Fig. 9.8) and SRS systems.

Another technique of federation is to construct queries over multiple databases without touching the databases themselves. You can create query processor which can map query to individual search capabilities of individual databases. Kleisli and OPM systems are implementations of this type of federation.

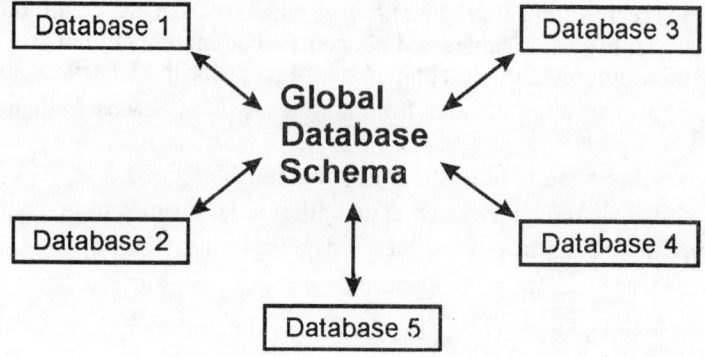

Fig. 9.7. Method to create global schemas.

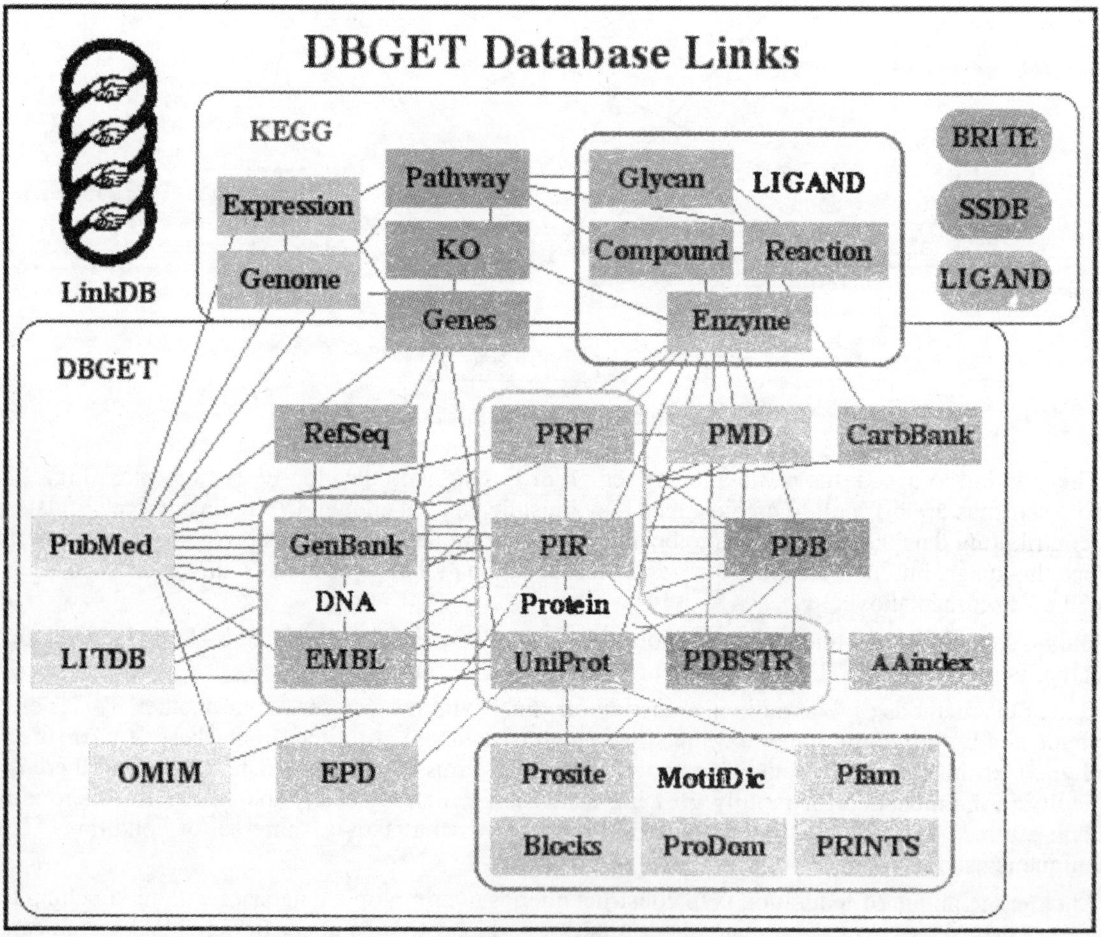

DBGET Database Links

Fig. 9.8. DBGET database links.

Another technique is used to develop a global schema for all the data in the databases. Data are transformed into this common schema and loaded in central repository on a regular basis in central repository. Query facilities are provided by central repository. There is a need to update global schema when local databases change their data formats/schemas. This technique is similar to consolidation strategy, but different in the way that local databases remain and are synchronized in the global database. Entrez uses this technique of federation.

9.6 MINING OF DATABASES

Data mining is an important step in an overall knowledge discovery process (Fig. 9.9). Knowledge discovery process involves selection and sampling of the appropriate data from the databases; preprocessing and cleaning of the data to remove redundancies, errors, and conflicts; transforming and reducing data to a format more suitable for the data mining; data mining; evaluation of the mined data; and visualization of the evaluation results.

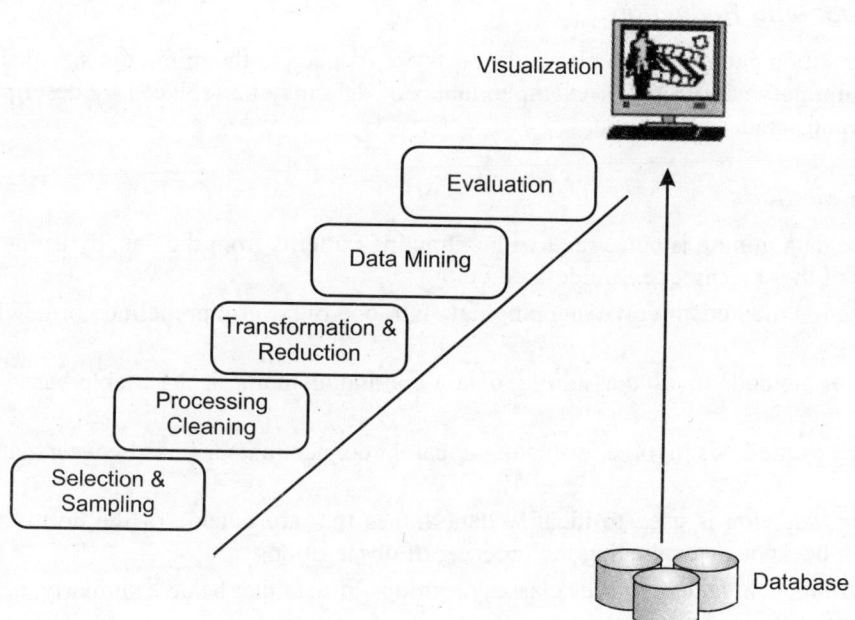

Fig. 9.9. Knowledge discovery process.

Usually many iterations of the knowledge discovery process are required. Similarly, each phase of the knowledge discovery process has associated challenges, as outlined here.

Selection and Sampling

The evaluation of the relationships that are revealed in the sampling can be used to determine which relationships in the data should be mined further using the complete data warehouse.

Preprocessing and Cleaning

Major part of the work is in preparing the data for the actual analysis associated with data mining. The major preparatory activities include the following activities :

1. Data Characterization — creating a high-level description of the nature and the content of the data to be mined.
2. Consistency Analysis — determining the statistical variability in the data, independent of the domain.
3. Domain Analysis — validating the data values in the larger context of the biology.
4. Data Enrichment — drawing from multiple data sources to minimize the limitations of a single data source.
5. Frequency and Distribution Analysis — weighing values as a function of their frequency of occurrence.
6. Normalization — transforming data values from one representation to another.
7. Missing Value Analysis — detecting, characterizing, and dealing with missing data values.

Transformation and Reduction

In the transformation and reduction phase, data sets are reduced to the minimum size possible through sampling or summary statistics. For example, tables of data may be replaced by descriptive statistics such as mean and standard deviation.

Data Mining Methods

The process of data mining is concerned with extracting patterns from the data by using various techniques. Some of these techniques are defined below :

1. *Classification* methods involve mapping data into one of several predefined or newly discovered classes.
2. *Regression* methods involve assigning data a continuous numerical variable based on statistical methods.
3. *Link analysis* methods involve evaluating apparent connections or links between data in the database.
4. *Deviation detection* is used to identify data values that are outside of the norm, as defined by existing models or by evaluating the ordering of observations.
5. *Segmentation* technique identifies classes or groups of data that behave similarly, according to an established metric.

Evaluation

In the evaluation phase of knowledge discovery, the patterns identified by the data mining analysis are interpreted. Evaluation ranges from simple statistical analysis and complex numerical analysis of sequences and structures to determining the biological implications of the findings.

Visualization

Visualization of evaluation results can range from simple pie charts to 3-D virtual reality displays.

Methods of Data Mining

Infrastructure needs

The infrastructure in a data mining laboratory data includes high-speed Internet and intranet connectivity, a data warehouse with a data dictionary that defines a standard vocabulary and data format, several databases, and high-performance computer hardware. Database management systems (DBMS) are required to support queries and ensure data integrity.

Pattern Recognition

Data mining involves identifying patterns and relationships in data that often are not obvious in large, complex data sets. This pattern recognition is most often concerned with the automatic classification of character sequences representative of the nucleotide bases or molecular structures, and of 3-D protein structures. From an information processing perspective, pattern recognition can be viewed as a data simplification process that filters extraneous data from consideration and labels the remaining data according to a classification scheme.

Machine Learning Techniques

The pattern matching and pattern discovery components of data mining are often performed by using machine learning techniques. Machine learning encompasses a variety of methods that represent the convergence of statistics, biological modeling, adaptive control theory, psychology, and artificial intelligence (AI). Some of the machine learning techniques are defined below :

1. *Inductive logic programming* uses a set of rules or heuristics to categorize data.
2. *Genetic algorithms* are based on evolutionary principles wherein a particular function or definition that best fits the constraints of an environment survives to the next generation, and the other functions are eliminated.
3. *Neural networks* learn to associate input patterns with output patterns in a way that allows them to categorize new patterns and to extrapolate trends from data.
4. *Statistical methods* used to support data mining are generally some form of feature extraction, classification, or clustering.
5. *Decision trees* are hierarchically arranged questions and answers that lead to classification.
6. *A Hidden Markov Model (HMM)* is a stochastic model for studying transition made from one state to the next.

Text Mining

The primary store of functional data that links clinical medicine, pharmacology, sequence data, and structure data is in the form of biomedicine documents in online bibliographic databases such as PubMed. Mining these databases is expected to reveal the relationships between structure and function at the molecular level.

The technologies available are :

1. *LISP (LISt Processing)*, a programming language that has been developed for handling free text.
2. *Natural language processing (NLP)*, a technology that encompasses a variety of computational methods ranging from simple keyword extraction to semantic analysis. The simplest NLP systems work by parsing documents and identifying the documents with recognized keywords such as "protein" or "amino acid". The contents of the tagged documents can then be copied to a local database and later reviewed.

9.7 MANAGEMENT OF WORKFLOW

Large scale biological analysis is a complex task that involves the integration of results from numerous bioinformatics tools. For high-throughput data analysis, these tools must be tied together in a coordinated system that can automate the execution of a set of analyses in sequence or in parallel. Workflow systems involve data integration as a sequence of tasks which use a variety of web services. An illustration of workflow in bioinformatics is given in Fig. 9.10 information flows from left to right entering at a workflow input (in this case called 'swissprotID'), passing through two operations and with the result exiting on the right at the workflow output 'DNASequence'. The operations in the middle are shown with all possible inputs, although in this case only some of them are being used (the rest will be left at their default settings). In this instance the two operations are tools from the EMBOSS package.

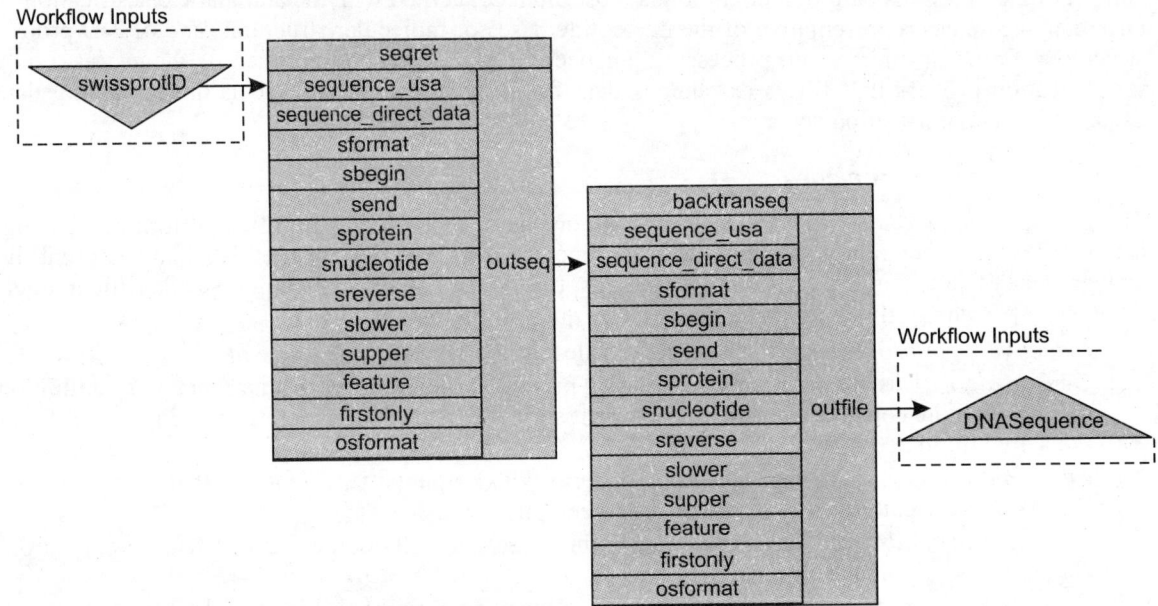

Fig. 9.10. A simple workflow example.

Kepler (http://www.kepler-project.org/) is a tool to produce a workflow system that allows scientists to design workflows and execute them efficiently using Grid-based approaches to distributed computation. Kepler is currently based on the Ptolemy II system for heterogeneous, concurrent modeling and design. A sample workflow from Kepler is shown in Fig. 9.11.

Examples of workflow services are as follows :

myGRID project, Taverna tool for workflow construction (http://www.mygrid.org.uk/)

Kepler, at UCSD Supercomputing Centre (http://kepler-project.org/)

The myGrid ontologies provides a controlled vocabulary of concepts with which to describe the kinds of data being manipulated and the nature of the services and workflows which are preforming the manipulation. For example, it provides the concept DNA sequence data along with which is specified in a machine interpretable way that this is kind of data that "encodes the sequence of a deoxyribonucleotide molecule which is a kind of nucleotide molecule".

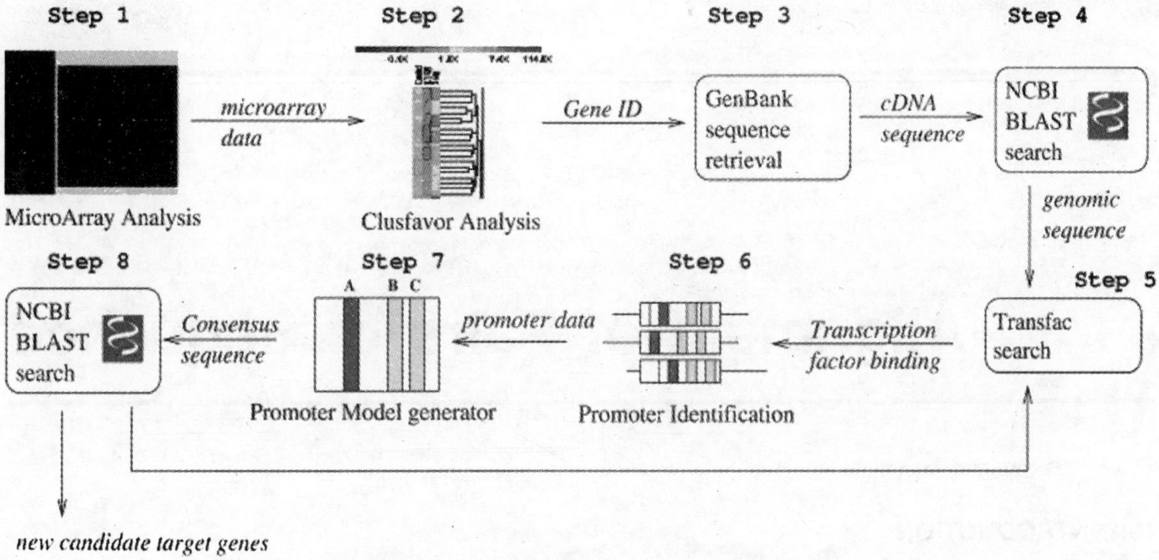

Fig. 9.11. Sample workflow output from Kepler.

10

Alignment of Pairs of Sequence

10.1 INTRODUCTION

One of the most powerful methods for inferring the biological function of a gene (or the protein that it encodes) is by *sequence similarity search* on protein and DNA sequence databases. This method has resulted in discoveries based solely on sequence homology e.g. the identification of a new tumor suppressor gene in humans that is related to yeast and *E. coli* DNA repair enzymes.

It has been hypothesized that sequence determines shape, and shape determines function. Hence when we study sequence similarity, we eventually hope to discover or validate similarity in shape and function. Sequences, for convenience of understanding and performing various mathematical functions, are seen as strings of characters.

Similarity in the sequences has both a quantitative and a qualitative aspect: A *similarity measure* gives a quantitative answer, saying that two sequences show a certain degree of similarity. An *alignment* is a mutual arrangement of two sequences, which is a sort of qualitative answer; it exhibits where the two sequences are similar, and where they differ. An *optimal alignment* is one that exhibits the most correspondences, and the least differences.

10.2 SEQUENCE ANALYSIS OF BIOLOGICAL DATA

Some of the relevant definitions are described here.

1. *Identical*, when a corresponding character is shared between two species or populations, that character is said to be identical.
2. *Similar*, the degree to which two species or populations share identities.
3. *Analogous* , when characters are similar due to convergent evolution, they are analogous.
4. *Homologous*, when characters are similar due to common ancestry, they are homologous. Homologous sequences can be *orthologous* (when characters are homologous with conserved function), or *paralogous* (when characters are homologous with divergent function).

Homology is not synonymous with similarity. Homology is a judgment (qualitative) and similarity is a measurement (quantitative).

The resemblance of two DNA sequences taken from different organisms of today can be explained by the theory that all contemporary genetic material has one ancestral ancient DNA. During the evolutionary process, mutations occurred that created differences between families of the then contemporary species. Most of these changes were due to local mutations, each modifying the DNA sequence at a specific manner. These local modifications between nucleotide sequences can be of following types:

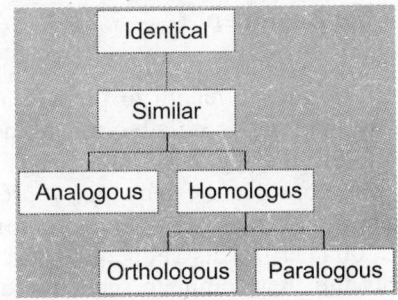

Fig. 10.1. Similarity and Homology.

1. *Insertion* - an insertion of a letter or several letters to the sequence.
2. *Deletion* - deleting a letter (or more) from the sequence.
3. *Substitution* - replacing a sequence letter by another.

For example, transformation of accgta to agcta is illustrated below :

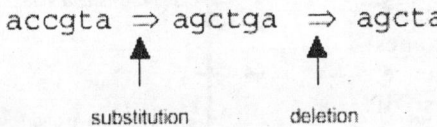

Insertion and deletion are the reverse of one another: given two sequences, if the insertion of a character (or more) into one yields the other, then equivalently its deletion from the latter sequence transforms it to the first one. Due to this reciprocity between insertion and deletion, they are usually called *indel* for short.

The notion of *distance* derives its definition from the concept of mutations: by assigning weights to each mutation. Given two strings, the *distance* between them is the minimal sum of weights for a set of mutations transforming one into the other. The notion of *similarity* derives its definition from the concept of one ancestral ancient DNA: by assigning weights corresponding for resemblance. Given two strings the *similarity* between them is the maximal sum of such weights.

Similarly, for protein sequence comparison, one can take protein sequence (e.g. from a human chromosome), and search a protein database to find *homologous* sequences, often from very divergent organisms. A representation of evolutionary tree is shown in Fig. 10.2. For example, if a yeast protein is homologous to one found in *E. coli*, that sequence must have existed in 2 billion years ago in the primordial organism that gave rise to bacteria and fungi.

10.3 MODELS FOR SEQUENCE ANALYSIS

The important models for sequence analysis are described here.

1. Global alignment
2. Local alignment
3. Gap penalty

Global Alignment

Global alignment is done across the entire sequence length to include as many matches as possible up to and including the sequence end. For example, consider the sequence representing RefSeq accession NC_0047110. This sequence represents the first complete sequence of the SARS Coronavirus (determined by the BC Cancer Agency Genome Sciences Centre, Canada). This sequence was submitted to GenBank prior to publication as an unannotated nucleotide sequence and assigned GenBank accession number AY274119. The sequence subsequently was processed through the NCBI viral genome annotation pipeline and is available in Entrez Genomes as the *SARS-CoV* reference sequence. Pair-wise global alignments of NC_0047110 with other viral genomic sequences are shown in Fig. 10.3.

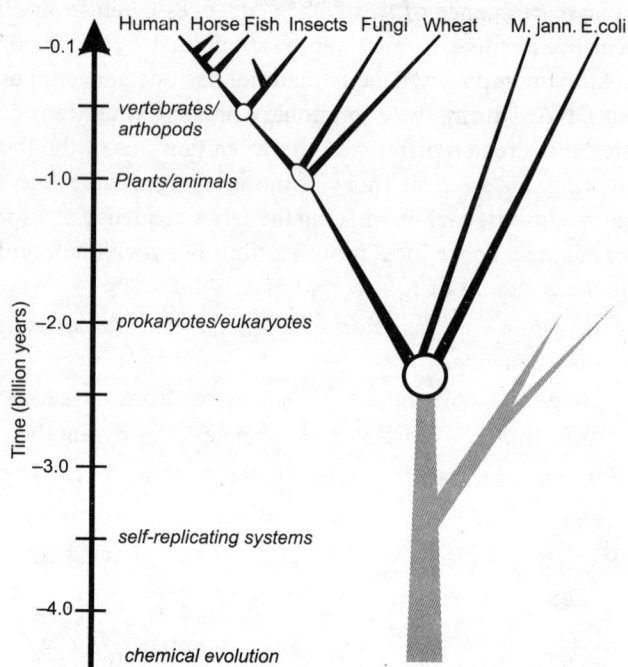

Fig. 10.2. Evolutionary tree of life.

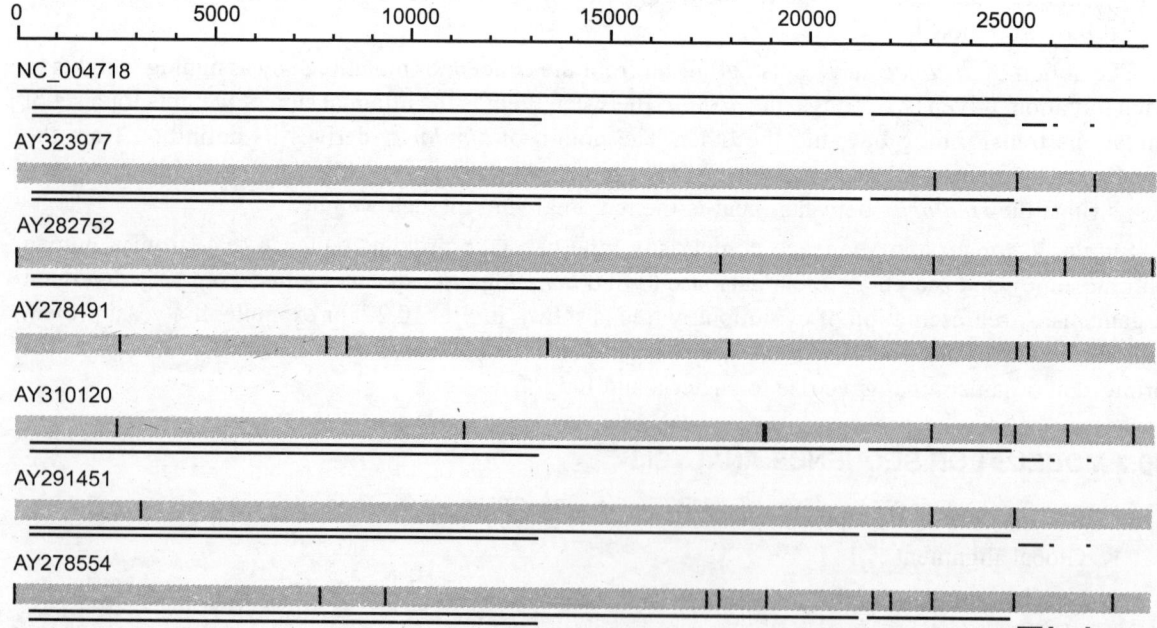

Fig. 10.3. Graphical representation of global alignment of NC_0047110 with other viral genome sequences.

Semiglobal alignment is a global alignment with no end gap penalties. Usually semiglobal alignment takes in two sequences - one short and one long. The objective is to find out if the shorter string is a part of the longer one. Biological applications include finding overlaps between fragments for sequence assembly and aligning cDNA's or EST's with genomic DNA to identify gene structure.

Local Alignment

In many applications two strings may not be highly similar as a whole, but many contain regions that are highly similar. The task is to find and extract pair of regions, one from each of the two given strings that exhibit high similarity. This is called the *local alignment* or *local similarity* problem.

For example, consider the two strings:

$$S = a\ b\ c\ x\ d\ e\ x$$
$$T = x\ x\ x\ c\ d\ e$$

If we give each match a value of 2 and each mismatch a value of -1, then the two substrings: alpha = cxde and beta = c-de of S and T respectively have the optimal alignment.

Consider the global alignment shown in Fig. 10.4. An alignment is forced across the whole table and each position is scored. The score in one particular section is higher than others. The goal is to find out the best possible local alignment.

In many biological applications local similarity is far more meaningful than global similarity. This is particularly true when long stretches of non-coding DNA are compared, since only small regions within those strings may be related. When comparing protein sequences, local alignment is also critical because proteins from very different families often share the same structural or functional sub-units, and local alignment is an appropriate tool for searching such modules.

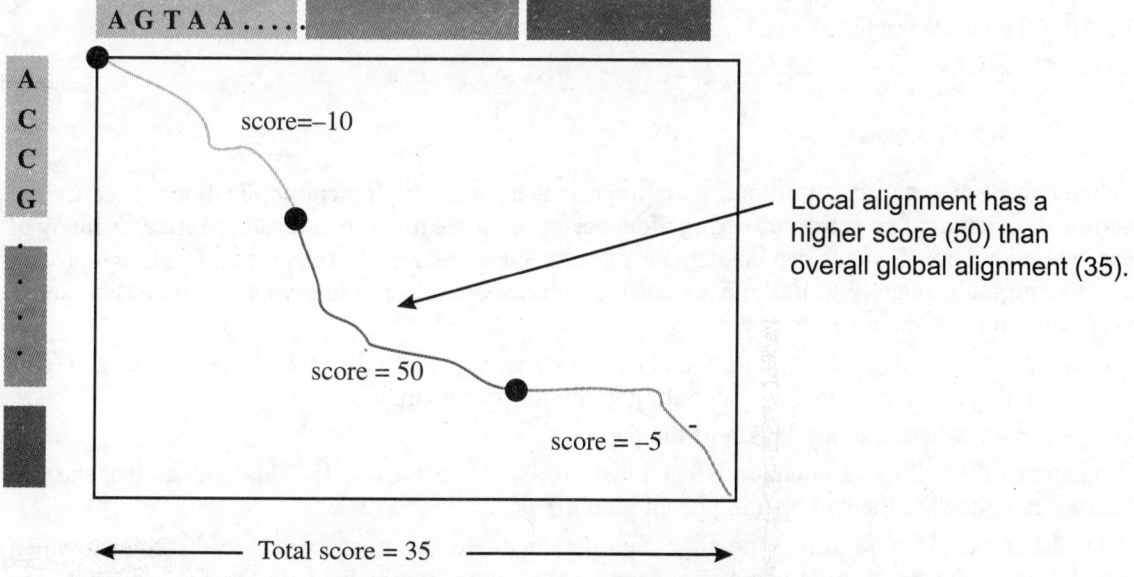

Fig. 10.4. Global and local alignments.

Examples of local alignment problems include finding regulatory elements in non-coding DNA and identifying functional or structural domains in protein sequences.

Gap penalty

A gap is any maximal, consecutive run of spaces in a single string of a given alignment. Gaps help create alignments that better conform to underlying biological models and more closely fit patterns that one expects to find in meaningful alignment. The idea is to take in account the number of continuous gaps and not only the number of spaces when calculating an alignment.

For example, consider the alignment:

$$S = a\,t\,t\,c\,-\,-\,g\,a\,-\,t\,g\,g\,a\,c\,c$$
$$T = a\,-\,-\,c\,g\,t\,g\,a\,t\,t\,-\,-\,-\,c\,c$$

This alignment has four gaps containing a total of eight spaces. That alignment would be described as having seven matches, no mismatch, four gaps and eight spaces. The length of the gap will be the number of indel operations in it. The number of gaps in the alignment will be denoted as number of gaps.

Gaps can occur in the following ways :

1. Before the first character of a string

    e.g.   CTGCGGG—GGTAAT

           |||| || ||

           —GCGG-AGAGG-AA-

2. Inside a string

    e.g.   CTGCGGG—-GGTAAT

           |||| || ||

           —GCGG-AGAGG-AA-

3. After the last character of a string

    e.g.   CTGCGGG—GGTAAT

           |||| || ||

           —GCGG-AGAGG-AA-

The concept of a gap in an alignment is important in many biological applications, because the insertion or deletion of an entire sub-string often occurs as single mutational event. Moreover, many of these single mutational events can create gaps of quite varying sizes. At the protein level, two protein sequences might be relatively similar over several intervals but differ in intervals where one contains a protein sub-unit that the other does not.

A gap opening penalty for any gap (g) and a gap extension penalty for each element in the gap (r) is used to give the total gap score (w_x) according to the following equation :

w_x = g + rx, where x is the length of the gap

Sometimes the following equation is used instead : w_x = g + r(x − 1). This implies that the gap penalty is not added to the gap opening penalty until x is 2.

This difference does not affect the alignment obtained. However, one needs to distinguish which method a particular program is using if correct results are to be obtained. In the first equation, the penalty for a gap of size 1 is g + x and in the second equation it is g. The values for these penalties have to be chosen to balance the scores in the scoring matrix that is used. For example, PAM 250 is represented in units of $\log_{10}$, which is approximately 1/3 bits. If this matrix were converted to 1/2 bits, the same gap penalties would no longer be appropriate.

If the gap penalty is too low, then a high sequence alignment score is achievable even between unrelated or random sequences. If too high a gap penalty is used relative to the range of scores in the substitution matrix, gaps will never appear in the alignment.

The relationship among match score, mismatch score and gap penalty is as follows:

1. If the gap penalty is large compared to the mismatch and match scores, then the alignment is determined by the match and mismatch scores and the score can be checked for significance i.e. the alignment will not get "out of control" with too many gaps.

2. If both mismatches and gaps are heavily penalized, then only see exact matches that can also be checked for significance.

3. If the mismatch score is much greater then the match score and the gap penalty is zero, then the longest common subsequence is found, but it is very difficult to test this subsequence for significance.

Scores should be a metric. If sequence A and B are aligned, and then B and C, then the score of A and C aligned should not be greater then the sum of A with B and B with C.

From an evolutionary point of view, the gap penalty scheme used in Needleman-Wunsch algorithm is simplistic. Although single point insertions or deletions ("indels") are probably more common than large indels, it is not obvious that any sort of linear relation exists between frequency of indels and length. That is, it's just as easy to delete 4 bases as to delete 2. Most alignment programs deal with this problem by having an "open gap" penalty to begin an indel, and an "extend gap" penalty for each subsequent gap character inserted into the alignment. Typically, the "open gap" penalty is much larger than the "extend gap" penalty.

10.4 METHODS OF ALIGNMENT

Graphic similarity comparisons

Similarity between two sequences can be detected as a diagonal on an identity matrix. Graphic similarity comparisons present relationships between sequences in a form so that the patterns in the data can be easily discerned. If you wish to determine whether two sequences are similar, you need to compare all parts of one sequence with all parts of the other. This can be accomplished by sliding one sequence along the other and noting the number of identities at each alignment. The alignment with the greatest number of identities would be the optimal alignment. This is shown in Fig. 10.5.

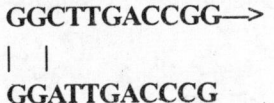

```
GGCTTGACCGG—>          GGCTTGACCGG—>          GGCTTGACCGG—>
 |  |                  || |||||| |             ||| |
GGATTGACCCG            GGATTGACCCG            GGATTGACCCG
```

```
GGCTTGACCGG-->        GGCTTGACCGG-->        GGCTTGACCGG-->
   |    |              || |||||| |            |  |  |
   GGATTGACCCG         GGATTGACCCG          GGATTGACCCG
```

Fig. 10.5. "Sliding" of one sequence along the other to observe alignment.

	G	G	C	T	T	G	A	C	C	G	G
G	A	A				A				A	A
G	A	A				A				A	A
A							A				
T				A	A						
T				A	A						
G	A	A				A				A	A
A							A				
C			A					A	A		
C			A					A	A		
C			A					A	A		
G	A	A				A				A	A

Fig. 10.6. Matrix to represent two sequences.

This can also be accomplished by placing both sequences on the X and Y axes of a matrix, and printing a character at each X,Y coordinate at which both sequences have identical bases. This matrix is shown in Fig. 10.6.

Dot-plots

Dot plots are used to visually compare two sequences and detect of regions of close similarity between them. In Fig. 10.7, two sequences are arranged along the axes of a simple graph. At every point where the two sequences are identical, a dot is placed (i.e. at the intersection of every row and column that have the same letter in both sequences). A diagonal stretch of dots will indicate regions where the two sequences are similar. A filter can be used to place a dot only when a group of successive bases match. In Fig. 10.8, the same dot plot is shown with a filter such that a dot is printed only if in a window of 4 bases, 3 of these 4 bases match.

To detect more distant similarities, it may be better to use a much larger window (i.e. 20, 30, or even 50 bases) and some suitable percentage of identities (e.g. 50%).

Generalisation of the dot-matrix algorithm

The dot-matrix algorithm can be generalized for sequences s and t of sizes m and n, respectively, and

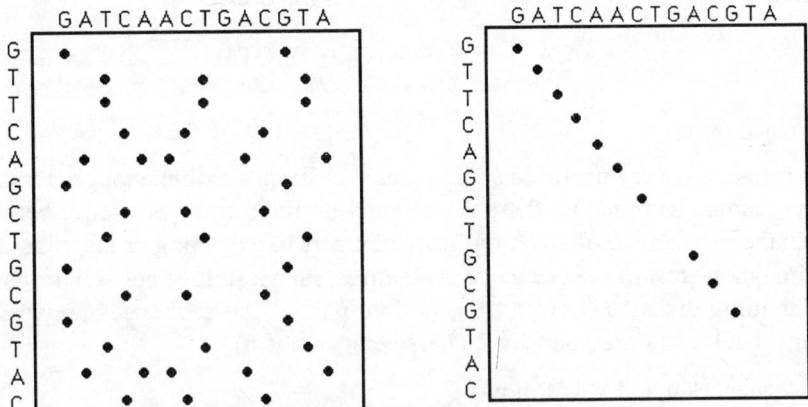

Figs. 10.7 and 10.8. Representations of dot plots.

window size l. For each position in sequences, compare a window of l nucleotides centered at that position with each window of l nucleotides in sequence t. Conceptually, it can be thought of as windows of length l sliding along each axis, so that all possible windows of l nucleotides are compared between the two sequences.

For sequences of realistic length, it's not practical to write both the sequences on the axes, so instead numbers are used to represent position in each sequence. Also for longer sequences, a window size of length = 2 is too small, because as sequences increase in length, the frequencies of dinucleotide matches will increase.

Using lookup tables

Similarity comparisons can be speeded up using lookup tables containing positions of short words (oligomers) from one of the sequences. The efficiency of the dot-matrix similarity search algorithm can be stated as $O(lmn)$. This notation means that the time required to compare two sequences is proportional to the product of the lengths of the sequences times the length of the search window. For example, a comparison of two 5000 nt sequences using a window size of 20 would require 5000 × 5000 × 20 = 5 × 10^{10} nucleotide comparisons.

10.5 SCORING MATRICES

Scoring matrices are used for computing alignment scores. Scoring matrices are often based on observed substitution rates, derived from the substitution frequencies seen in multiple alignments of sequences.

Quantification of similarity of two sequences can be done using *similarity measure*. A similarity measure is a function that associates a numeric value with a pair of sequences. A higher value indicates greater similarity.

Quantification can also be done using a *distance measure*. The notion of distance treats sequences as points in a metric space. A distance measure is a function that associates a numeric value with a pair of sequences, but with the idea that the larger the distance, the smaller the similarity, and vice-versa. Distance values are never negative.

The simplest notion of distance is the Hamming distance. In this schema, for two sequences of equal length, we need to count the character positions in which they differ.

For example:

Sequence s :	AATA	TGCATG	GTA
Sequence t :	TAAT	AGCATA	ATA
Hamming distance (s,t) :	3	2	1

This distance measure is very useful in some cases, but is not flexible enough. First, the sequences may have different length and second, there is generally no fixed correspondence between their character positions. In the mechanism of DNA replication, errors like deleting or inserting a nucleotide are not unusual. Although the rest of the sequence is identical, such a shift of position leads to exaggerated values in the Hamming distance. Look at the middle part of the sequences above. The Hamming distance 2 implies that s and t are apart by 2 characters (out of 6).

Consider the sequences u and v as follows :

Sequence u : AAT AGCAA AGCACACA

Sequence v : TAA ACATA ACACACTA

Let us instead model the distance of u and v by considering the simple, one-character edit operations that turn u into v . We introduce a gap character "-" and say that the pair :

    (a,a) denotes a match (no change from u to v),

    (a,-) denotes deletion of character a (in u),

    (a,b) denotes replacement of a (in u) and b (in v), where a is not equal to b,

    (-,b) denotes insertion of character b (in u)

Since the problem is symmetrical, an insertion in u can be seen as a deletion in v and vice versa. An alignment of two sequences u and v is an arrangement of u and v by position, where u and v can be padded with gap symbols to achieve the same length:

    u : AGCACAC—A or AG—CACACA

    v : A—CACACTA or ACACACT—A

If we read the alignment column-wise, we have a protocol of edit operations that lead from u to v.

Left :	Match (A,A)	Right :	Match (A,A)
	Delete (G,—)		Replace (G,C)
	Match (C,C)		Insert (—,A)
	Match (A,A)		Match (C,C)
	Match (C,C)		Match (A,A)
	Match (A,A)		Match (C,C)
	Match (C,C)		Replace (A,T)
	Match (—,T)		Delete (C,—)
	Match (A,A)		Match (A,A)

The left-hand alignment shows one Delete, one Insert, and the other edit operations are Matches. The right-hand alignment shows one Insert, one Delete, two Replaces, and some trivial ones. The above edit protocol can be converted into a measure of distance by assigning a "cost" to each operation. The *cost of an alignment* of two sequences u and v is the sum of the costs of all the edit operations that lead from u to v. An *optimal alignment* of u and v is an alignment which has minimal cost among all possible alignments. The *edit distance* of u and v is the cost of an optimal alignment of u and v.

The above scheme is known as the *Levenshtein distance*, also called *unit cost model*. Unlike Hamming distance, it is defined for strings of arbitrary length. It counts the differences between two strings, where we would count a difference not only when strings have different characters but also when one has a character whereas the other does not.

In general, more sophisticated cost models must be used. For example, replacing an amino acid by a biochemically similar one should weight less than a replacement by an amino acid with totally different properties.

The number of possible alignments between two sequences is gigantic, and unless the weight function is very simple, it may seem difficult to pick out an optimal alignment. The problem can however be reduced to the task of finding the optimal path through a graph. The "best-path strategy" is called "dynamic programming". The basic idea is that any partial optimal subpath that ends at a point along the true optimal path must itself be the optimal path leading upto that point.

Let us take the example of two sequences s and t,

Sequence s : AGCACACA and Sequence t : ACACACTA

The two sequences may be rewritten in the form of a scoring matrix as below (Fig. 10.9):

In the second diagram in Fig. 10.3, we have drawn a path through the distance matrix indicating which case was chosen when taking the minimum. A diagonal line means Replacement or Match, a vertical line means Deletion, and a horizontal line means Insertion.

In this discussion we have treated the gap symbol "–" as yet another character, denoting an individual insertion or deletion. This may not always be valid. Sometimes we want *no-gap alignments*. For example, in a family of proteins there may be a strongly conserved subunit that is the site of some protein-protein interaction. Any deletion/insertion in the chain of amino acids would be likely to destroy its biochemical function. Such regions need to be aligned using matches or replacements only.

Sometimes, when comparing proteins, we can increase sensitivity to weak alignments using a substitution matrix. Some amino acids, because of similar properties, can substitute easily for one another. Hence identical (or similar) amino acids need to be given higher values than substitutions.

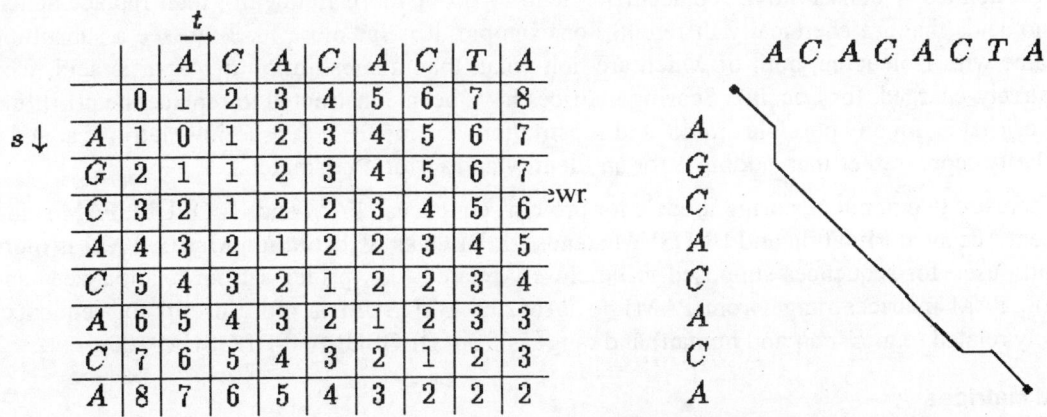

Fig. 10.9. Representation of a scoring matrix.

Sometimes, from an evolutionary point of view, it is more realistic to assume that nature inserts or deletes entire substrings as a unit. This is called the *block-indel-model*. It means that we charge a certain set-up cost for introducing a new gap, whereas extending an existing gap is less expensive.

The biological equivalence of a scoring matrix is an implicit particular theory of evolution (see PAM and BLOSUM matrices discussed later in this chapter). All analysis involving sequence comparisons can be done by using scoring matrices. The choice of matrix (model used to build the matrix) can strongly influence the outcome of the analysis.

Similarity versus Distance

Elements of the matrices specify the weight to assign a given comparison by either the cost of replacing one residue with another (*distance*); or a measure of the *similarity* for the replacement.

Similarity is used for database searching, while distance is more applicable for phylogenetic tree reconstruction. Maximizing a similarity is fundamentally the same as minimizing a distance. Hence distance and similarity matrices are inter-convertible by some mathematical transformation appropriate for the given application.

Similarity versus Homology

A database search is a frequently, but incorrectly, referred to as homology searching. The term homology implies a common evolutionary relationship between two traits -whether they are DNA sequences or bristle patterns on a fly's nose. Just because two sequences share a stretch of nearly identical nucleotides (or amino acids), does not mean that they are directly descended from a common ancestor. A very high level of similarity is a strong indication of homology. As a general rule, 25% identity over a stretch of 100 amino acids can be considered to be good evidence of common ancestry for two sequences.

Construction of scoring matrices

Construction of biologically significant alignments should take into account the fact that protein evolution is constrained by the chemical properties of amino acids, and by the degeneracy of the genetic code. Chemically conservative replacements tend to occur more frequently than replacements with amino acids that are chemically different. For example, it is far more likely to see a substitution of Leucine with Isoleucine, both of which are non-polar, than a substitution of Aspartic acid, which is negatively-charged, for Leucine. Scoring matrices have been constructed to replace the $p(i,j)$ function above. That is, for any possible amino acid substitution, a value from the scoring matrix is added to the similarity score, rather than adding 1 for an identity and -1 for a mismatch.

There are two popular scoring models for protein sequences : PAM and BLOSUM. PAM stands for Percent Accepted Mutation and BLOSUM stands for BLOcks SUbstitution Matrix. PAM is more frequently used for sequences supposed to be closely related (e.g. proteins from chimpanzees and human). PAM matrices range from PAM1 to PAM250. BLOSUM is more useful for sequences not closely related (e.g. *E. coli* and human) and range is from BLOSUM 10-BLOSUM 100.

PAM Matrices

Margaret Dayhoff et. al. proposed PAM model (1 PAM = 1 point mutation/100 amino acids). PAM

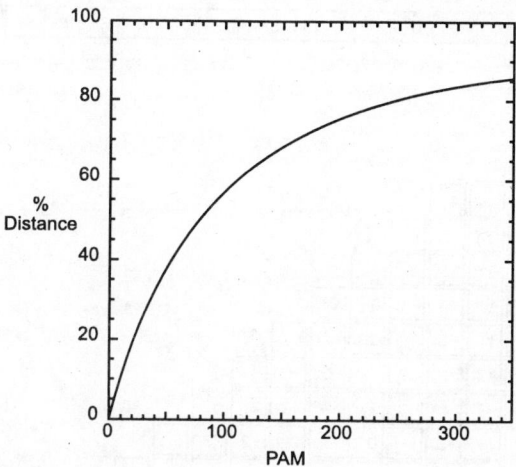

Fig. 10.10. Relationship between % difference and PAM distance.

matrices are based on global alignments of closely related proteins. The relationship between % difference and PAM distance was obtained by statistical analysis of two randomly aligned sequences as in Fig. 10.10. PAM- 1 therefore is a scoring system for sequences in which 1% of the residues have undergone mutation and PAM- 250 represents 250% mutation, i.e., an average of 2.5 accepted mutations per residue. PAM tries to model what happens at long evolutionary distances based on a simple Markov model derived from closely related sequences.

One of the most commonly used scoring matrices is the PAM250 matrix, shown in Fig. 10.11.

Substitution of an Aspartic acid for Glutamic acid (both acidic) adds 3 to the score. Substitution of the positively-charged Lys for the non-polar Pro adds -1 to the score. Generally, the more conservative the replacement, the higher the value that will be added to the score.

Substitution matrices like PAM250 are constructed by observing the frequencies of amino acid replacements in large samples of protein sequences. For a given replacement, the PAM value is proportional to the natural log of the frequency with which that replacement was observed to occur. One PAM unit is defined as the amount of sequence divergence corresponding to a 1% amino acid replacement rate. For closely-related sequences, it is appropriate to use a PAM100 matrix, in which PAM units have been extrapolated to 100% replacement. For most database searches, a PAM250 matrix is preferred, since larger databases will tend to have sets of more distantly-related sequences.

PAM approach can be summarised as follows:

- Carefully examine the kinds of mutations that occur in closely related protein sequence, i. e., at short evolutionary times.
- Extrapolate these differences to greater mutational distance/ longer times
- Accepted point mutations - tabulate actual mutations by looking at proteins that are sufficiently closely related that there is no ambiguity in alignment
- Sequences no more than 15% different so that changes can be thought of as a single evolutionary step
- Consider a tree to correctly count changes

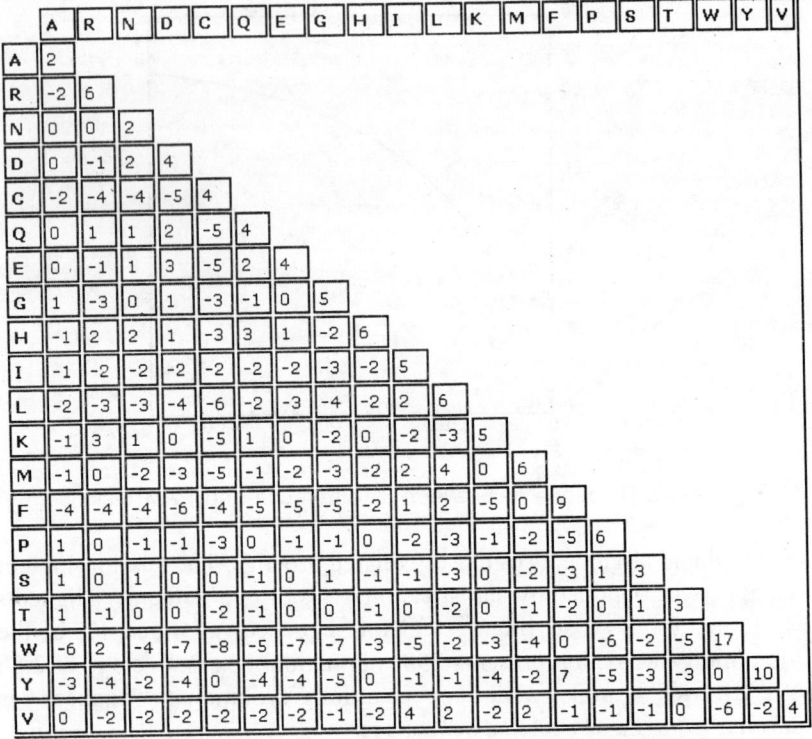

Fig. 10.11. PAM 250 Amino Acid Similarity Matrix.

Two types of matrix can be constructed: *Mutation probability matrix* - probability that residue in column j will be replaced by residue in row i after some amount of evolution and *relatedness odds matrix* – log- odds form of the mutation probability matrix.

Problems with the PAM approach are as follows:

- Not all positions are the same
- Evolutionary rates vary greatly within a sequence
- Each position has a unique three dimensional environment
- Environment changes over evolutionary time
- The most mutable positions were inadvertently selected as the basis for the calculation
- Proteins change more rapidly at the least constrained positions and most slowly at buried "core" positions

BLOSUM Matrices

Henikoff and Henikoff as a way to explicitly represent those important distant relationships developed BLOSUM matrices. They used blocks of sequence fragments from different protein families, which can be aligned without the introduction of gaps. These sequence blocks correspond to the more highly conserved regions (Fig. 10.12). Amino acid pair frequencies can be compiled from these blocks simply

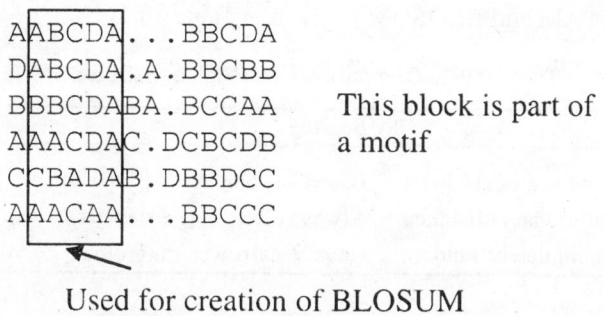

Used for creation of BLOSUM
matrix

Fig. 10.12. Conserved regions in blocks.

by summing over all possible pairs of the block. These frequencies can be written down in a frequency table, and the odds for relatedness calculated in a similar way as described for the Dayhoff matrix.

Different evolutionary distances are incorporated into this scheme with a clustering procedure: two sequences that are identical to each other for more than a certain threshold of positions is clustered. More sequences are added to the cluster if they are identical to any sequence already in the cluster at the same level. All sequences within a cluster are then averaged. A consequence of this clustering is that the contribution of closely related sequences to the frequency table is reduced, if the identity requirement is reduced. This leads to a series of matrices, analogous to the PAM series of matrices. The index denoting the level of clustering, e.g. BLOSUM 100 is derived from sequence blocks clustered at the 100% identity level.

BLOSUM approach can be summarised as follows :

1. Locally align each feature to get blocks.
2. To build the BLOSUM 62 matrix one must replace sequences that are identical in more than 62% of their amino acid sequences by a single representative sequence.
3. Dealing with bias and distance
   – Cluster all sequences with less than X% identities
   – Clustered sequences count as 1 sequence
   – If X is 100% it simply removes identical sequences
   – If X < 100% it reduces the weight on closely related sequences

Calculate substitution frequencies and log- odds matrix. The probability for a pair of amino acids to be in the same column is calculated. In the previous page this would be the probability of replacement of A with A, A with B, A with C, and B with C. This gives the value qij. Then calculate the probability that a certain amino acid frequency exists, fi. Then, calculate the log odds ratio $s_{i,j} = \log_2(q_{ij}/f_i)$. This value is entered into the scoring matrix.

1. This gives a BLOSUM X table. For example :
   a. BLOSUM 62 - sequences greater than 62% identical are clustered
   b. BLOSUM 100 - sequences greater than 100% identical are clustered

Comparison between PAM and BLOSUM is given in Table 10.1.

Table 10.1. Comparison of PAM and BLOSUM

Pam	Blosum
Based on explicit evolutionary model	Based on empirical frequencies
Represents a specific evolutionary distance	Always a blend of distances as seen in the database (PROSITE)
Ranges from identical to completely random	Have a narrower range than PAM matrices

However scoring matrices are difficult to compare because they reflect different target frequencies and evolutionary distances.

Blosum 45 Amino Acid Similarity Matrix is shown in Fig. 10.13.

Scoring Matrices for Nucleic acids

Nucleotide scoring matrices have been developed for scoring DNA sequence alignments, on similar lines as amino acid scoring matrices. DNA matrices can include ambiguous DNA symbols and information from mutational analysis. Typical information about mutation included is that transitions (substitutions between the purines and pyrimidines themselves) are more probable than transversions (substitutions between purine to pyrimidine or vice versa).

A series of nucleic acid PAM matrices based on a Markov transition model similar to that used to generate PAM scoring matrices have been developed. The scoring matrices at large evolutionary provide little information per aligned nucleotide pair. When sequences have so little similarity, a much longer alignment is necessary to be significant.

```
Gly   7
Pro  -2   9
Asp  -1  -1   7
Glu  -2   0   2   6
Asn   0  -2   2   0   6
His  -2  -2   0   0   1  10
Gln  -2  -1   0   2   0   1   6
Lys  -2  -1   0   1   0  -1   1   5
Arg  -2  -2  -1   0   0   0   1   3   7
Ser   0  -1   0   0   1  -1   0  -1  -1   4
Thr  -2  -1  -1  -1   0  -2  -1  -1  -1   2   5
Ala   0  -1  -2  -1  -1  -2  -1  -1  -2   1   0   5
Met  -2  -2  -3  -2  -2   0   0  -1  -1  -2  -1  -1   6
Val  -3  -3  -3  -3  -3  -3  -3  -2  -2  -1   0   0   1   5
Ile  -4  -2  -4  -3  -2  -3  -2  -3  -3  -2  -1  -1   2   3   5
Leu  -3  -3  -3  -2  -3  -2  -2  -3  -2  -3  -1  -1   2   1   2   5
Phe  -3  -3  -4  -3  -2  -2  -4  -3  -2  -2  -1  -2   0   0   0   1   8
Tyr  -3  -3  -2  -2  -2   2  -1  -1  -1  -2  -1  -2   0  -1   0   0   3   8
Trp  -2  -3  -4  -3  -4  -3  -2  -2  -2  -4  -3  -2  -2  -3  -2  -2   1   3  15
Cys  -3  -4  -3  -3  -2  -3  -3  -3  -3  -1  -1  -1  -2  -1  -3  -2  -2  -3  -5  12
     Gly Pro Asp Glu Asn His Gln Lys Arg Ser Thr Ala Met Val Ile Leu Phe Tyr Trp Cys
```

Fig. 10.13. BLOSUM 45 matrix.

10.6 METHODS FOR OPTIMAL ALIGNMENTS

While dot-matrix searches provide a great deal of information in a visual fashion, they can only be considered semi-quantitative, and therefore do not lend themselves to statistical analysis. Also, dot-matrix searches do not provide a precise alignment between two sequences. Dynamic programming can provide global or local sequence alignments.

A summary of methods of optimal alignments is given in Table 10.2.

Table 10.2. Summary of alignment methods.

Method	Value calculated	Gap penalty	Time required
Needleman-Wunsch	Global similarity	Penalty/gap q	$O(n^2)$
Sellers	(Global) distance	Penalty/residue rk	$O(n^2)$
Smith-Waterman	Local similarity	Affine q+rk	$O(n^2)$
BLAST	Maximum segment score	Multiple segments	$O(n^2)/K$
FASTA	Approx. local similarity	Limited gap size q+rk	$O(n^2)/K$

Global sequence alignment by dynamic programming

Basically, dynamic programming is a method for breaking down the alignment of sequences into small parts where one considers all the possible changes in moving from one pair of characters in the alignment to the next. It is comparable to moving across a dot matrix and keeping track of all the matching pairs, adding up those pairs that are along a diagonal and the subtracting when insertions are necessary to maintain an alignment.

Sequence alignment methods predate dot-matrix searches, and all of the alignment methods in use today are related to the original method of Needleman and Wunsch. Needleman and Wunsch wanted to quantify the similarity between two sequences. Over the course of evolution, some positions undergo base or amino acid substitutions, and bases or amino acids can be inserted or deleted. Any measurement of similarity must therefore be done with respect to the best possible alignment between two sequences. Because insertion/deletion events are rare compared to base substitutions, it makes sense to penalize gaps more heavily than mismatches when calculating a similarity score. As an example, a very simple scoring scheme would add +1 for each match, -1 for each mismatch, and -2 for each gap inserted. That is, the larger the gap, the more we subtract.

The similarity between two sequences would then be

Sim = +1(# identities) -1(#mismatches) -2(#gaps)

For example:

GCTGGAACCAG

‖‖‖‖‖ ‖‖‖

ACTGGAT-CAG

Sim = 1(10) - 1(2) -2(1) = 4

By definition, the alignment that gives the highest similarity score is the optimal alignment. However, the number of alignments that must be checked increases exponentially with the lengths of the sequences. Allowing gaps also results in as exponential increase in the computation time required. The problem seems intractably large for all but very small sequences. Needleman and Wunsch conceptualized alignment as a problem in dynamic programming, in which the solution to a large problem is simplified if we first know the solution to a smaller problem that is a subset of the larger problem. Think of an alignment occurring in matrix, where sequence s of length m is written on the Y-axis, and sequence t of length n is written on the X-axis. The alignment can then be accomplished in two steps:

a. All possible alignments of **s** and **t** are contained in array a[0..m,0..n] (the component a[0,0] represents a gap at the beginning of each sequence).

b. The optimal alignment will be the path through the array that has the highest score (the largest number of matches and fewest mismatches and gaps.)

Needleman and Wunsch realized that all parts of the alignment problem boiled down to the same decision made at every position **i** in sequence **s**, when compared with every position **j** in sequence **t**.

If we want to calculate the score at any position **a[i,j]** in the alignment matrix **a**, we only have to look at three adjacent cells in the matrix to calculate that score, **a[i,j-1]**, **a[i-1,j-1]**, or **a[i-1,j]**. These are the positions in the alignment that represent the part of the alignment just prior to **a[i,j]**, at which point either:

1. A gap penalty was subtracted for an insertion in **t** (e.g. -2)
2. An identity or a mismatch was scored (+1 or -1)
3. A gap penalty was subtracted for an insertion in **s** (e.g. -2)

This formula can be used to calculate partial alignment scores at all parts of the alignment matrix.

Step 1: Calculation of the alignment matrix (Fig. 10.14)

The first step is the trivial calculation of the case in which one or more terminal gaps are added to the beginning of either sequence (Fig. 10.15). This is done by running across the top of the array and progressively adding a gap penalty (e.g. -2) to the score in each cell, and doing the same to the leftmost column. Next, we apply the three scoring rules to each cell in the matrix.

At cell a[1,1], the score is the largest of three possible scores

(i)   a[1,0] -2 = -2 - 2 = -4
(ii) a[0,0] + p(1,1) = 0 + 1 = 1
(iii) a[0,1] - 2 = -2 - 2 = -4

where **p(i,j)** is a function that returns +1 if **s[i]** = **t[j]** (match) or -1 if **s[i]** ¬ = **t[j]**.

This process is repeated down the matrix until all cells are filled (Fig. 10.16).

Step 2 : Construction of the optimal alignment

The final example (Fig. 10.17) shows the completed array, with arrows pointing from each cell to one adjacent cell (i.e. the cell that gave the highest score) or more than one adjacent cell in case of a tie. Since the path to the highest scoring adjacent cell (s) is always known, we can start at the last position in the alignment, a[m,n], and work backwards to the beginning, a[1,1], adding scores along a fairly limited number of alternative paths.

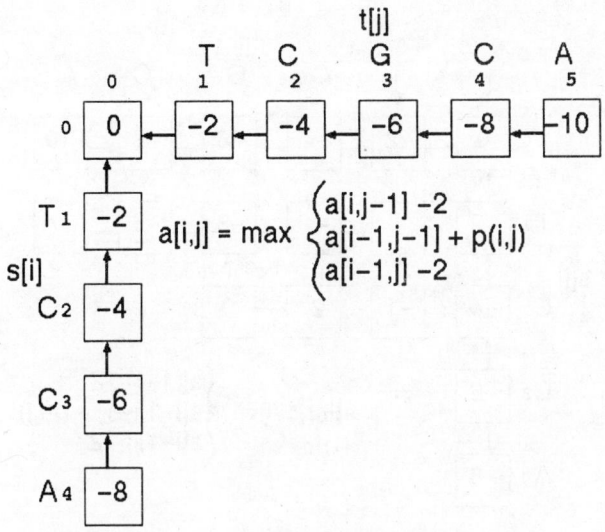

Fig. 10.14. Calculation of the alignment matrix.

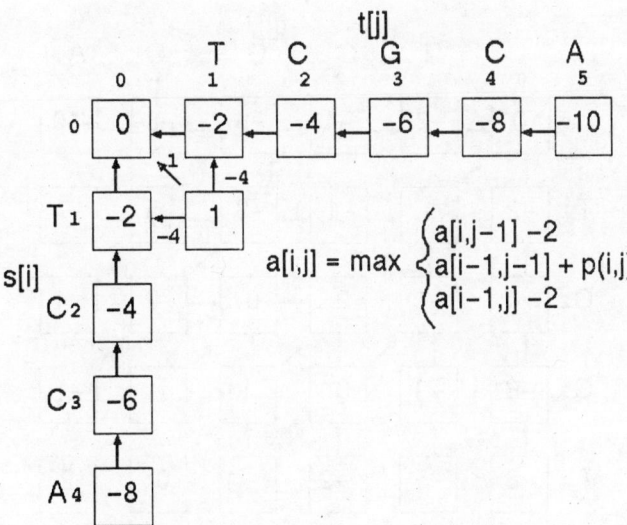

Fig. 10.15. Applying the scoring rules

The optimal alignment will be the path that gives the highest total score. In the example, the optimal alignment would be

    TCGCA
    || ||
    TC-CA

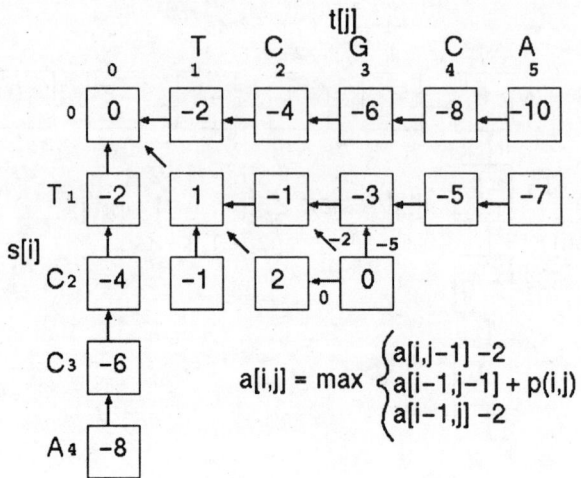

Fig. 10.16. Filling up the matrix using scoring matrix.

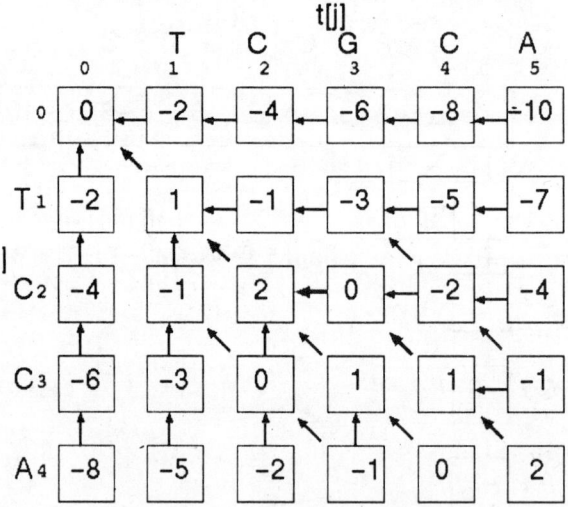

Fig. 10.17. Completed array.

and the similarity score is simply the score at cell a[i,j], the last cell in the alignment. We can check the score by using the written alignment: 4(+1) + 0(-1) + 1(-2) = 2.

The DP and other alignment methods provide a sequence alignment from which the following calculations may be made:

1. Percent identity.
2. Percent similarity for protein sequences is percent identity plus percent conservative substitutions.

3. Similarity score which is the sum of all the scores of all the identities and similarities in the alignment minus the sum of all the gap penalties. The similarity scores for amino acids are taken from a comparison table such as the PAM250 and BLOSUM62 matrices.

Variations of the DP method may be used to determine either global or local alignments, multiple sequence alignment or database searches. Sometimes passing back through the matrix in the reverse direction one or more times refines the local alignment found in one sweep through the sequences.

Local Alignment

The algorithm developed by Needelman and Wunsch calculates global similarity score between the entire lengths of the sequences being compared. Global algorithms are not sensitive for highly diverged sequences and it is better (and faster) to focus on local similarity. The three most widely used local similarity algorithms are : Smith-Waterman, BLAST and FASTA.

Smith-Waterman is a dynamic programming algorithm. The Smith-Waterman algorithm is a rigorous "dynamic programming" approach that does not make use of heuristic shortcuts. The algorithm gives the highest-scoring local match between two sequences. Smith-Waterman can be used instead of Needleman-Wunsch algorithm for matching two sequences that have a matched region that is only a fraction of their lengths, that have different lengths, that overlap, or where one sequence is a fragment of the other.

The rules for calculating scoring matrix values are slightly different in this case, most important being :

1. The scoring system must have negative scores for mismatches.
2. When a scoring matrix value becomes negative, that value is set to zero, which effectively terminates the alignment up to that point.

The alignments are arrived at by starting at the highest-scoring positions in the scoring matrix and following a trace path from those positions up to a box that scores zero.

Smith Waterman is not generally used for routine database searching because although it is more sensitive than BLAST and FASTA, it runs much slower. For some DNA-DNA searches, FASTA may be more sensitive than BLAST, but in most cases both programs should be tried to insure the most comprehensive search.

FASTA (developed by Lipman and Pearson), considers exact matches between short substrings, for a given paramter. If a significant number of such exact matches are found, FASTA uses the dynamic programming algorithm to compute optimal alignments. This approach allows to trade-off speed for precision: the larger we choose the parameter, the smaller is the number of exact matches. This makes the program faster, but loses precision: it becomes less likely that the optimal alignment contains enough *exact* matches of length , and the procedure may find nothing. Nevertheless, experience shows that with sensibly chosen parameters, FASTA misses very few cases of significant homology.

BLAST (developed by Altschul et al.), is another heuristic based on a similar idea. BLAST focuses on no-gap alignments of a certain, fixed length . Rather than requiring exact matches, BLAST uses a scoring function to measure similarity (rather than distance). In particular for proteins, one can argue that segment pairs with no gaps and a high similarity score indicate regions of functional similarity. For a given threshold parameter, BLAST reports to the user all database entries which have a segment pair with the query sequence that scores higher than the threshold parameter. If the scoring function used has a probabilistic interpretation, BLAST can also give an assessment of the statistical significance of the matches it reports.

10.7 SENSITIVITY AND SPECIFICITY

How can we measure how good a pattern is at detecting a particular sequence feature? There are two different, complementary measures that can be used to describe how well a pattern performs. Sensitivity is the fraction of the true matches that actually are correctly predicted as matches by the pattern. If the pattern is too stringent (to avoid junk), then too few of the true matches will be identified by it. Specificity is the fraction of the sequences predicted as matches that really are true matches. If the pattern is too inclusive (to catch as many as possible), then a lot of junk will also be falsely identified by it.

Definitions of Parameters and Measures

Some of the important parameters and measures are defined below :

True Positives (TP) are entries that were reported and are true hits, i.e. homologues.

False Positives (FP) are entries that were reported and are not homologues.

True Negatives (TN) are entries that were not reported and are not homologues.

False Negatives (FN) are entries that were not reported but are actually true hits, i.e. homologues.

There are some measures of how poorly the program did. These are given below :

1. *Overprediction (OP)* : OP is the measure of False Positives and is defined as follows : OP = FP/ (TP + FP)
2. *Underprediction (UP)* : UP is the measure of False Negatives and is defined as follows : UP = FN / (TP + FN)

Measures of how well the program did are defined as follows :

1. *Overlap Quality (OQ)* : OQ is the measure of True Positives, as defined as follows: OQ = TP / (TP + FP + FN)
2. *Correlation Coefficient (CC)* : CC is the overall performance indicator and is defined as follows:
   CC = (TP*TN - FP*FN) / SqRt[(TP + FP) * (TN + FN) * (TP + FN) * (TN + FP)]

Thus CC = 1 when FP = 0 and FN = 0. FN is treated like FP and TN is treated like TP.

Sensitivity

Sensitivity measure attempts to report all "real" hits (homologues), i.e. FN = 0. This implies that the program is "sensitive" to reporting true homologues. It is measured by Underprediction. The lower the False Negatives or Underprediction, the higher is the sensitivity.

It can also be measured directly as follows : sensitivity = 1 - UP = TP / (TP + FN). Thus, sensitivity = 1 when FN = 0 or UP = 0.

Specificity

Specificity attempts to report only "real" hits (homologues), i.e. FP = 0. This means that the program is "specific" for reporting only true homologues. It is measured by Overprediction. The lower the False Positives or Overprediction, the higher the specificity.

It can also be measured directly: Specificity = 1 - OP = TP / (TP + FP**).**

Thus, specificity = 1 when FP = 0 or OP = 0. "Selectivity" is sometimes used as a synonym for "Specificity" (program "selects" and reports only true homologues).

10.8 ILLUSTRATIVE EXAMPLES

1. What is the edit distance of the words "INDUSTRY" and "INTEREST"? What of "CCT" and "ACGCTT"? Show an optimal alignment for each case.

   The edit distances are 6 and 3, respectively.

   For the first case, optimal alignments are

   INDUSTRY

   ||

   INTEREST

   or

   IN—DUSTRY

   || ||

   INTEREST—

   For the second case, an optimal alignment is

   -C-C-T

   |||

   ACGCTT

2. Calculate a dynamic programming matrix and alignment for the sequences ATT and TTC. How many optimal alignments are there ?

   Matrix:

   0 1 2 3

   1 1 2 3

   2 1 1 2

   3 2 1 2

   Alignment:

   ATT

   |

   TTC

   The other optimal alignments is,

   ATT-

   ||

   -TTC

3. The number of possible alignments is often described as "something close to the possible movements in chess". How many are there for the sequences ATT and TTC ? Also, devise a formula for the number of alignments which can be used to enumerate them systematically

There are 63 possible Alignments, and this is the number of paths through the matrix :

```
0  1  2  3
1  1  2  3
2  1  1  2
3  2  1  2
```

One can arrive at this value by considering alignments with a varying number of gaps:

0 gaps: 1 alignment, which corresponds to the diagonal.

1 gap : 12 alignments. There are 4 placements of a gap in sequence 1, making it look like -XXX, X-XX, XX-X, or XXX-. For each of these, there are 3 possible placements of the gap in the second sequence. Note that a gap may not align to a gap.

2 gaps: 30 alignments. (From 5 possible positions in XXXXX, we need to select 2 positions which may have a gap. There are 10 of these, namely —XXX, -X-XX, -XX-X, -XXX-; X—XX, X-X-X, X-XX-; XX—X, XX-X-; XXX—. For all 10 possibilities, 2 gaps are selected for the second sequence, from 3 admissible positions. For example, if the first sequence is —XXX, then the gaps in the second sequence can be set as follows, YY-YY, YYY-Y, or YYYY-. There are 3 possibilities for any of the 10 settings of gaps in the first sequence.

3 gaps: 20 alignments. From 6 possible positions in XXXXXX, we need to select 3 positions which may have a gap. There are 20 of these, namely —XXX, —X-XX, —XX-X, —XXX-;-X—XX, -X-X-X, -X-XX-, -XX—X, -XX-X-, -XXX—;X—XX, X—X-X, X—XX-, X-X—X, X-X-X-, X-XX—;XX—X, XX—X-, XX-X—, XXX—. For any of these, there is only one way to set the gaps in the second sequence.

To derive a formula, note that the dynamic programming recursive formula can be used to reason about the number of alignments (which is equal to the number of paths thru the matrix).

For sequences of length m and n, the number of alignments, #Alignments, is :

#Alignments(m,n) = #Alignments(m-1,n) + #Alignments(m,n-1) + #Alignments(m-1,n-1)

In the above example, we have

#Alignments(3,3) = #Alignments(2,3) + #Alignments(3,2) + #Alignments(2,2)

= 2 * #Alignments(2,3) + #Alignments(2,2)

= 2 * [#Alignments(1,3) + #Alignments(2,2) + #Alignments(1,2)] + #Alignments(1,2) + #Alignments(2,1) + #Alignments(1,1)

= 2 * [1+5+1 + 5+5+3 + 1+3+1] + 1+3+1 + 1+3+1 + 1+1+1 = 63.

3. Consider the three alignments of CAAAAGAT and CGAGGGGT shown below. Calculate the cost of each under :

a) The unit cost model

b) The unit cost model with block-indels, with g_i=1 and g_e=0.2.

   (1) GAAAAGAT

       CGAGGGGT

   (2) GAAAAGA—T
        C—GAGGGGT
   (3) GAAAAGA——T
        C——GAGGGGT
   (1) GAAAAGAT
        CGAGGGGT   cost a) = 4   cost b) = 4
   (2) GAAAAGA—T
        C—GAGGGGT   cost a) = 6   cost b) = 4.4
   (3) GAAAAGA——T
        C——GAGGGGT   cost a) = 10   cost b) = 3.2

5. Design the dynamic programming (recursive) formula for the block-indel case.

   The standard recursive formula takes the minimum over 3 values, representing Match/Replacement, Deletion, and Insertion, respectively, as the last edit operation giving rise to the alignment of the sub-sequences considered thus far.

   Since Deletions and Insertions may now extend beyond one gap, the costs for introducing them has to be calculated by minimizing over all possible lengths of such an indel, as follows:

   I(i,j) = min {d_w(0:s:k,0:t:j) + g_i+(i-k)*g_e}, where k=0,...,i-1

   D(i,j) = min {d_w(0:s:i,0:t:k) + g_i+(j-k)*g_e}, where k=0,...,j-1

   "i" in "g_i" stands for "Insertion" (of a gap), and it has got nothing to do with the index variable i.

   The overall minimization then looks like this:

   d_w(0:s:i,0:t:j) = min { d_w(0:s:i-1,0:t:j-1) + w(s_i,t_j),I(i,j), D(i,j) }

6. Calculate a dynamic programming matrix and local alignment for the sequences ATT and ATCTTC.

   A T C T T C
   0 0 0 0 0 0 0
   A 1 0 1 1 1 1 1
   T 2 1 0 1 1 1 2
   T 3 2 1 1 1 1 2

   There are 5 possible optimal local alignments, i.e.

   ATCTTC
   ||
   —ATT-
   ATCTTC
   ||
   ATT—
   ATCTTC
   || |
   AT-T—

AT-CTTC
||
ATT——
A-TCTTC
| |
ATT——

11

Tools for Sequence Alignment

11.1. INTRODUCTION

While the previous chapter focussed on the concepts and the applications of database searching and sequence alignment, this chapter focuses on the "real-life" tools and techniques. The most famous of the tools : FASTA and BLAST are discussed with their most useful versions. These tools are applied extensively in bioinformatics. Although these tools are discussed in detail here, the focus is on "how they work" and most of the syntax used by these tools has not been discussed in detail. The documentation related to the syntax for these tools is readily available on the various sites with extensive "help".

11.2. FASTA (Fig. 11.1)

Introduction

FASTA is a powerful tool for scanning databases to find sequences that are similar to a query sequence. It is generally best to make protein-protein comparisons, but FASTA can also compare DNA sequence to DNA databanks.

The related program TFASTA allows a protein query sequence to be compared to DNA databanks. Each DNA sequence in the databank is translated in all six reading frames, then six protein-protein comparisons are made with FASTA. This is generally the best way to scan the EST databases.

FASTA starts by making a generalization from the idea of dot plots. In a dot plot, regions of similarity between two sequences show up as diagonals. FASTA essentially calculates the sum of the dots along each diagonal. The "FAST" in fasta comes from the method of calculating those diagonal sums. If it were necessary to actually construct a dot plot matrix and then add along the diagonals for every sequence in the database, then FASTA wouldn't be any quicker than Smith-Waterman. Instead, FASTA uses a "word" based method - it looks for matching sequence patterns or words, called k-tuples, and then attempts to build a local alignment based upon these word matches.. It makes a list of all words, (1 or 2 amino acids, or 5 or 6 nucleotides) in each sequence. It matches identical words from each list, and then creates diagonals by joining adjacent matches, but it only counts non-overlapping words. It then re-scores the highest scoring regions using a replacement matrix such as the PAM250 - the best of these scores is called "init1". It then tries to join together the high scoring diagonals, allowing for gaps.

The best score from that is called "initn". Finally, it makes an optimal local alignment around the regions it has discovered using the Smith-Waterman algorithm. This last alignment step is only applied to a small number of "hit" sequences, which had high "initn" values after the database search.

FASTA Algorithm

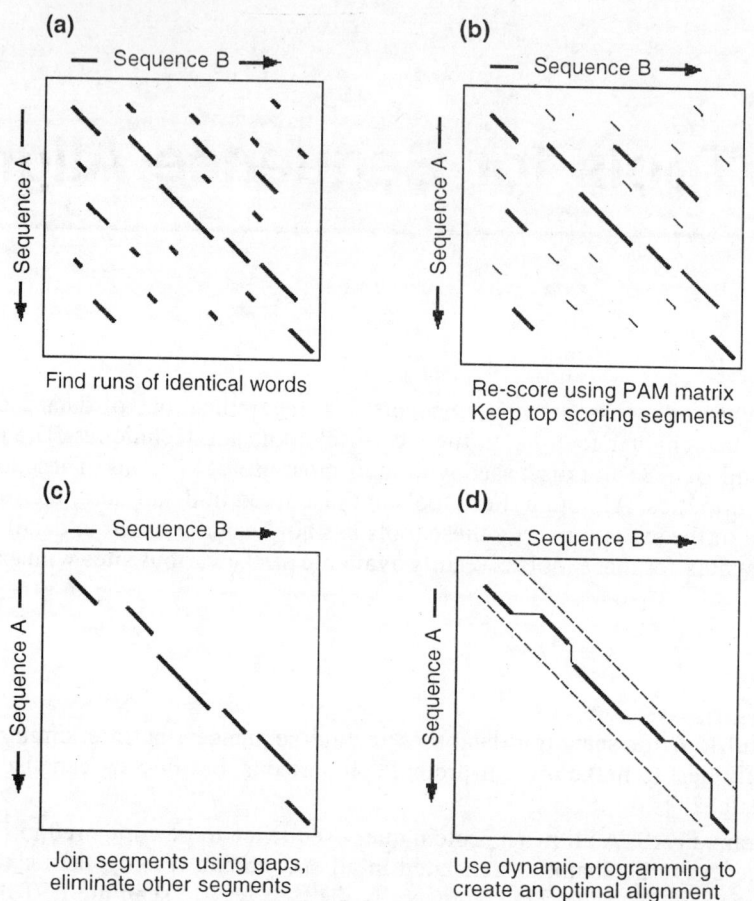

(a)

— Sequence B →

Sequence A

Find runs of identical words

(b)

— Sequence B →

Sequence A

Re-score using PAM matrix
Keep top scoring segments

(c)

— Sequence B →

Sequence A

Join segments using gaps,
eliminate other segments

(d)

— Sequence B →

Sequence A

Use dynamic programming to
create an optimal alignment

Fig. 11.1.

FASTA compares an input DNA or protein sequence to all of the sequences in a target sequence database, and then reports the best matched sequences and local alignments of these matched sequence with the input sequence. The input sequence and database are usually in FASTA format.

FASTA uses four steps to calculate similarity scores between a pair of sequences:

1. Identify regions shared by the two sequences that have the highest density of single residue identities (ktup=1) or two-consecutive identities (ktup=2)

2. Re-scan the best regions identified in step 1 using the PAM-250 matrix. The single best score is stored as init1 for reporting later.

3. Determine if gaps can be used to join the regions identified in step 2. If so, determine a similarity score for the gapped alignment, which is reported as initin.

4. Construct an optimal alignment of the query sequence and the library sequence (Smith-Waterman algorithm). This score is reported as the optimized score (opt.)

In the initial search for regions of similarity, FASTA uses a method known as hash coding. In this method, a lookup table showing the positions of each sequence word of length k (a k-tuple), is constructed for each sequence. The relative position of each word in the two sequences is then calculated by subtracting the position in the first sequence from that in the second. Words that have the same offset position reveal a region of alignment between the two sequences. The number of comparisons increases linearly in proportion to average sequence length. In contrast, the time taken in dot matrix and dynamic programming methods increases as the square of the average sequence length. The k-tuple length is user-defined and is usually 1 or 2 for protein sequences (i.e. either the positions of each of the individual 20 amino acids or the positions of each of the 400 possible dipeptides are located). For nucleic acid sequences, the k-tuple is 5-20, and is much longer because short k-tuples are much more common due to the 4 letter alphabet of nucleic acids. The larger the k-tuple chosen, the more rapid but less thorough, a database search.

Lookup method for finding an alignment

```
position        1    2    3    4    5    6    7    8    9   10   11
protein 1       n    c    s    p    t    a    .    .    .    .    .
protein 2       ..   .    .    .  ac  s pr   k
```

amino acid	position in protein 1	position in protein 2	offset pos A - pos B
a	6	6	0
c	2	7	-5
k	-	11	
n	1	-	
p	4	9	-5
r	-	10	
s	3	8	-5
t	5	-	

Amino acids c,s and p have the common offset for the 3 amino acids c,s and p. A possible alignment is thus:

```
    protein 1     n    c    s    p    t    a
                       |    |    |
    protein 2     a    c    s    p    r    k
```

This procedure may also be performed as quickly by searching for 2-mers, 3-mers or higher i.e. a table would be made for finding 2-mers such n c, c s, etc in the above sequences, or 3-mers such as n c s, c s p, etc. The speed will be increased but the sensitivity decreased as the n-mer length is increased. For proteins, an n-mer of 1 or 2 is fine, but for nucleic acids, the n-mer must be much higher 7-10 or so. Compressing the DNA sequences into a more compact binary form can also speed up the process.

Significance of Fasta matches

FASTA calculates an E()-value (expectation of significance). The final output plots the initial scores of each library sequence in a histogram ranked by the z-score which is derived from the opt score corrected for differences in sequence length. The general idea of this graph is to show a normal curve of z-scores and E() values that allows you to see the typical values of these statistics for random matches versus the more significant matches at the very bottom of the graph. A list of the most significant scores follows the histogram and then the optimal alignments are displayed for these matches (the cutoff can be set by the user). The list of matches also contains, for each database sequence, the beginning and end positions of the region of significant similarity to your query sequence. It is also possible to force FASTA to show global alignments between the best hits and your query sequence rather than the local alignments used in its similarity calculations [you can use the "/SHOWALL" option on the FASTA command line].

Fasta3 (version 3 of Fasta) uses the extreme value distribution to calculate the significance of similarity scores found in a database search. The steps are as follows :

1. The average score for sequences in the same length range is determined
2. The average score is plotted against logarithm of average sequence l
3. The points are fitted to a straight line by linear regression
4. A z score, the number of standard deviations from the fitted line, is calculated for each score
5. High scoring, presumably related or low complexity sequences, and also of very low scoring alignments that do not fit the straight line are removed from consideration
6. Steps 1 through 5 are repeated one or more times
7. z scores are used to calculate the probability that a score greater than z would be found between unrelated sequences, using the extreme value distribution equation:

$$P\ (Z > z) = 1 - \exp\ (-e^{-\ 1.2825\ z - 0.5772})$$

The expected value of a database search for similar sequences is this score times the number of sequences in the database (approx. 80,000) : $E\ (Z > z) = D \times P\ (Z > z)$

Fasta plots a distribution of the scores found and shows how well the scores with unrelated sequences match the extreme value distribution. Normalized similarity scores are calculated for each score by the formula $z' = 50 + 10z$. Thus an alignment score with a standard deviation of 5 has a normalized score of 100.

Recommended steps for a Fasta search

The following strategy is recommended for searches with Fasta for finding the most homologous sequences in a database search while avoiding false negative matches :

1. Always compare protein sequences if possible by translating DNA sequences
2. Search two non-redundant protein databases like PIR or Swiss-prot with ktup = 2. These two are recommended since these databases are carefully annotated and updated. The GenPet database, for example, has a problem of having many duplicate sequences from automatic translation of DNA sequences which affects the E() scores.
3. Look for agreement between the real and theoretical distribution of scores. If the probe sequence has a low-complexity, repeated domain or if the gap penalties are set too low, then there may be an excess of unrelated sequences with E() less than 0.1. If there is an excess of 3-5 fold more

sequences than expected in the score range of 80-110, repeat the search after removing the low complexity region from the query sequence or increase the gap penalties from -12/-2 to -14/-4. Another test to apply is to examine the number of high-scoring unrelated sequences with E() smaller than 1.0. If there are more then 5-10 such sequences, then the analysis is suspect.

4. E() of a database match is the number of times that an unrelated database sequence would obtain a score higher than z' just by chance. For a match to be significant, E() should be < 0.05. If the search has correctly identified homologous sequences, then the corresponding E() values should be much less than 0.02, while scores between unrelated sequences should be much greater than this value e.g at least 0.5. If there are no E() less than 0.1 then the search has not found any sequences with significant similarity to the probe sequence.

5. If there are no matches with E() less than 0.1 then repeat the search with Fasta with ktup = 1, or else use the Smith-Waterman Dynamic Programming method with a program such as Ssearch. If Fasta now finds matches with E() less than 0.02, then the sequences may be homologous, if there is not a low complexity region in the probe sequence. Sequences with score of 0.2 to 10 may also be homologous but have marginal sequence similarity. For further study of this possibility select some of these marginal sequences and use them as probe sequences for additional database searches with Fasta. Additional family members with significant similarity may then be found.

6. Confirm homology of marginal matches by shuffling the probe or database sequence many times to calculate the significance of the real alignment. The program Prss performs this task.

7. Protein sequence alignments with 50% identity in a short 20-40 amino acid region are common in unrelated proteins. To be truly significant, the alignment should extend over a longer region.

Implementations and extensions of FASTA

There are several implementations of the FASTA algorithm (as given by Pearson):

FASTA - compares a protein sequence to another protein sequence or a protein library or a DNA sequence to another DNA sequence or to a DNA sequence library.

TFASTA - compares a protein sequence to a DNA sequence or DNA sequence library by translating each DNA sequence into all 6 possible reading frames and then comparing each frame to the protein sequence.

LFASTA - identifies one or more regions of similarity between two sequences.

PLFASTA - presents a dot matrix plot of regions of sequence similarity between two sequences.

The following are newer versions of Fasta that are designed to align a DNA sequence with a protein sequence allowing gaps and frame shifts. If a DNA sequence has a high possibility of errors such as EST sequences, then the translated sequence may be inaccurate due to amino acid changes or frame shifts. These programs are designed to go around such errors by matching substituted amino acids and incorrect reading frames. Fastx and Tfastx allow only frame shifts between codons whereas Fasty and Tfasty allow substitutions and frame shifts within a codon.

FASTX and FASTY - translate a probe DNA sequence in three reading frames and compares all three frames to a protein sequence database.

TFASTX and TFASTY - compare a probe protein sequence to a DNA sequence database, calculating similarities with frameshifts to the forward and reverse orientations.

The Fasta algorithm has also been adapted for searching through a pattern database instead of a sequence database. The Fasta algorithm normally identifies sequence similarity very rapidly by a method for finding common patterns or k-tuples in the same order in two sequences. In Fasta-pat and Fasta-swap, the same rapid method is used to find common patterns. Fasta-pat performs a faster method of comparing sequences to patterns by means of a lookup table as described above. Fasta-swap performs a more rigorous search for the most significant matches of sequence to patterns. This combination of program and pattern database has been found to be useful for finding distant relatives of the probe sequence that may be missed in a search for sequence similarity. For example, if a conserved domain has many substitutions, then it may be missed by Fasta or Blast, but could be found by the pattern searching method. Thus, if a search with Fasta or Blast, then with Ssearch has not found any matches, then Fasta-pt and Fasta-swap should be tried also.

Other Fasta programs and related programs in the Pearson Fasta package are as follows :

Lalign - provides a specified number of best set alignments of a pair of sequences using the Smith-Waterman dynamic programming algorithm with subsequent improvements

Plalign - a version of Lalign that provides a dot matrix type plot of the best alignments between two sequences.

Lfasta - provides a specified number of best alignments of a pair of sequences using the Fasta algorithm.

Plfasta - a version of Lfasta that provides a dot matrix type plot of the best alignments between two sequences.

Prss - when a match of query sequence to database sequence has been found, there is the possibility that the score is artificially inflated due to the low complexity of the one or both sequences such as repeats of the same amino acid. Prss creates a library of a specified number of shuffled sequences of the same length and amino acid composition as the library sequence. These sequences are aligned with the query sequence using the Smith Waterman Dynamic Programming algorithm and the resulting alignments scores are fitted to the extreme value distribution to estimate the parameters l and K of the distribution. The significance of the alignment score between the query sequence and the library sequence may then be evaluated using these parameters.

Prdf - this program performs the same task as Prss except that the Fasta algorithm is used to align the sequences. The program will therefore run much faster than Prss.

The databases available for FastA searching (at the RCR) are:

Peptide (protein) Sequence Databases

sp:* = SwissProt - Amos Bairoch's protein sequence database
gp:* = GenPept - Translations of all GenBank DNA seqs (according to exons in features tables)
pir:* - Protein Information Resource
pir1:* - Annotated PIR entries
pir2:* - New PIR entries
pir3:* - Unverified PIR entries
pir4:* - Unencoded or untranslated
nrl_3d:* - sequences from 3-dimensional structure Brookhaven Protein Data Bank
Prosite - consensus seqs of conserved protein domains
TFD - Transcription Factor database

Nucleotide Sequence Databases VECTOR - vector sequences

MALARIA - malaria genomic sequences

gb:* - all of GenBank (includes EMBL, DDBJ, PDB) updated daily

GenBank Subdivisions

gb_ba:* Bacterial

gb_in:* - Invertebrate

gb_om:* - Other Mammalian (non-rodent, non-primate)

gb_ov:* - Other Vertebrate (non-mammalian vertebrates)

gb_or:* - Organelle

gb_pat:* - Patents

gb_ph:* - Phage

gb_pl:* - Plant

gb_pr:* - Primate

gb_ro:* - Rodent

gb_st:* - Structural RNA

gb_sy:* - Synthetic sequences (recombinant constructs, etc.)

gb_un:* - Unannotated

gb_vi:* - Viral

gb_est*:* - Expressed Sequence Tags (short cDNAs) - now has sections est1 to est 9 with more added each quarter.

gb_sts:* - Sequence Tagged Sites

gb_gss:* - Genomic Survey Sequences (large genomic contigs)

gb_htg:* - High Throughput Genomic sequences (single pass sequences churned out by the genome projects, unannotated and filled with errors)

gb_tag:* - ESTs + STS + GSS + HTG

11.3 BLAST

Introduction

BLAST (Basic Local Alignment Search Tool) is a similarity search program developed by the research staff at NCBI/GenBank. It is available as a free service over the Internet that provides very fast, accurate, and sensitive database searching.

BLAST, like FASTA, is a word based method. However, one major difference is that BLAST requires a pre-formatted search database.

BLAST goes through the following 3 steps :

1. It takes each word from the query sequence (3 amino acids or 11 nucleotides), and locates all similar words in the current test sequence.
2. If similar words are found, BLAST tries to expand the alignment to the adjacent words (but it does not allow gaps).
3. After all words are tested, a set of HSPs (High-scoring Segment Pairs) are chosen for that database sequence. Several short, non-overlapping HSPs may be combined in a statistical test to create a larger, more significant match.

BLAST Algorithm

BLAST algorithm is given below:

1. Find the list of high scoring words w
2. Compare the word list to the database and identity exact matches
3. For each word, match extend the alignment in both directions to find alignments that score greater than a threshold of value S

(1) Find the list of high scoring words w

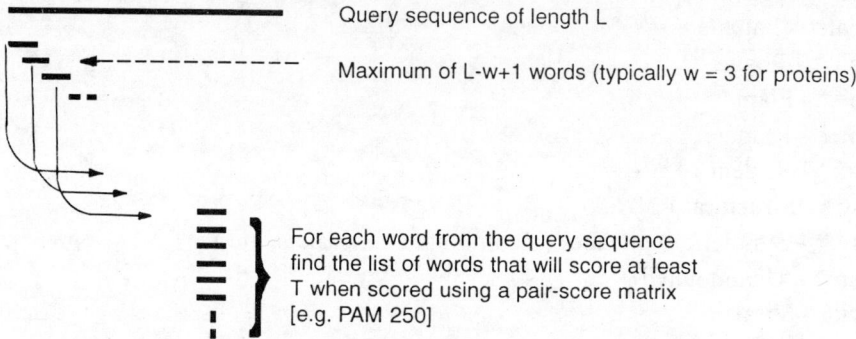

Query sequence of length L

Maximum of L-w+1 words (typically w = 3 for proteins)

For each word from the query sequence find the list of words that will score at least T when scored using a pair-score matrix [e.g. PAM 250]

(2) Compare the word list to the database and identify exact matches

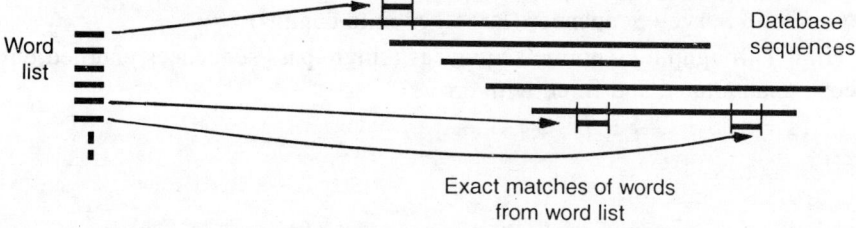

Word list

Database sequences

Exact matches of words from word list

(3) For each word match, extend the alignment in both directions to find alignments that score greater than a threshold of value S

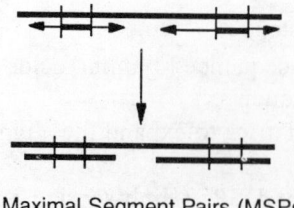

Maximal Segment Pairs (MSPs)

BLAST Considerations

BLAST is a complex tool. The default (non-redundant) database does NOT include the EST database. BLAST is fast because it initially throws away all database sequences that do not have a significant match without gaps to the query sequence. If two sequences are generally similar over a long region, but do not have a single highly conserved region, BLAST might miss the similarity. BLAST works much better for proteins than for nucleotides. Mostly this arises from the requirement for 11 consecutive identical nucleotides to start a HSP. The estimate is that BLAST can find protein sequences that have diverged by as much as 250 substitutions per 100 amino acids, but only 50 substitutions for 100 nucleotides. If you need to search nucleotide sequence against nucleotide databases, and you are looking for something remote, as opposed to an overlapping clone, then use FASTA instead. BLAST is particularly sensitive to short repeats and low complexity sequences (GC or AT rich). If you have them in your query sequence, you may get a couple of thousand bogus hits. You can remove both from your query sequence with the option "/FILTER=XS" (filtering is now the default). If this is applied, such regions are removed from the query sequence. If your sequence comes from a system that does not use the standard genetic code, be sure to use option "/TRANSLATE=N" to specify the proper translation table. For instance, yeast mitochondrial is 3, and vertebrate mitochondrial is 2.

BLAST Output

The output from BLAST can be enormous. For first runs, you might want to restrict the number of hits returned with /LISTSIZE and /SEGMENTS The first restricts the summary of hits at the top of the BLAST output, the second restricts the detailed alignments that follow. BLAST and FASTA produce similar output files. First there is a short description of the program and a list of the databases and program options chosen. Then there is a list of all of the database sequences that matched your query sequence. Several numbers are assigned to each of these sequences that represent the quality of the match. The list is presented in descending order,so that the best matches are at the top of the list. However, the most biologically significant matches are not always the ones ranked highest in the list.

The P-value is an indicator for the quality of a match. P-value smaller than e-100 (represents negative exponents) is exact matches (same gene, same species). P-values in the range of e-50 to e-100 are nearly identical genes (alleles, mutations, related species). P-values in the range of e-10 to e-50 are interesting closely related sequences. P-values between 0.1 and e-5 are still interesting but usually represent distant relationships. P-values greater than 0.1 are generally uninteresting or totally bogus matches.

Significance of Blast results

The probability p of observing a score S equal to or greater than x is given by the equation,

$$p\,(\,S > x) = 1 - \exp(-e^{-\lambda(x-u)})$$

where $u = [\log (Km'n')]/\lambda$ (K and λ are parameters that are calculated by Blast for the amino acid substitution scoring, n' is the effective length of the query sequence and m' is the effective length of the database sequence). The expect value E, the number database sequences not related to m but which by chance would give a score x with the query sequence is given by,

$$E = 1 - e^{-Dp}$$

where D is calculated as the length of the database divided by m and and E ~ Dp for small p, as in the Fasta calculation.Specifically, p is the average probability for a Poisson distribution of scores where 0,1,2,3... scores can be found. $E = 1 - e^{-Dp}$ is the probable number of sequences giving the score. E is roughly significant at 0.02-0.05

Recommended steps in the Blast algorithm

1. Sequence is filtered to remove low complexity regions
2. List of words of length 3 in the query protein sequence is made (length 11 for DNA sequences).
3. Words are evaluated for matches with any other combination of 3 amino amino acids using Blosum 62 scoring matrix as default. Matches of PQG to PEG would score 15, to PRG 14, to PSG 13 and to PQA 12
4. For DNA words, a match score of +5 and a mismatch score of -4 is used corresponding to the changes expected in sequences separated by a PAM distance of 40
5. A cutoff score T called a neighborhood word score threshold is selected to reduce the number of matches.
6. The above procedure is repeated for each 3-letter word in the query sequence. For a sequence of length 250 amino acids, the total number of words to search for is approximately 50 x 250 = 12,500.
7. Words organized into an efficient search tree for comparing them rapidly to the database sequences.
8. Each database sequence is scanned for an exact match to one of the 50 high scoring amino acid words corresponding to the first query sequence position
9. In Blast2 or gapped Blast, short matched regions called HSPs or high scoring segment pairs lying on the same diagonal and within a certain distance of each other are extended in each direction as long as the score keeps rising.
10. HSPs of score greater than a cutoff score S are kept.
11. In earlier versions of Blast and some of the later ones, the statistical significance of each HSP score is determined and if two or more HSP regions are found, thereby providing additional evidence that the query and database sequences are related, these scores will be combined to form a combined score.
12. In Blast 2, a local gapped alignment of the sequences is made and the significance of the score is determined

Blast programs

Program	Query sequence	Database	Type of alignment
Blastp	protein	protein	gapped
Blastn	nucleic aci	nucleic acid	gapped
Blastx	translated nucleic acid	protein	each frame gapped
Tblastn	protein	translated nucleic acid	each frame gapped
Tblastx	translated nucleic acid2	translated nucleic acid1	ungapped

Comparison between Fasta and Blast algorithms

- Fasta searches for all matching words of length k; Blast searches for the most unusual or high scoring words (proteins of length 3, nucleic acids of length 11
- Fasta3 calculates statistical parameters from unrelated sequences during databases search; Blast2 calculates parameters for the scoring matrix and gap penalty combination and uses in database search. Other versions of Blast calculate significance of matching regions rather than of a local alignment with gaps.

- Low complexity regions can give high scoring matches with sequences that are not related to the query sequence. Fasta3 does not remove low complexity regions - Blast2 does. Fasta3 provides the program Prss3 to shuffle one sequence by individual amino acids or by a window of amino acids. Scores based on low complexity will then score with less significance against this background.

Databases

Some of the databases available for BLAST searching (at NCBI) are:

Peptide (protein) Sequence Databases

nr = All non-redundant GenBank CDS translations+PDB+SwissProt+PIR

month = All new or revised GenBank CDS translation+PDB+SwissProt+PIR released in the last 30 days.

swissprot = The SWISS-PROT protein sequence database

yeast = Yeast (Saccharomyces cerevisiae) protein sequences.

pdb = Sequences derived from the 3-dimensional structure Brookhaven Protein Data Bank

kabat = Kabat's database of sequences of immunological interest

alu = Translations of select Alu repeats

Nucleotide Sequence Databases

nr = All Non-redundant GenBank+EMBL+DDBJ+PDB sequences (but no EST's or STS's)

month = All new or revised GenBank+EMBL+DDBJ+PDB sequences released in the last 30 days.

dbest = Expressed Sequence Tags dbsts = Sequence Tagged Sites

yeast = Yeast (Saccharomyces cerevisiae) genomic nucleotide sequences

pdb = Nucleotide sequences derived from 3-dimensional protein structures in the Brookhaven Protein Data Bank

kabat = Kabat's database of sequences of immunological interest

vector = Vector subset of GenBank

mito = Database of mitochondrial sequences

alu = Select Alu repeats

epd = Eukaryotic Promoter Database

gss =Genome Survey Sequence, includes single-pass genomic data, exon-trapped sequences, and Alu PCR sequences.

11.4. FILTERING AND GAPPED BLAST

Filtering and related definitions

1. Filter is the process of removing the undesired sequences from the query sequence prior to the search
2. Masking is the process to "mark" regions of the query sequence so that they will be skipped in the search. GCG programs can do this process.

3. Annotation is the process of adding comments to a "feature table" associated with the query sequence; information from this feature table then dictate to the search program which regions of the query sequence to skip.

Types of sequences one may wish to filter

1. Vector Sequences: these often end up in sequences as a result of sequencing procedures in the lab.
2. Repeated Sequences: low c_ot DNA sequences, highly repetitive sequences, VNTRs (variable Number of Tandem Repeats), STRs (Short Tandem Repeats) etc.
3. Low information content sequences: runs of a single amino acid or few amino acids; runs of pyrimidines or purines in DNA etc.
4. Structural Nucleic Acid sequences: DNA sequences that encode structural RNAs (tRNA, rRNA, snRNA, etc) that do not encode proteins.

Filtering in BLAST

One of the parameters for the BLAST programs is the FILTER parameter. This parameter attempts to handle two cases that yield HSPs which are real but which are usually non-interesting. These two cases are: Direct repeats and Low information content sequences.

The SEG filter is used for Low Information Content or Low Complexity Sequences. A similar filter called Dust is used for DNA sequences specifically. In SEQ, the complexity K for each Word w or "window" of the sequence is defined as:

$$K_w = (1 / L) \log_A (L! / PI[n_i!])$$

where L is the window size (length of word w), PI means the product of each of the n_i factorials, the n_i in turn are the number of each residue present in a Window or Word, and A is the size of the residue alphabet (A = 4 for DNA, A = 20 for proteins). The expression L! / PI[n_i!] is sometimes called (Omega)i.

Examples for DNA sequences

1. The word AAAA ... one of 4 possible "least complex" DNA words (same base at each position):
   L = 4; L! = 4 x 3 x 2 x 1 = 24; $n_G = 0$, $n_A = 4$, $n_T = 0$, $n_C = 0$;
   Thus: PI[n_i!] = 4!0!0!0! = 4 x 3 x 2 x 1 x 1 x 1 x 1 = 24
   And: $K_w = (1/4) \log_4 (24 / 24) = (1/4) \log_4 1 = 0$

2. The word GATC ... one of 24 "most complex" DNA words (different base at each position):
   L = 4; L! = 4 x 3 x 2 x 1 = 24; $n_G = 1$, $n_A = 1$, $n_T = 1$, $n_C = 1$;
   Thus: PI[n_i!] = 1!1!1!1! = 1 x 1 x 1 x 1 = 1
   And: $K_w = (1/4) \log_4 (24 / 1) = (1/4) \log_4 24 = 2.292 / 4 = 0.573$

3. The word GATT ... one of many words of intermediate complexity:
   L = 4; L! = 4 x 3 x 2 x 1 = 24; $n_G = 1$, $n_A = 1$, $n_T = 2$, $n_C = 0$;
   Thus: PI[n_i!] = 1!1!2!0! = 1 x 1 x 2 x 1 x 1 = 2
   And: $K_w = (1/4) \log_4 (24 / 2) = (1/4) \log_4 12 = 1.792 / 4 = 0.448$

SEQ uses an algorithm that requires that given Words must have a complexity above some value. Direct repeats will appear in Dot Plots as "hits" in diagonals that parallel the main diagonal, but are displaced to one side or the other. The lengths of these "hits" is the same as the length of the repeats.In the XNU filter, only HSPs within a bandwidth of 10 of the main diagonal are reported.

Gapped-BLAST

Gapped BLAST is also known as BLAST 2.0. It represents BLAST plus a new heuristic for gapped alignments. It runs approximately 3-fold faster than BLAST.

The various programs available are as follows:

Query	Sequence	Database
BLASTN	DNA	DNA
BLASTP	Protein	Protein
BLASTX	DNA	Protein
TBLASTN	Protein	DNA

Translates of the query seq in each of the 6 reading frames are used in BLAST 2.0. Like TFASTA, each database entry is translated into its 6 reading frames.

Major parameters for using BLAST 2.0 are as follows:

DATALIB: Database, or group of databases, chosen

MATRIX: Distance Matrix used: BLO62 (default), PAM40, PAM120, PAM250

CUTOFF: Score S_G, chosen to limit Gapped Extensions to about 2% of the database entries

EXPECT: Number of Random Hits expected to be found (default = 10) E-value

FILTER: Option to use one of two "filters", to ignor highly repeated sequences or sequences of "low information content", e.g. runs of a given amino acid.

Output of BLAST 2.0 is as follows:

1. Information on Query sequence and Databases used
2. Histogram like the FASTA histogram
3. Descriptions (default = 100) of Hits found in the Databases
4. Scores in bits- E-value: number of hits expected to be reported by chance.
5. Alignments found (default = 50)
6. Parameters used in the BLAST search

Need for BLAST improvements:

1. Tradeoff between speed and sensitivity via word parameter T. The higher the threshold T, the faster the speed of the run. But also implies lower sensitivity in finding all true homologues - it would miss out the weak similarities.
2. Speed is also inversely proportional to the product of the length of the input sequence and size of database. This has significant implications as databases continue to increase in size exponentially.

Objective of modifications are to improve speed and maintain (or improve) sensitivity.

Three major refinements have been included :

1. Two-Hit
2. Non-Gapped Extension
3. Gapped Alignment

1. Modified procedure for extension of Word Pairs

The original "extension of Word Pairs" procedure in BLAST is the main time-consuming step. The 'Two-hit' method has the following characteristics:

   a. It requires two non-overlapping Word Pairs on same diagonal (no gaps) within distance A of each other. Based on the observation that HSPs are much longer than Word Pairs - identify best HSP in nearly all cases has at least two Word Pairs.

   b. Decrease T to achieve comparable sensitivity.

2. Do Non-Gapped Extension

   a. Do this only for the cases where two diagonal "Word Pairs" are within distance A of each other

   b. Find only the best Non-Gapped Extension. This local region consists of "Two Word Pairs + Non-Gapped (Ungapped) Extension".

   c. Proceed with Step 3(the Gapped Alignment), only if the Score S of the Ungapped Extension is above some Cutoff Score S_G

3. Generate Gapped Alignments

Original BLAST calculates combined P(N) probability for all local regions found. Here, we have one "local region", which is the best of the Non-Gapped Extensions.

   If this best of the Non-Gapped Extensions has a Score S greater than the Cutoff S_G, then:

   a. Apply Dynamic Programming to extend the Non-Gapped Extension in both directions.

   b. In this Dynamic Programming alignment, consider only alignments that drop the score no more than an amount.X_G below the best score seen. This limits the region of the two sequences over which the dynamic programming alignment is done

   c. Choose the score S_G so as to limit Gapped Extensions to about 2% of the database entries.

The 'Two-Hit' Method : Central BLAST

Any HSP will contain at least one "Word Pair". However, most HSPs contain more than one Word Pairs. This is because HSPs are normally long compared with Word Pairs.

Algorithm

   1. Find all Word Pairs satisfying w and T criteria.

   2. Choose a Distance A, for example, A = 40 residue

   3. Extend a Word Pair ONLY IF a second Word Pair is on the same Diagonal within this distance A

Diagonal

The Diagonal of a dot plot is defined by position x_1 in one sequence and x_2 in the other sequence such that the DIFFERENCE $x_1 - x_2$ is constant. Similarly here, the diagonal for the two words in a Word Pair, one word from the query sequence starting at position x_1 and the other word from a database entry starting at position x_2, is defined by all Word Pairs where $x_1 - x_2$ is constant. This requirement for the presence of twoWord Pairs before an Extension is performed decreases computation time some 2- to 3-fold.

Modeling Experiments using BLAST statistics and 100,000 HSPs have shown that the 2-hit method is somewhat more sensitive than the original BLAST algorithm for HSP scores of 33 or higher (correct range for protein homologues):

Summary of Gapped Alignment Procedure

Gapped extension includes 5 HSPs, with E-value of 0.5. Original BLAST finds only 2 of these, with combined E-value of 31. Dynamic Programming used for Gapped extension begins with a seed pair of aligned residues and proceeds in both directions, using all diagonals such that the alignment score does not fall below the best alignment score yet found by more than X_G units. X_G default is set at 40. The "Gap Cost" is $10 + k$, where k is the length of the gap. Choice of "Seed Pair" for extension is based on the central residue pair in the 11-mer of the HSP with highest Alignment Score.

11.5 PSI-BLAST

Introduction

Psi-blast is an implementation of Blast for finding protein families. It is a method of finding related sequences in a database that is just as powerful as sequence-by-sequence comparison is to use a profile of a group of sequences for the search. Instead of using a single amino acid at a given position in the query sequence, it is better to use a combination of amino acids known to be present at the same position in that protein and related ones. The search of sequence databases will thereby be expanded to include additional related sequences that might otherwise be missed. The major difficulty with such an expanded search is that an alignment of related sequences must already be available in order to know the variations at each position in the query sequence. An extension of Blast called position-specific-iterated blast or Psi-blast has been designed to provide information on this variation starting with a Blast search by a single query sequence.

The method used by Psi-blast involves a series of repeated steps or iterations as follows:

1. A database search of a protein sequence database is performed using a query sequence.
2. The results of the search are presented and can be assessed visually to see if any database sequences that are significantly related to the query sequence are present.
3. If such is the case, user decides to go through another iteration of the search.
4. The high scoring sequence matches found in the first step are aligned and from the alignment a sequence motif which indicates the variations at each aligned position is produced. The database is then searched with this motif. The search has thus been expanded to include sequences that match the variations found in the motif at each sequence position.
5. The results are again displayed, indicating any newly discovered sequences that are significantly related to the motif sequences in addition to those found in the previous iteration.
6. Again, an opportunity is given to go through another iteration of the program, but this time including any newly recruited sequences to refine the motif. In this fashion, a new family of sequences that are significantly similar to the original query sequence can be found.

It is noteworthy that this new method was made possible by the development of the gapped blast program which increased the speed of the Blast algorithm by over one-half so that more sophisticated search routines of Psi-blast could be added without an overall loss of speed. Psi-blast may not be as sensitive as other motif generating and searching programs but the simplicity and ease-of-use of this program are very attractive options for exploring protein family relationships. In a comparison of the ability of Psi-blast with the Smith-Waterman program Ssearch to identify members of 11 protein families defined by sequence similarity, Psi-blast found more sequences, in some case many-fold more sequences, than Ssearch but at a 40-fold greater speed.

Searching motifs with PSI-BLAST

Psi-blast is a blast program that will search a protein sequence database with a query sequence motif, a matrix with rows representing sequence positions and columns representing variations in that position. The motif represents the observed variations in the alignment of a set of related proteins. Psi-blast has been engineered to find database matches almost as rapidly as blastp finds matches to a query sequence. There are some differences between the motifs found by Psi-blast. First, the motif covers the entire sequence length whereas motifs usually cover only a short stretch of the sequences. Second, the same gap penalties are used throughout the procedure and there is no position specific penalty as in other programs. Third, each subsequent motif is based on using the query sequence as a master template for producing a multiple sequence alignment of the same length as the query sequence. Columns in the alignment involve varying numbers of sequences depending on the extent of the local alignment of each sequence with the query, and columns with gaps in the query sequence are ignored. Sequences >98% similar to the query are not included in order to avoid biasing the motif. Thus, the alignment is a compilation of the pairwise alignments of each matching database sequence with the query sequence and is not a true multiple sequence alignment.

Problems with PSI-BLAST Approach

The main difficulty with searching for subtle sequence relationships based on similarity is determining the significance of the motifs that are found. Such similarities may be evidence of structural or evolutionary relationships but they could also be due to matching of random variations that have no common origin or function. Protein structures are in general comprised of a tightly packed core and outside loops. Amino acid substitutions within the core are common but only certain substitutions will work at a given amino acid position in a given structure. Thus, sequence similarity is not usually a good indicator of structural similarity and the motifs found need to be carefully evaluated before any firm conclusions are drawn.

Another difficulty with the Psi-Blast approach is that the procedure follows a "greedy algorithm". With greedy algorithm, once additional sequences which match the query are found, then these newly found sequences influence the finding of more sequences like themselves, and so on. If a different query sequence were initially used, a different group with the possible overlaps with the first may be found. Thus, there is no guarantee that the group finally discovered authentically represents a functional group.

Position Specific Scoring Matrices

Once the motif has been found, the frequencies of amino acids in each column are adjusted by using the following:
1. Weighting the sequences to reduce the influence of the more alike sequences.
2. Adding more counts (pseudocounts) representing other amino acid substitutions found among the observed types in to increase the statistical power of the matrix.

These procedures are called Position Specific Scoring Matrices (PSSM). The resulting scores in each column of the scoring matrix are scaled using the same scaling factor 1 as the Blosum62 scoring matrix in order that a threshold value T for HSP's and other statistical parameters used by Blastp may also be used by Psi-blast. At each iteration, previously matched sequences with an E value less than 0.001 are used to produce the next motif, but this value may also be changed.

Example of Psi-blast search

The sequence of the Arabidopsis XPF DNA repair gene was used to query the Swiss-Prot database, with an E setting of 0.01, requesting 10 descriptions and alignments with otherwise the recommended default program settings. The initial iteration found 3 matching sequences, and these were used to enter iteration 1. Iteration 1 did not produce any additional matches at the chosen level of significance, and the program indicated that the search had converged with no more sequences at the chosen level of significance. Therefore, for iteration 2, the sequences scoring worse than the threshold were used. Since only those lower scoring sequences that have an alignment with the query could influence the result, this option could potentially find additional sequences. A yeast transport protein was then reported. With another iteration using the 4 sequences above threshold, another set of sequences was now pulled into the high scoring group. This search therefore revealed that the Swiss-prot database has 3 other sequences strongly related to the query sequence but that other sequences of lower scoring similarity were also present.

Psi-blast initial iteration

sp|Q92889|XPF_HUMAN DNA-REPAIR PROTEIN COMPLEMENTING XP-F CELL ...   504   e-142

sp|P06777|RAD1_YEAST DNA REPAIR PROTEIN RAD1   300   6e-81

sp|P36617|RA16_SCHPO DNA REPAIR PROTEIN RAD16   231   3e-60

Psi-blast iteration 1

with sequences scoring better than E threshhold

Converged

sp|Q92889|XPF_HUMAN DNA-REPAIR PROTEIN COMPLEMENTING XP-F CELL ...   1020   0.0

sp|P06777|RAD1_YEAST DNA REPAIR PROTEIN RAD1   953   0.0

sp|P36617|RA16_SCHPO DNA REPAIR PROTEIN RAD16   897   0.0

Psi-blast iteration 2

with sequences scoring worse than E threshhold

sp|Q92889|XPF_HUMAN DNA-REPAIR PROTEIN COMPLEMENTING XP-F CELL ...   1020   0.0

sp|P06777|RAD1_YEAST DNA REPAIR PROTEIN RAD1   967   0.0

sp|P36617|RA16_SCHPO DNA REPAIR PROTEIN RAD16   939   0.0

sp|P25386|USO1_YEAST INTRACELLULAR PROTEIN TRANSPORT PROTEIN USO1   53   3e-06

Psi-blast iteration 3

with sequences scoring better than E threshhold

sp|Q92889|XPF_HUMAN DNA-REPAIR PROTEIN COMPLEMENTING XP-F CELL ...   1007   0.0

sp|P06777|RAD1_YEAST DNA REPAIR PROTEIN RAD1   950   0.0

sp|P36617|RA16_SCHPO DNA REPAIR PROTEIN RAD16   884   0.0

sp|P25386|USO1_YEAST INTRACELLULAR PROTEIN TRANSPORT PROTEIN USO1   294   5e-79

sp|Q08696|MST2_DROHY AXONEME-ASSOCIATED PROTEIN MST101(2)   52   4e-06

sp|Q62209|SCP1_MOUSE SYNAPTONEMAL COMPLEX PROTEIN 1 (SCP-1 PROT...   49   5e-05

sp|Q03410|SCP1_RAT SYNAPTONEMAL COMPLEX PROTEIN 1 (SCP-1 PROTEIN)   49   5e-05

sp|Q02224|CENE_HUMAN CENTROMERIC PROTEIN E (CENP-E PROTEIN)   45   5e-04

11.6. COMPARISON OF RUNNING TIME FOR VARIOUS PROGRAMS

Th e comparison of running time for various programs is shown below. This is based on the number of SWISS-PROT sequences yielding alignments with E-value <=0.01. To score and evaluate the significance of the alignments found, the original BLAST program uses BLOSUM-62 substitution scores and sum-statistics. The Smith-Waterman and gapped BLAST programs use BLOSUM-62 substitutions scores, 10+k gap costs and with the experimentally determined parameters $l_g = 0.255$ and $K_g = 0.035$. The normalised running times are the mean ratio of program running time to that of the original BLAST. The time for PSI-BLAST includes the time for the initial BLAST search. (Only one iteration is executed)

Protein family	Query	Smith-Waterman	BLAST	Gapped BLAST	PSI-BLAST
Serine protease	P00762	275	273	275	286
Serine protease inhibitor	P01008	108	105	108	111
Ras	P01111	255	249	252	375
Globin	P02232	28	26	28	623
Hemaglutinnin	P03435	128	114	128	130
Interferon a	P05013	53	53	53	53
Alcohol dehydrogenase	P07327	138	128	137	160
Cytochrome 450	P10635	211	197	211	224
Glutathione transferase	P14042	83	79	81	142
H-transporting ATP synthase	P20705	198	191	197	207
Normalised running time		36	1.0	0.34	0.87

12

Alignment of Multiple Sequences

12.1. INTRODUCTION

What is MSA

Multiple sequence alignment (MSA) is a tool to determine levels of homology, and hence relatedness, between members of a series of globally related sequences. While homologs are genes or proteins with the same function in different species and orthologs are related, but diverged genes or proteins resulting from gene duplication in the same species or functionally diverged genes or proteins from different species. MSA is very important for finding similar domains in a set of sequences and for doing phylogenetic analysis. (Phylogenetic analysis is dealt with in a separate chapter).

Motivation for MSA

What is the need for MSA? The answer lies in the limitations of pair-wise comparison tools. For many genes a simple database search will reveal a whole number of homologous sequences. However, this output given by pair-wise comparisons do not readily show positions that are conserved among a whole set of sequences and tend to miss subtle similarities that become visible when observed simultaneously among many sequences. If we have to find the evolution and the sequence conservation in such a group, we need to simultaneously compare several sequences. This is where MSA tools become very useful.

How is MSA done

The basic process is the same as pair-wise comparison. If one were to do it manually, it would mean arranging a set of sequences in a scheme where positions believed to be homologous are written in a common column. Like in a pair-wise alignment, when a sequence does not possess an amino acid in a particular position this is again denoted by a dash. Similarly, there are conventions regarding the scoring of a multiple alignment. The full set of optimal pair-wise alignments among a given set of sequences will generally over-determine the multiple alignment. To assemble a multiple alignment from pair-wise alignments, we put together pair-wise alignments as long as no new pair-wise alignment is included to a sequence which is already part the multiple alignment. In particular, pair-wise alignments can be merged when they align one sequence to all others, when a linear order of the given sequence is maintained, or when sequences pairs with pair-wise alignments form a tree. While all these schemes allow for the ready definition of algorithms that output multiple aligned sequences, they do not include any information stemming from the simultaneous analysis of several sequences.

Manual process cannot obviously done for large problems. The alternative approach is to generalize the dynamic programming optimization procedure applied for pair-wise alignment to the delineation of a multiple alignment that maximizes a score. The algorithm used is a generalization of the global alignment algorithm. This is easy to see, in particular, for the case of column-oriented scoring function avoiding gap penalty in favor of the simpler linear one. With this scoring, the arrangement of gaps and letters in a column can be represented by a Boolean vector indicating which sequences contain a gap in a particular column. Given the letters that are being compared, one needs to evaluate the scores for all these arrangements. However, the computational complexity of this algorithm is high: for n sequences it is proportional to 2n times the product of the lengths of all sequences.

Hence the DP algorithm in practice this algorithm can only be run for a small number of sequences. The real-life approach is use heuristics. There are software tools to compare three sequences with this algorithm that additionally implements a space-saving technique. For more than three sequences algorithms have been developed that aim at reducing the search space while still optimizing the given scoring function. These approaches are, however, dependent on the number of sequences to be aligned.

The approach to solve this problem is to reduce the multiple alignment problems to an iterated application of the pair-wise alignment algorithm. However, in doing so, one also aims at drawing on the increased amount of information contained in a set of sequences. A completely different approach of using profiles is used. Instead of simply merging pair-wise alignments of sequences, the notion of a profile is used to grasp the conservation patterns within subgroups of sequences. A profile is essentially a representation of an already computed multiple alignment of a subgroup. This alignment is kept constant for the remaining computation. Other sequences or other profiles can be compared to a given profile based on a generalize]d scoring scheme defined for this purpose.

Bioinformatics approaches to solving MSA problems

While the heuristics approach and DP algorithms are theoretically possible, the practical applications are built using profile approach, clustering and phylogenetic trees and statistical methods.

Profile scoring schemes respect conservation patterns. Given a profile and a single sequence, the two can be aligned using the basic dynamic programming algorithm together with the accompanying scoring scheme. The result will be an alignment between the two that can readily be converted into a multiple alignment now comprising the sequences underlying the profile plus the new one. Likewise, two profiles can be aligned with each other resulting in a multiple alignment containing all sequences from both profiles. With these tools various multiple alignment strategies can be implemented. Most commonly, a hierarchical tree is generated for the given sequences, which is then used as a guide for iterative profile construction and alignment.

Dialign uses clustering approach. This is different in that it aims at the delineation of regions of similarity among the given sequences. Since iterative profile alignment tends to be guided by a hierarchical tree, this step of the computation also influences the final result. Usually this tree is computed based on pair-wise comparisons and the resulting scores. Subsequently this score matrix is used as input to a clustering procedure like single linkage clustering or UPGMA. However, it is well understood that in an evolutionary sense such a hierarchic clustering does not necessarily result in a biologically valid tree. Thus, when allowing this tree to determine the multiple alignment there is the danger of directing further evolutionary analysis of this alignment into the wrong direction. Consequently, the question has arisen of a common formulation of evolutionary reconstruction and multiple sequence alignment.

The statistical methods are different in approach and include Gibbs sampling, expectation maximization and hidden Markov models.

Global and Local MSA

Global and local alignments have been discussed for pair-wise comparisons. The corresponding concept for MSA is given in the Fig. 12.1.

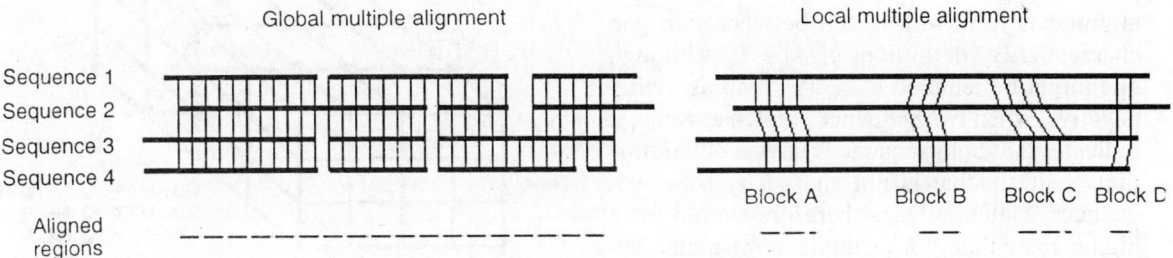

Fig. 12.1. Global and Local MSA

12.2. TOOLS FOR MSA

The following methods are discussed :
1. Sum-of-pairs method
2. Star alignment
3. Two-step method (Clustal and Pileup approaches)
4. Automated tools (Macaw, Meme etc.)

Sum-of-pairs method

DP approach is similar to that of DP for two sequences. However, instead of aligning two sequences at a time with dynamic programming, one needs to align three or more simultaneously. This is a little harder to visualise than for the two sequences case, but essentially one can imagine for 3 sequences lying along the edges of a cube and then filling up the cube with numbers which represent the matches with each sequence, plus allowing for deletions. For more sequences, more than 3 dimensions are needed. This approach is cumbersome and hence not practical.

Example - SP method

An optimal multiple alignment depends in all possible pairwise comparisons of all amino acids in each protein at each position. It is possible to extend the dynamic programming algorithm for pairwise comparisons from the special case of k=2 sequences to the more general case of k=n sequences.

Scoring is used for these comparisons. Consider the alignment

M1	Q	P	I	L	L	L
M2	L	R	-	L	L	-
M3	K	-	I	L	L	L
M4	P	P	V	L	I	L

The sum-of-pairs (SP) function scores each position in the protein, that is, each column, as the sum of the pairwise scores. For k sequences, there are k(k-1)/2 unique pairwise comparisons, excluding self comparisons. For example, in column 3, the score would be

SP-score(I,-,I,V) = p(I,-) + p(I,I) + p(I,V) + p(-,I) + p(-,V) + p(I,V)

where p(a,b) is the pairwise score of two amino acids. This function is valid regardless of the order of sequences in the alignment. Unlike pairwise alignments, it is legitimate in multiple alignments to have a match between two gap characters. By definition, p(-,-) = 0. Although one might be tempted to score a gap as highly negative, when two sequences match at a gap, it indicates that both sequences have a deletion at that position, that is not shared by other sequences. Matching gaps therefore should get a higher score than, for example, a mismatch between two very different amino acids, such as Proline and Lysine.

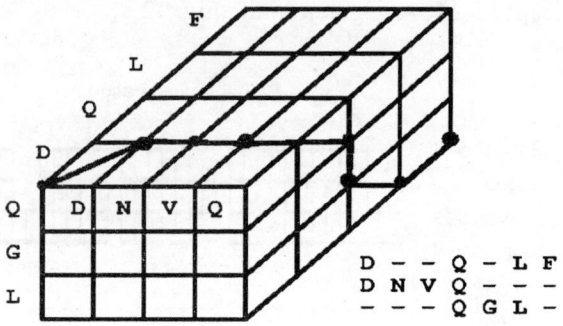

Fig. 12.2. Optimal alignment between k=3 sequences

Generalizing the pairwise dynamic programming algorithm to k sequences is, in essence, doing an alignment in k dimensions. For example, an optimal alignment between k=3 sequences could be visualized in 3 dimensions (Fig. 12.2):

The problem with the dynamic programming algorithm is size and speed. To start with, where k sequences of length n are compared, the storage required for the alignment matrix is $O(n^k)$. For 20 sequences of 500 amino acids each, it would require 500^{20} units of storage (e.g. bytes).

Recall that in a pairwise comparison, calculation of the similarity score in a given cell of the array For each cell in the 2-dimensional array the score was dependent on the 3 preceding adjacent cells. In a k-dimensional array, there are 2^k-1 preceding cells. (This makes sense: for k=2 ie. a pairwise comparison, 2^2-1 = 3). Finally, for each column, there are k(k-1)/2 pairwise comparisons. In summary, the time required for a truly exhaustive multiple alignment, using the most straightforward approach, is $O(k^2 2^k n^k)$.

Although some methods have introduced great efficiencies that bring global dynamic programming to a level that is practical for a handful of sequences, more efficient approximate methods are needed for typical alignment problems.

PIMA - pattern-induced multiple alignment ("Star Alignment")

Smith and Smith (1990) introduced a scoring method that progressively weights matches between classes of amino acids, according to chemical properties.

Example - Star alignment

For an alignment among 5 sequences:

S1	T	C	Y	G	I	F	V	L		
S2	T	C		G	I	F	V	L		
S3	S	C	Y	G	I	F	V	L	S	G
S4	T	C	F	G	I	F	V	L		
S5	A	C		G	I	F	V	L	S	G

All pairwise comparisons are performed, resulting in a matrix of scores.

	S1	S2	S3	S4	S5
S1		26	38	38	26
S2	26		26	26	32
S3	38	26		36	36
S4	38	26	36		26
S5	26	32	36	26	

The most closely-related pair of sequences is aligned, in this case S1 and S3 (S1 and S4 have the same score, so they could also be used as the first pair.)

S1	T	C	Y	G	I	F	V	L	-	-
S3	S	C	Y	G	I	F	V	L	S	G

S4 is added next:

S1	T	C	Y	G	I	F	V	L	-	-
S3	S	C	Y	G	I	F	V	L	S	G
S4	T	C	F	G	I	F	V	L	-	-

then S2

S1	T	C	Y	G	I	F	V	L	-	-
S3	S	C	Y	G	I	F	V	L	S	G
S4	T	C	F	G	I	F	V	L	-	-
S2	T	C	-	G	I	F	V	L	-	-

and finally S5

S1	T	C	Y	G	I	F	V	L	-	-
S3	S	C	Y	G	I	F	V	L	S	G
S4	T	C	F	G	I	F	V	L	-	-
S2	T	C	-	G	I	F	V	L	-	-
S5	A	C	G	I	F	V	L	S	G	-

The alignment can be thought of as occurring in a "star" configuration, where the sequence with the greatest total similarity to the others is at the center, and the rays of the star represent the pairwise distances to the remaining sequences. Each time a sequence is added, gaps are inserted in the either in the newly added sequence, or in the entire alignment, to optimize alignment. If you think of the addition step as a simple pairwise alignment between the current alignment and the next sequence, it is easy to see why this algorithm is fast. Its speed is roughly $O(kn^2 + k^2l)$ where l is an upper bound on alignment lengths.

One observation to make is the "once a gap always a gap" rule. That is, once a gap is entered into the alignment, it will always remain in that alignment, and all sequences added subsequently will also receive that gap.

Two Step Method

The problem is broken down into two steps:

1. Find which sequences are most similar by comparing all combinations of the sequences using the dynamic programming method to obtain similarity scores.
2. The most similar sequences are again locally aligned with dynamic programming. A consensus sequence is derived from each of these comparisons, the most alike consensus sequences are aligned with each other or with other sequences which are similar to them, and finally all the sequences are joined using the consensus sequences as a guide. The alignment obtained will favor the most alike sequences.

Examples of this method are the CLUSTAL program, and the GCG program PILEUP. CLUSTAL is recommended for local alignments. CLUSTAL also varies the gap penalties so that they are higher where the sequences are more alike. Thus, conserved regions are more likely to be found. PILEUP is a global alignment program and should only be used for an alike set of sequences with of the same approximate length. As with alignment of sequence pairs, the scoring matrix and gap penalty must be chosen carefully.

CLUSTAL - Neighbor-Joining Trees

The CLUSTAL family of program works on the hypothesis that sequences in an alignment will reflect their evolutionary history. That is, if one were to go from one sequence to the next most-closely related one, one would visit all nodes on the phylogenetic tree describing how these sequences evolved.

CLUSTAL begins by constructing a distance matrix, representing the sequence distances for each pairwise comparison between proteins. Next a phylogenetic tree is built using the Neighbor-Joining method (Fig. 12.3). Using this tree as a guide, sequences, again beginning with the most closely-related pair, are sequentially added to the alignment. Again, as in the star alignment, once a gap always a gap. The efficiency of a tree alignment is comparable to that of a star alignment.

The sequences to be aligned are the end nodes, the "leaves" of the tree. A subtle feature that distinguishes tree alignments from star alignments is that distances, between nodes (ie. between sequences) are calculated, rather than similarities. Distances are the amount subtracted from a score, due to amino acid substitutions, when amino acid sequence is transformed into another.

Pileup

Pileup creates multiple sequence alignment from a group of related sequences using progressive, pairwise alignment method of Feng and Doolittle. It can also plot a tree showing the clustering relationships used to create the alignment.

The input file for Pileup is a list of sequence file names or sequence accession numbers in the database. Pileup follows the general clustering strategy called UPGMA that stands for Unweighted Pair-Group Method using Arithmetic average. The clustering algorithm it uses initializes the clusters one sequence each, and iteratively constructs larger clusters. In each iteration, it merges the two clusters whose pairwise alignment distance is the smallest. Cluster pairwise alignment is a simple extension of sequence alignment: For a pairwise alignment of clusters of sequences, the comparison score between any two positions in those clusters is simply the arithmetic average of the scores for all possible symbol comparisons at those positions. When gaps are inserted into a cluster to produce an alignment, they are inserted at the same position in all of the sequences of the cluster. The full multiple alignment is obtained once all the sequences have been clustered into one cluster. This hierarchical clustering is naturally described by a dendrogram, which Pileup can plot.

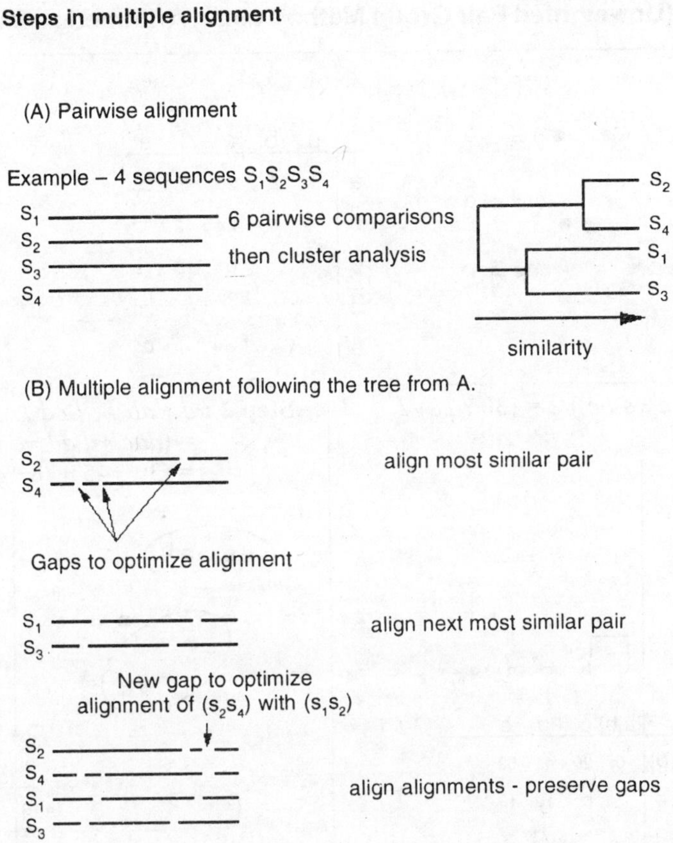

Steps in multiple alignment

(A) Pairwise alignment

Example – 4 sequences $S_1S_2S_3S_4$

S_1 ——————— 6 pairwise comparisons

S_2 ———————

S_3 ———————   then cluster analysis

S_4 ———————

S_2

S_4

S_1

S_3

similarity

(B) Multiple alignment following the tree from A.

S_2 ——————— —

S_4 —— ——————   align most similar pair

Gaps to optimize alignment

S_1 —— ——————— ——

S_3 —— ———— ——— ——   align next most similar pair

New gap to optimize
alignment of (s_2s_4) with (s_1s_2)

S_2 ——————— —-—

S_4 —— —————— ——   align alignments - preserve gaps

S_1 —— ——————— ——

S_3 —— ———— ——— ——

Fig. 12.3. Multiple alignment method

Since the alignment is calculated on a progressive basis, the order of the initial sequences can affect the final alignment. In addition, anything that affects the calculation of the dendrogram such as different comparison matrixes or gap weights will also affect the multiple alignment. PILEUP has an option to output a figure of the dendrogram it created. It's usually a good idea to look at it, just to make sure that the order of alignment makes some sort of sense - it can help you catch misnamed sequences, for instance.

As a general rule, Pileup can align up to 500 sequences, with any single sequence in the final alignment restricted to a maximum length of 7000 characters (including gap characters inserted into the sequence by Pileup to create the alignment). However, the longer are the sequences in the alignment, the number of sequences Pileup can handle decreases.

PILEUP is very sensitive to gaps, so if a set of sequences are of different lengths, gaps will be added to the ends of all shorter sequences to make them equal to the longest one in the set. If one tries to align five 300 nucleotide EST's with a single 20,000 nucleotide cosmid, one is adding 5 X 19,700 gaps to the alignment - and PILEUP might crash. Instead, do a pairwise alignment between one of the ESTs and the cosmid (using GAP). Then, identify the region of similarity in the longer sequence and copy that short region to a new file. Next, align six 300 nucleotide sequences. If you are aligning a bunch of different proteins, and you know some regions are just not at all similar, cut those regions out before you do the alignment. If you are interested just in some particular repeat or motif, extract it from the original sequence as best you can and then do the alignment.

Illustration of UPGMA (Unweighted Pair Group Method using Arithmetic averages) (Fig. 12.4)

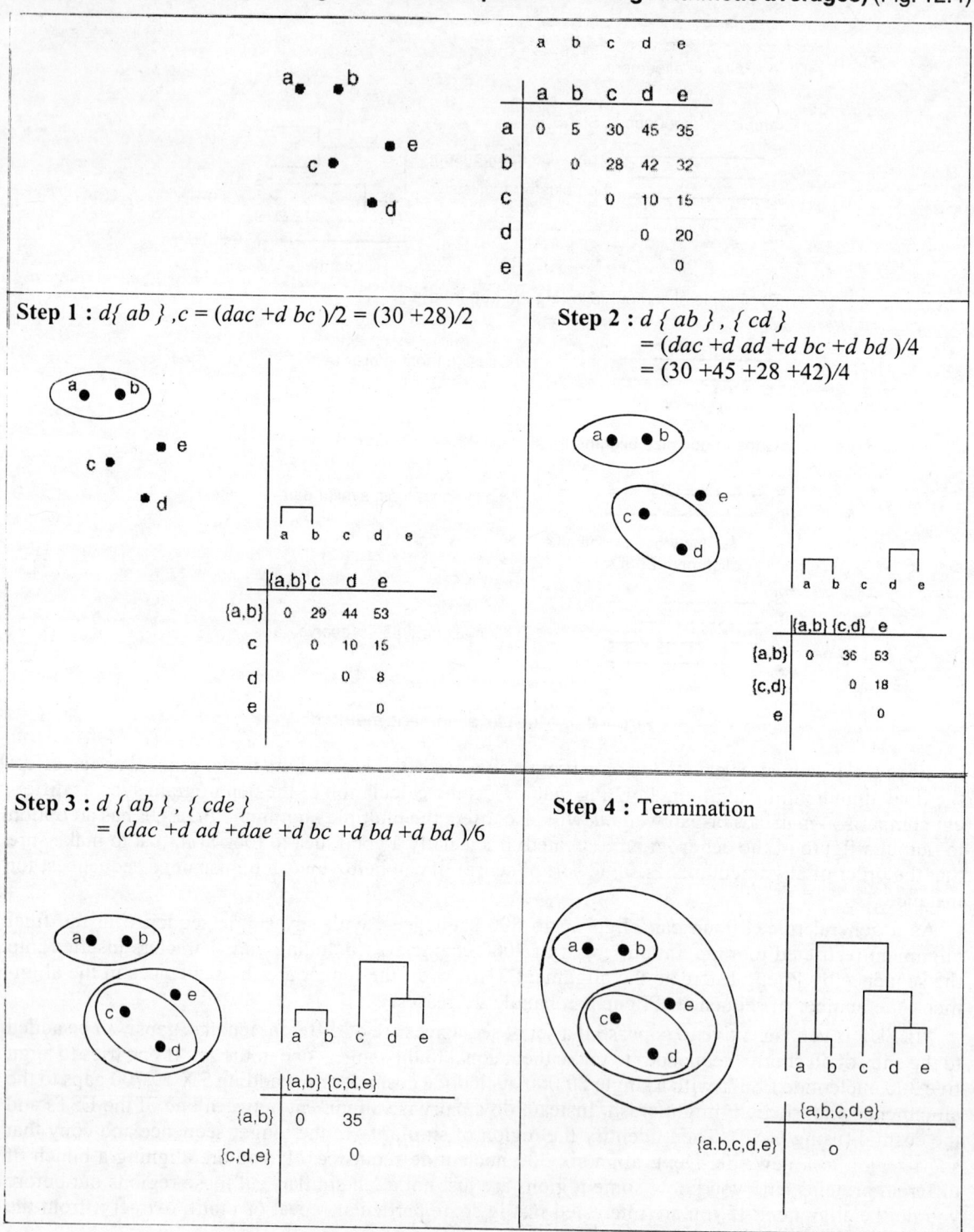

Fig. 12.4. Illustration of UPGMA procedure

ClustalW

As discussed above, this is a fully automatic program for global multiple alignment of DNA and protein sequences. The alignment is progressive and considers the sequence redundancy. Trees can also be calculated from multiple alignments. The program has some adjustable parameters with reasonable defaults. ClustalW improves the sensitivity of progressive multiple sequence alignment through sequence weighting, positions-specific gap penalties and weight matrix choice. It can create multiple alignments, manipulate existing alignments, perform profile analysis and create phylogenetic trees. Alignment can be constructed either slow but accurate or by fast but more approximated. The input file for clustalW is a file containing all sequences in one of the formats: NBRF/PIR, EMBL/SwissProt, Pearson (FastA), GDE, Clustal, GCG/MSF, RSF.

BlockMaker

It is a system for finding ungapped local multiple alignments (blocks) in protein sequences. Two sets of blocks, made by different alignment methods, are returned. The system is fully automatic and sets all parameters. The system assumes a model where all sequences contain all blocks and blocks are in the same order in all sequences. If some blocks are not found in some sequences than either these blocks or these sequences are not used in the alignment. The resulting blocks can be used with the BLIMPS, MAST and LAMA search programs. A consensus sequence (cobbler) for database searches, PCR primers, a tree and graphical representation of the blocks are also included in the output. BlockMaker is available on the WWW and on an e-mail server.

MEME

Meme is a program for local multiple alignments of DNA and protein sequences. The user must specify how many motifs are expected and how are they expected to occur. The returned motifs in each sequence do not overlap but do not necessarily have the same order. The program handles repeated motifs. Each block as a whole and each motif occurrence are given values to approximate their significance. MEME output can be used with the MAST search program. The program receives input through the WWW and returns it by e-mail. MEME is available for installation on UNIX systems.

MACAW

This is a program for semi-manual local multiple alignment of DNA and protein sequences. The user delimits the sequences and regions in which to search for blocks and decides which blocks to keep. Blocks can also edited or even defined by the user. The significance of each block is given a statistical value. The program has two different methods to search for blocks, the more accurate one is the Gibbs procedure. MACAW is available for Mac and Windows operating system.

12.3 CONSIDERATIONS IN CONDUCTING MSA

Analysing related proteins

As discussed before, homology or convergence can relate protein sequences. In both cases multiple alignment can be useful. Homologous proteins have a common ancestor and typically a common function. Converged proteins independently evolve to have common sequence features that typically preform a common function or have a common structure. Examples of convergence are the various hydrolase enzymes that cleave ester and polypeptide bonds by a common catalytic triad structure and the different archaeal, eubacterial and eukaryotic proteins that have a helix-turn-helix DNA binding domain.

Sequences either have or not have a common ancestor. Thus, sequences can either be homologous or not, but they cannot be "70% homologous". However, sequences can be similar by different degree and therefore be "70% similar". In addition, a statement like that is not informative unless we know what is the significance of this similarity, is it across the whole sequence/region or just in conserved regions, and by what method (program) was it found. Proteins that have significant sequence similarity are most often homologous.

Finding sequences of related proteins

Frequently we only have a single protein sequence. Querying sequence databases with the sequence we have can identify other members. The search should be repeated with every found member until no more sequences are found. A keyword search of the database can be done when only the protein name is known and when we wish to verify that all sequences were found. Scientific literature is also a source for identifying related sequences, especially very diverged members that might be missed in a single sequence search. Deciding if a sequence belongs to a group relies on the significance of its similarity to other members, on whatever is known about the protein, and most importantly on the researcher's knowledge of the proteins.

How many sequences are needed?

The more sequences we have the better. Multiple alignments of two and three sequences have limited usefulness. Try to use as many sequences as you have (but see below about the redundancy issue). If you think your sequences form sub-groups than try to also separately align these.

Excluding redundant sequences

Redundant sequences are separate sequences that are highly similar to each other. The extreme example is a set of identical sequences. Obviously only one sequence of the set should be used, the rest do not contribute to finding the alignment. Worse, the redundant sequences will bias the alignment toward their own features. Ideally all sequences in the aligned group should have a comparable similarity to each other. (This similarity can be assessed from the single sequence database searches.) A good rule of thumb in cases of varied similarities is to leave only a single sequence from each set with more than 70-80% intra-sequence similarity. This threshold could be modified for different cases and the results evaluated. Sequences removed from the alignment step can later be joined to the alignment if they have any difference in the aligned regions and if the resulting alignment can be sequence weighted.

Evaluating multiple alignments

Some programs give quantitative measures for the significance of the alignment. These are usually based on the chance occurrence of such alignments and depend on the size and composition of the aligned sequences. Empirical measures are also extremely useful for deciding the 'correctness' of the multiple alignment. Consistency is a powerful measure for correct multiple alignments. If the same alignment is found in the sequence-to-sequence searches and various multiple alignment methods it is most probably correct. One pitfall to avoid is biased sequence composition that may lead to trivial alignments.

Experimental data can be used in evaluating, and even constructing, multiple alignments. For example, if we know the catalytic site in the aligned proteins we expect the sites to be aligned together and may 'force' that alignment. Such manual alignments can serve as a seed to an alignment with more sequences. Local multiple alignments (blocks) from different programs can be joined or used together. Another approach is 'divide and conquer' (Fig. 12.5). Blocks present in all sequences divide them into separate parts, in each of which more blocks can be searched for.

12.4. APPLICATIONS OF MULTIPLE ALIGNMENT

The principal applications of MSA are as follows :

1. Alignment of amino acid and nucleotide sequences
2. Searching for sequences
3. PCR primer design

1. Aligning amino acids and nucleotides

MSA is the process of aligning 3 or more sequences with each other so as to bring as many similar sequence characters (nucleotides or amino acids) into register as possible. The resulting alignments can be used for two purposes:

1. To find regions of similar sequence in all of the sequences that define a conserved consensus pattern or domain
2. To use the aligned positions to try and derive the possible evolutionary relationships among the sequences, if the alignment is particularly strong,

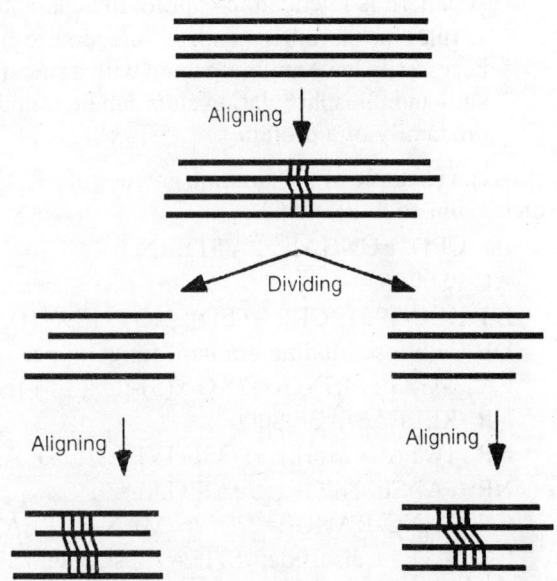

Fig. 12.5. Divide and conquer approach for MSA

When dealing with a sequence of unknown function, the presence of similar domains in several similar sequences implies a similar biochemical function or structural fold that may become the basis of further experimental investigation. A group of similar sequences may define a protein family that may share a common biochemical function or evolutionary origin.

Similar proteins have been organized by several methods into protein families. The major ones are as follows :

1. The sequence families used by PAM matrices used for sequence comparisons.
2. Patterns called MOTIFS used by PROSITE tool. This approach is based on identification of a large number of protein families called the PROSITE catalog and which defines the active sites of these proteins. These motifs may have more than one amino acid at each position and may include gaps. Once motifs have been defined, the sequence databases may be searched for additional sequence entries with the same motif.
3. BLOSUM approach involved the alignment all of these families, addition of more members from the databases, and then definition of conserved patterns of amino acids called blocks. Blocks are present in all members of the family and are approximately 4-60 amino acids long with no gaps or substitutions. The BLOSUM amino acid comparison tables were derived from these aligned blocks.

PROSITE

PROSITE aims at describing characteristic patterns for some domain families using regular expressions, and contains about 1400 patterns, rules and profile/matrices. Pfam is a more modern tool and has superseded PROSITE.

PROSITE makes a distinction between patterns and rules, which are both described by regular expressions:

- A pattern is intended to capture the characteristic fingerprint of a protein domain family.
- A rule, on the other hand, is intended to highlight features in a protein sequence that does not necessarily have anything to do with a specific protein family. For example, potential glycosylation sites and phosphorylation sites can be found in many protein sequences, and have little to do with the family of a protein.

As an example of the notation and use of PROSITE, let us use the PROS!TE pattern CBD_FUNGAL (accession code PS00562).

```
ID  CBD_FUNGAL; PATTERN.
AC PS00562;
DT DEC-1991 (CREATED); NOV-1997 (DATA UPDATE); JUL-1998 (INFO UPDATE).
DE Cellulose-binding domain, fungal type.
PA C-G-G-x(4,7)-G-x(3)-C-x(5)-C-x(3,5)-[NHG]-x-[FYWM]-x(2)-Q-C.
NR /RELEASE=38,80000;
NR /TOTAL=21(18); /POSITIVE=21(18); /UNKNOWN=0(0); /FALSE_POS=0(0);
NR /FALSE_NEG=1; /PARTIAL=0;
CC /TAXO-RANGE=??E??; /MAX-REPEAT=4;
CC /SITE=1,disulfide; /SITE=7,disulfide; /SITE=9,disulfide;
CC /SITE=16,disulfide;
DR Q00023, CEL1_AGABI, T; Q12714, GUN1_TRILO, T; P07981, GUN1_TRIRE, T;
DR P07982, GUN2_TRIRE, T; P43317, GUN5_TRIRE, T; P46236, GUNB_FUSOX, T;
DR P46239, GUNF_FUSOX, T; P45699, GUNK_FUSOX, T; P15828, GUX1_HUMGR, T;
DR Q06886, GUX1_PENJA, T; P13860, GUX1_PHACH, T; P00725, GUX1_TRIRE, T;
DR P19355, GUX1_TRIVI, T; Q92400, GUX2_AGABI, T; P07987, GUX2_TRIRE, T;
DR P49075, GUX3_AGABI, T; P46238, GUXC_FUSOX, T; P50272, PSBP_PORPU, T;
DR O59843, GUX1_ASPAC, N;
DO PDOC00486;
//
```

The central line is the PA line, which contains the pattern.

PA   C-G-G-x(4,7)-G-x(3)-C-x(5)-C-x(3,5)-[NHG]-x-[FYWM]-x(2)-Q-C.

This is what these elements mean:

- Each non-x letter defines one particular type of amino-acid residue in that position in the pattern. Here, we must have a tripeptide Cys-Gly-Gly in the beginning of the matching segment of a protein chain. The dash characters '-' add no information to the pattern, and are added to make the pattern slightly easier to read.
- The notation x(4,7) means that at least 4 and at most 7 residues of any type may occur at this position.

- The notation [NHG] means that any of the residues within the brackets may be chosen. One and only one such residue must be at this position.
- The notation x(2) means that exactly two residues of any type may occur at this position.
- The notation {GP} means that all residues except Gly and Pro are allowed in this position.
- The lines marked DR are the protein sequence entries in SWISS-PROT that match (character T) or do not match (character N) the regular expression. In this case, the protein GUX1_ASPAC does not match the PROSITE rule, although it should; it is a false negative.

2. Searching

Multiple alignments are powerful tools for identifying new members of the aligned group. It is possible to query databases of multiple alignments with single sequences and to query sequence databases with multiple alignments. It has been shown that such searches are more sensitive and selective than sequence-to-sequence searches. A simple 'hybrid' approach is to use a properly made consensus sequence.

Some of the automated tools are as follows:

Blimps

It is a program to query both protein and nucleotide sequence databases with protein blocks and vice versa. The queries are single sequences or blocks. The program is available on the WWW and by e-mail server for searching multiple alignment databases with single sequences. It is available for installation on UNIX systems.

MAST

This is a program to query sequence databases with blocks. Protein or nucleotide databases are queried with protein blocks. The query can be obtained from the MEME or BlockMaker programs. The query can be a single block or all the blocks of a protein family. The program receives input through the WWW and returns it by e-mail. It is available for installation on UNIX systems.

LAMA

A tool to search blocks databases with block queries. Queries can be obtained from the Blocks database, BlockMaker program or by reformatting multiple alignments. The program receives input through the WWW and returns it interactively or by e-mail.

3. PCR primer design

Design of degenerate PCR primers is emerging as a major use for multiple alignments. PCR can identify the sequence of a gene in genomic or other DNA from two short flanking segments (primers). Conserved sequence regions are (by definition) a good source for primer design. When designing primers the conservation of the regions, the degeneracy of the genetic code and parameters of the PCR reaction must be considered. The Blocks WWW server designs PCR primers for each family in the database, for sequence groups submitted to be aligned and for multiple alignment submitted to be reformatted. These primers are degenerate at the 3' end and consensus at the 5' end (codehop- COnsensus DEgenerate Hybrid Oligonucleotide Primers). The design is fully automatic but the user can set the requested Tm, genetic code and bias the primers toward some of the sequences. codehop primers were shown more effective than simple degenerate primers in various cases.

12.5. VIEWING MSA

Multiple alignments of many sequences and those with different sequence weights are difficult to visualize. Sequence logos are a graphical way for presenting multiple alignments.

```
ID    ADH_IRON_1; BLOCK
AC    BL00913C; distance from previous block=(56,76)
DE    Iron-containing alcohol dehydrogenases proteins.
BL    HHG motif; width=22; seqs=11; 99.5%=492; strength = 1428
ADHE_CLOAB  (720)  CHSMAIKLSSEHNIPSGIANAL    66
FUCO_ECOLI  (262)  VHGMAHPLGAFYNTPHGVANAI    44
GLDA_BACST  (259)  HNGFTALEGEIHHLTHGEKVAF   100
GLDA_ECOLI  (269)  VHNGLTAIPDAHHYYHGEKVAF   100
MEDH_BACMT  (259)  VHSISHQVGGVYKLQHGICNSV    78
ADH1_CLOAB  (258)  CHSMAHKTGAVFHIPHGCANAI    47
ADHE_ECOLI  (721)  CHSMAHKLGSQFHIPHGLANAL    47
ADH2_ZYMMO  (261)  VHAMAHQLGGYYNLPHGVCNAV    36
ADH4_YEAST  (263)  VHALAHQLGGFYHLPHGVCNAV    41
ADHA_CLOAB  (266)  CHPMEHELSAYYDITHGVGLAI    50
ADHB_CLOAB  (266)  VHLMEHELSAYYDITHGVGLAI    49
//
```

A graphical view of multiply aligned sequences is by a tree relating their sequence similarity. This is very useful when the aligned sequences are of several functional subtypes and we wish to know to which one does our sequence/s belong. A way to estimate the significance of a tree is by bootstrap values. Simply put, these values show how many times was each bifurcation (branching point) observed with different models of the input data. The higher the fraction of the bootstrap value (number of observations/ number of trials) the more confident we can be that the sequences emerging from that branch point cluster together. A tree is made from the three blocks in the iron containing alcohol dehydrogenases family. Bootstrap values are for 100 trials. The tree was calculated from the blocks with the ClustalW program and drawn with the TreeView program (Fig. 12.6).

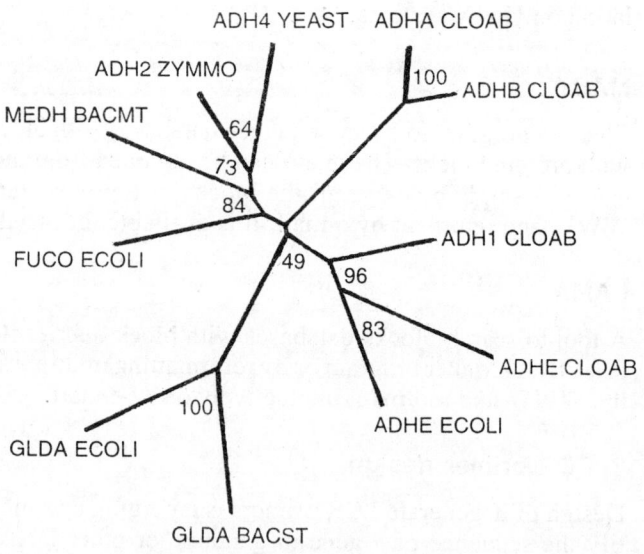

Fig. 12.6. Tree representation of MSA

12.6 SEQUENCE DETECTION EFFICIENCY MEASURES : SENSITIVITY AND SPECIFICITY

A regular expression can easily be designed that has 100% sensitivity: just use the wild card expression that matches anything: .* (dot, star). Everything will be identified as matching this expression, so all true positives will also be identified, and none will be left out (i.e. no false negatives). Conversely, it is easy to prepare a regexp that is 100% specific: just use a regexp that exactly matches one of the known members of the domain family. Only one member will be predicted, and no others, (i.e. no false positives).

Sequence patterns using regular expressions (such as PROSITE) have a problem with large-scale multiple alignments of divergent families. As more sequences are added, the probability that there will be even a few constant or even strongly conserved sites will diminish. There will always be an exception to the rule. In order to avoid missing a known member of a family, the regexp has to be made more general, but then the danger of including garbage increases. This is the typical sensitivity-specificity problem.

13

Phylogenetic Analysis

13.1. INTRODUCTION

Similarity searches and multiple alignments of sequences naturally leads to the question: "How are these sequences related?" And more generally: "How are the organisms from which these sequences come related?". While sequence alignment methods lead to identification of similar sequences, multiple sequence alignment methods are applied to a set of related sequences before a phylogenetic analysis can be performed. After working with sequences for a while, one develops an intuitive understanding that for a given gene, closely related organisms have similar sequences and more distantly related organisms have more dissimilar sequences.

Also, it seems logical that given a set of sequences, it should be possible to reconstruct the evolutionary relationships (ancestral relationships) among genes and among organisms. This involves creating a branching structure, termed a phylogeny or tree that illustrates the relationships between the sequences. Hence a phylogenetic analysis of a family of related nucleic acid or protein sequences is a determination of how the family might have been derived during evolution. Placing the sequences as outer branches on a tree represents the evolutionary relationships. Two sequences that are very much alike will be located as neighbouring outside branches and would be joined to a common branch beneath them. Usually phylogenetic analysis methods assume that each position in the protein or nucleic acid sequence changes independently of others.

13.2. CONCEPT OF TREES

Definitions

A tree is a 2-dimensional graph showing evolutionary relationships among organisms, or in our case, in certain genes from separate organisms. We refer to these separate sources of sequences as taxa (singular taxon), defined as phylogenetically distinct units on the tree. The tree is composed of nodes (a point where branches bifurcate) representing the taxa and branches representing the relationships among the taxa. The lengths of the branches are often drawn proportional to the number of sequence changes in the branch and hence can represent the divergence.

A clade is a monophyletic taxon. Clades are group of genes that include the most recent common ancestor of all of its members and all the descendents of that most recent common ancestor.

Basic properties of Trees

Some of the important properties of trees are as follows :

- The root is the common ancestor of all taxa. It is defined by including a taxon that we are reasonably sure branched off earlier than the other taxa under study but should be related to the remaining taxa a unique path leads from the root node to any other node and the direction indicates evolutionary time (Fig. 13.1).
- If we do not have taxa to define the root, we can predict relationships by an uprooted tree as shown below (Fig. 13.2).
- Leaves represent things (genes,species) being compared.
- Internal nodes are hypothetical ancestral units.
- In a rooted tree, path from root to a node represents an evolutionary path.
- An unrooted tree specifies relationships among things, but not evolutionary paths.
- Paralogues are genes that diverged within the same species. They are multiple genes (tree leafs) per species.
- Orthologues are genes that diverged with species.

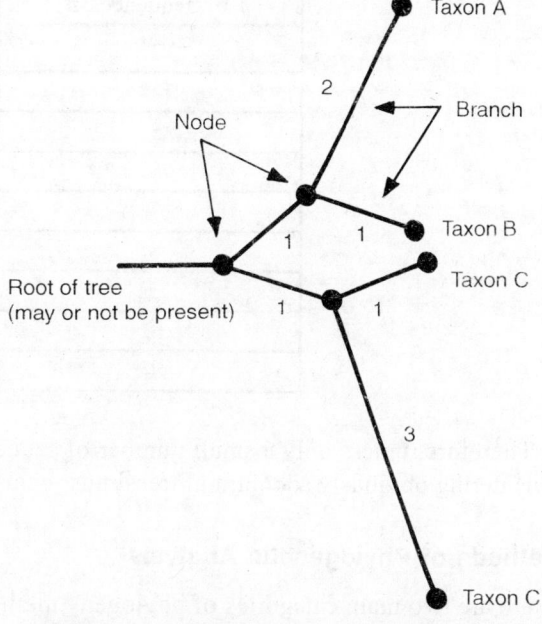

Fig. 13.1. Example of a rooted tree of 4 taxa showing branch lengths proportional to number of changes in branch.

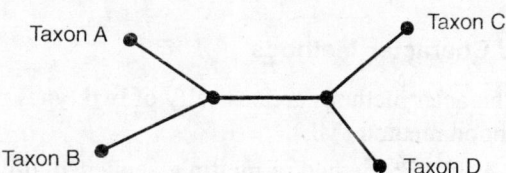

Fig. 13.2. Example of an uprooted tree for 4 taxa

13.3. PHYLOGENETIC TREES AND MULTIPLE ALIGNMENTS

Steps in Phylogenetic Analysis

The phylogenetic analysis in general is a four-step method:

1. Alignment strategy
2. Determination of the substitution model
3. Tree builiding
4. Tree evaluation

For n sequences, the number of possible trees is given in the Table below :

# of sequences n	# of trees
3	1
4	3
5	15
6	105
7	945
8	10,395
9	135,135
10	1,027,025
50	2.8×10^{74}

Therefore, unless only a small number of sequences are to be included in a tree, methods to avoid considering obviously suboptimal trees must be used to reduce the total number of trees considered.

Methods of Phylogenetic Analysis

There are two main categories of phylogeny methods: distance methods and character methods.

1. Distance methods

All possible pairs of sequences are aligned to determine which pairs are the most similar or closely related. These alignments provide a measure of the genetic distance between the sequences. These distance measurements are then used to predict the evolutionary relationship.

2. Character Methods

Character methods are basically of two types : maximum parsimony method(MP) and maximum likelihood method (ML).

- In MP method, a multiple sequence alignment is produced in order to predict which sequence positions are likely to correspond. These positions will appear in vertical columns in the multiple sequence alignment. For each aligned position, phylogenetic trees that require the smallest number of evolutionary changes to produce the observed sequence changes are identified. This analysis is continued for every position in the sequence alignment. Finally, those trees which produce the smallest number of changes overall for all sequence positions are identified.
- ML method depends upon first obtaining a reliable multiple sequence alignment and then examining the changes in each column in the alignment. In this case, however, the likelihood of a particular tree miscalculated using an expected model of change in the sequences. For example, all nucleotides are assumed to be equally frequent and the probability of change of any nucleotide to any other nucleotide is assumed to be the same in the Jukes-Cantor model. For each possible tree, the likelihood of finding the actual sequence changes at each column in the aligned sequences is calculated. The probabilities for each aligned position are then multiplied to provide likelihood for each tree. The tree that provides the maximum likelihood value is the most probable tree.

Alignment strategy using Phylogenetic analysis

The aim is to reduce the problem of a multiple alignment to an iteration of pairwise alignments. The strategy is hence an interative one. The procedure works as follows:

- Compute all pairwise distances between given sequences
- Compute a tree by single linkage clustering
- Align the sequences in bottom up order (see Fig. 13.3):

The bottom up alignment requires comparing groups of pre-aligned sequences. This is achieved by using profile alignment. Profile alignment relies on a NW like algorithm, however with scores defined as average scores among columns of pre-aligned sequence groups. Again the concept of the edit matrix is used to obtain a dynamic programming algorithm. A possibility to treat the gaps in profile alignments is to look into the profiles and to overtake gap-penalties to the edit matrix.

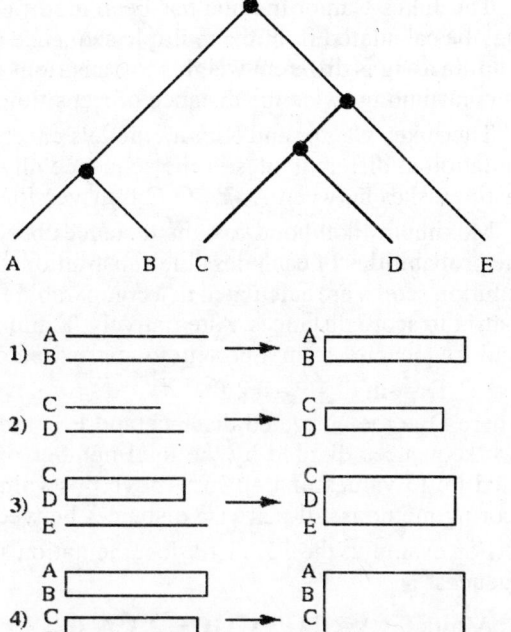

Fig. 13.3. Iterative alignment

Advantages of iterative alignment procedure:

- profile alignment reflects the conservation within a group (biologically relevant)
- it's fast and scales to large numbers of sequences

Disadvantages :

- unclear objective function
- misalignments introduced during the procedure are kept

13.4. DISTANCE MATRIX METHODS (MD)

Methods of calculation of distance matrices

In general, DNA distance matrices are calculated such that each mismatch between two sequences adds to the distance, and each identity subtracts from the distance. Scoring matrices include values for all possible substitutions.

General substitution matrix

	A	C	G	T
A	-(a1+a2+a3)	a1	a2	a3
C	a4	-(a4+a5+a6)	a5	a6
G	a7	a8	-(a7+a8+a9)	a9
T	a10	a11	a12	-(a10+a11+a12)

The simplest scoring method is that of Jukes and Cantor, in which all-possible nucleotide substitutions are of equal value. The model also assumes that each base will eventually have the same frequency in DNA sequences (0.25) once equilibrium has been reached.

The Jukes-Cantor method has been modified to take into account unequal base frequencies, which may be calculated from the multiple sequence alignment of the sequences. The 2-parameter method of Kimura assigns different weights to transitions and transversions. Typically, transversions are weighted as contributing twice the distance of transitions, since transitions occur more frequently.

The Jukes-Cantor and Kimura models can be modified to take into account variations in the rates of mutation at different sites in the sequence alignment. There is also a Kimura 3-parameter model that distinguishes between A -T / G-C transversions with A-C/G-T transversions.

Maximum likelihood assigns distances based on the Kimura formulae, but weighted according to the probabilities of each possible substitution, as determined from nucleotide frequencies. Protein substitution scores are calculated in a comparable fashion. One common method is to use Dayhoff's PAM1 matrix to score distances. Alternatively, Kimura's protein distance metric simply uses observed amino acid frequencies from a protein to approximate a PAM distance:

$$D = -\ln (1 - P - 0.2\, P^2)$$

where D is the corrected distance and P is the observed distance (number of exact matches between two sequences divided by the total number of matched residues in alignment). This formula can be used up to values of P=0.75. Above this value, Dayhoff PAM model is used. Using the appropriate scoring methods, all pairwise distances between sequences are calculated.

For example, the PHYLIP documentation gives the example of a set of 5 short aligned DNA sequences

Alpha	A A C G T G G C C A C A T
Beta	. . G . . C C
Gamma	C . G T . C . . . . . . A
Delta	G . G A . T T . . G . C .
Epsilon	G . G A . C T . . G . C C

The corresponding distance matrix using the Kimura 2 parameter model is

	Alpha	Beta	Gamma	Delta	Epsilon
Alpha	0.0000	0.2997	0.7820	1.1716	1.4617
Beta	0.2997	0.0000	0.3219	0.8997	0.5653
Gamma	0.7820	0.3219	0.0000	1.4481	1.0726
Delta	1.1716	0.8997	1.4481	0.0000	0.1679
Epsilon	1.4617	0.5653	1.0726	0.1679	0.0000

The Neighbor-Joining method (NJ)

The Neighbor-Joining method is one of the simplest distance methods. It begins by choosing the two most closely-related sequences, and then adding the next most distant sequence as a third branch to the tree (Fig. 11.4). Fitch and Margoliash give a simple example for a tree with 3 sequences A,B and C and the distances between nodes x, y and z:

	B	C
A	24	28
B		32

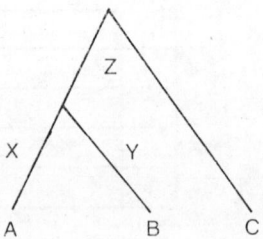

Fig. 13.4. Neighbour-joining method.

Simultaneous linear equations can be used to calculate the branch lengths:

A to B: x + y = 24
A to C: x + z = 28
B to C: y + z = 32

Thus with 3 equations and 3 unknowns we can calculate that x = 10, y = 14 and z = 18.
Addition of branches is iterative. Branches are added until all sequences are included in the tree.

Advantages

- fastest tree building method   high-throughput
- can use empirical substitution scoring methods   these high-throughput technologies.

Disadvantages

- tests only a single tree
- does not consider intermediate ancestors, meaning that there is no requirement for an internally-consistent evolutionary model
- misses homoplasies, especially over long distances; long evolutionary distances will be underestimated.

The Fitch/Margoliash method

The Neighbor-Joining method only attempts to build one tree. However, the raw pairwise distances may not always be perfectly additive. The ideal example shown above was internally consistent. In the example, the sums of the 3 simultaneous equations (i.e. 2 × the sums of the branch lengths) were precisely equal to the sums of the pairwise distances. This will not always be true for real data. In part this is due to undetected homoplasy. Fitch and Margoliash showed that different sets of internal branch lengths could be obtained by considering alternate trees which moved one or more branches to different parts of the tree. Consider a distance matrix for four sequences with pairwise distances D_I :

D_{ij}

	A	B	C	D
A	0	0.16	0.38	1.18
B	0.16	0	0.49	0.93
C	0.38	0.49	0	0.91
D	1.18	0.93	0.91	0

The Neighbor-Joining tree for these sequences is :

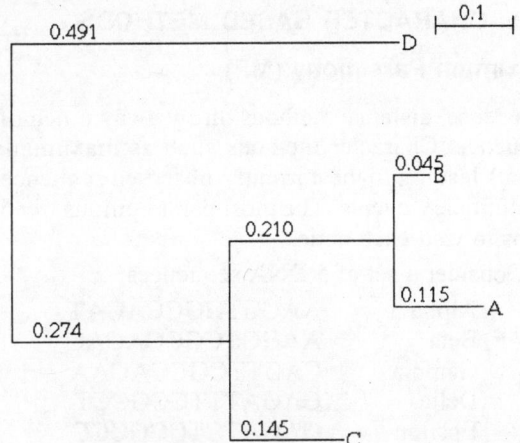

If we recalculate the pairwise distances $\mathbf{d}_{ij}$ from the tree, they are different from the original distances:

$$\mathbf{D}_{ij}$$

	A	B	C	D
A	0	0.16	0.47	1.09
B	0.16	0	0.40	1.02
C	0.47	0.40	0	0.91
D	1.09	1.02	0.91	0

The least squares method of Fitch and Margoliash tries different tree topologies, swapping branches among closely-related sequences, and recalculating the distances. For each tree considered, a different matrix of distances will be generated (dij). The best tree is defined as that tree which minimizes:

$$\sum_{ij} \frac{(D_{ij} - d_{ij})^2}{D^2_{ij}}$$

Advantages

- tests more than one tree
- still pretty fast
- can use empirical substitution scoring methods
- global optimization of tree by statistical criteria

Disadvantages

- Requires longer execution time than Neighbor Joining, but still quite practical on most computers, for typical data sets.
- Does not consider intermediate ancestors, meaning that there is no requirement for an internally-consistent evolutionary model misses homoplasies, especially over long distances; long evolutionary distances will be underestimated.

13.5. CHARACTER BASED METHODS

Maximum Parsimony (MP)

In a sense, distance methods throw away much of the data by only considering the end states for each sequence. Character methods such as maximum parsimony (MP) attempt to reconstruct mutational events leading to the currently-observed sequences. Therefore, each tree is a hypothetical model of the evolutionary events. The most parsimonious tree is therefore that tree which requires fewer mutational steps to visit each node.

Consider a set of 5 DNA sequences:

Alpha	AACGTGGCCACAT
Beta	AAGGTCGCCACAC
Gamma	CAGTTCGCCACAA
Delta	GAGATTTCCGCCT
Epsilon	GAGATCTCCGCCC

The output from the PHYLIP DNAPARS program lists 3 most parsimonious trees, each requiring a total of 13 substitutions to traverse the entire tree. One such tree is:

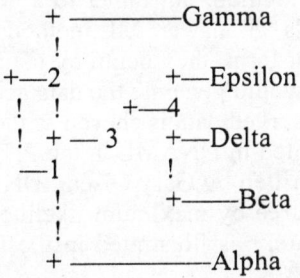

```
   + ——————Gamma
   !
 +—2         +—Epsilon
 ! !     +—4
 ! + — 3     +—Delta
 —1         !
   !         +——Beta
   !
   + ——————Alpha
```

requires a total of   13.000 steps in each site:

```
 0 1 2 3 4 5 6 7 8 9
 *   ———————————————————————————
 0! 2 0 1 2 0 2 1 0 0
 10! 1 0 1 3
```

	1		AASGTSGCCACAH
1	2	maybe	. . G . . C . . . .
2	Gamma	yes	C . . T . . . . A
2	3	maybe	. . . . Y
3	4	yes	G . . A . . T . . G . C .
4	Epsilon	maybe	 C
4	Delta	yes	. . . . . T . . . . . . T
3	Beta	maybe	 C
1	Alpha	maybe	. . C . . G . . . . . T

Internal nodes in the tree are given numbers. Five sequences require four ancestral nodes. For example, to go from Epsilon to 4 may require one mutation. To go from 4 to Delta requires 2 mutations. To go from 4 to 3 requires 5 mutations, and to go from 3 to Beta may require 1 mutation.

Examination of the other trees in testphyl.dnapars.outfile shows that Delta and Epsilon always cluster together, but that the positions of Alpha, Beta and Gamma are more variable.

The point of maximum parsimony is that, although sequences could be placed at any position on the tree, the number of steps required to interconvert one sequence to another changes each time branches are moved. Thus, the most parsimonious tree is the tree whose topology requires the fewest total mutations.

Advantages

- reconstructs ancestral nodes, thereby using all the evolutionary data
- has been to perform better than distance methods using simulated data & real data from pedigrees
- provides numerous "most parsimonious trees"

Disadvantages

- branch lengths can not be determined, only topology
- slower than matrix methods
- provides numerous "most parsimonious trees"
- sensitive to order in which sequences are added to tree

Maximum Likelihood (ML)

The term Maximum Likelihood does not refer to a single statistical method, but rather to a general approach. Most analytical methods begin with data and work towards an answer. ML methods take what has been described as an "inside out" approach. In their simplest form, they begin by listing all possible models, and then calculating the probability that each model would generate the data actually observed. The model with the highest probability of generating the observed data is chosen as the best model. Joe Felsenstein's application of ML to phylogeny is implemented in DNAML in the PHYLIP package, and in a modified version of DNAML called fastDNAml, written by Gary Olsen . DNAML works by successive addition of sequences to a tree, optimizing the tree by maximum likelihood at each step. Each site (position) in the alignment is considered separately as illustrated in the figure below:

DNAML output using the same five sequences Alpha - Epsilon as in the previous example, is shown:

```
Nucleic acid sequence Maximum Likelihood method, version 4.0
Empirical Base Frequencies:

    A           0.24615

    C           0.36923

    G           0.21538

  T(U)          0.16923

Transition/transversion ratio = 2.000000
```

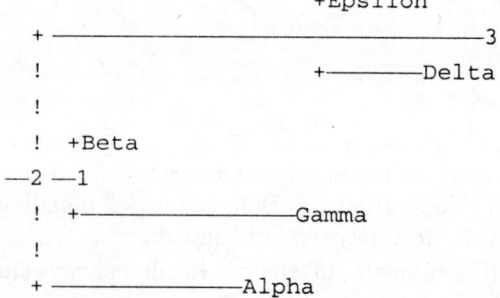

```
Ln Likelihood = -60.05644
```

Between	And	Length	Approx.	Confidence	Limits	
2	Alpha	0.30389	(	zero,	0.68289)**	
2	3	0.61975	(	zero,	1.28978)**	
3	Epsilon	0.00006	(	zero,	0.26048)	
3	Delta	0.16586	(	zero,	0.40674)**	
2	1	0.00006	(	zero,	infinity)	
1	Beta	0.00006	(	zero,	infinity)	
1	Gamma	0.33972	(	zero,	0.77181)**	

```
    *  = significantly positive, P < 0.05
   ** = significantly positive, P < 0.01
```

Advantages

- reconstructs ancestral nodes, thereby using all the evolutionary data
- generates branch lengths
- generates statistical estimate of significance of each branch
- has been to perform better than distance methods using simulated data and real data from pedigrees

Disadvantages

- It is very slow. Time required increases roughly with the fourth power of the number of sequences. Only practical with small numbers of sequences.

13.6. METHODS OF EVALUATING PHYLOGENIES

It is important to remember that the output from phylogenetic analysis is one answer obtained using one set of conditions. Even when an alignment has been carefully crafted and conditions such as substitution matrices or scoring methods are carefully chosen, it is possible to generate a meaningless tree. All other reasons aside, the input data may simply not be robust. That is, the data itself may contain more noise than evolutionary signal. Two ways to test phylogenies are described below.

1. Jumbling sequence addition order

Most methods for phylogeny construction are sensitive to the order in which sequences are added to the tree. Consequently, the simplest way to test a phylogeny is to repeat the analysis several times with different addition orders. All PHYLIP programs, and most other phylogeny programs, have an option called JUMBLE, that uses a random number generator to choose which sequence to add at each step, rather than adding them in the order in which they appear in the file. The user is asked to supply a random number to use as a "seed" in generating a random number chain.

It is especially important to remember that the order in which sequences appear in a file is often not random. For example, a sequence file used in an alignment might contain sequences from each species grouped together in the file. Non-random sequence order might therefore introduce a bias into the data set. Therefore, even when doing only one run on a phylogeny, it is probably a good idea to jumble the order of sequences.

2. Bootstrap and Jacknife replicates

One of the fundamental problems with phylogenetic inference is that we are stuck with a single set of data, of finite length. We have no way of knowing whether the tree inferred from the data is truely representative of the evolutionary history of the gene family. To make matters worse, not all positions in an alignment are informative. That is, some positions are invariant, and therefore make no contribution to the phylogenetic tree. In particular, when sequences are short or polymorphism is minimal, we can have little confidence that the tree inferred from that data is the correct one.

Ideally, we would like to have a very long alignment with many polymorphic sites, so that no one site, or small number of sites in the alignment, would be heavily weighted in constructing the tree. Put another way, the more data, the less likely it is for an artifactual phylogeny to be produced.

The statistical method of bootstrapping is based on the assumption that the statistical properties of a sample should be similar to the statistical properties of the population from which that sample was drawn. The larger the sample, the more representative it should be of the population. If the original sample was large enough, it should also be possible to take smaller samples from the larger sample, and expect that the smaller samples would also retain most of the statistical properties of the original population.

This is the assumption upon which the method of Jacknife resampling is based. If we repeatedly took random samples of the data set, the resultant small data subsets should give us the same answer as the original large data set. In the case of phylogenies, if we create smaller alignments containing only some of the positions from the total alignment, and use these mini-alignments to construct a tree, we should still get the same tree each time. This gives us a way of assessing how strongly a tree is supported by the data. If we get a different tree each time the data is sampled, then we are strongly confident that all the data is consistent with the tree. If we get a different tree with each sample, then we can conclude that no tree is strongly supported by the data.

Jacknife resampling has the drawback that the sub-replicates are of a smaller size than the original data set, which may change the statistical properties of the samples. For that reason, Jacknife resampling has largely been replaced by bootstrap resampling. Bootstrap resampling is sampling with replacement. In the case of a multiple sequence alignment, sites are sampled at random until the data set is equal in length to the original alignment.

In each of the bootstrapped replicates, most sites are sampled once, some sites are sampled twice, and a small number of sites are sampled three times. Some sites are never sampled. For bootstrap resampling of a sequence alignment, it is best to create at least 100 bootstrapped data sets, and redo the phylogeny for each one. A consensus tree can then be built which indicates, for each branch in the tree, how often it occurs in the population of replicate samples. Certain positions are biased in each replicate, while others are underrepresented. However, with enough replicates, all sites will be weighted equally.

The disadvantage of bootstrap resampling is that it drastically increases the time required to construct a phylogeny. For example, doing 100 bootstrap replicates for a tree means essentially, increasing the execution time by a factor of 100. You are making 100 trees instead of 1. Bootstrap sampling is therefore typically only practical with distance methods where large numbers of sequences must be used.

13.7. SUMMARY OF THE PHYLOGENETIC METHODS

Assumptions of multiple alignment

The following are the assumptions of doing any multiple alignment process:
- All sequences are homologous
- No duplicate sequences are present
- In each column, amino acid residues are homologous
- The alignment is optimal, with minimal gaps

Assumptions of phylogeny

The following are the assumptions of the phylogenetic analysis process:
- All sequences are homologous
- No duplicate sequences are present
- In each column, amino acid residues are homologous
- The alignment is optimal with minimal gaps
- No back mutation has occurred (some methods take this into account)
- All sequences are the same length

Using the phylogenetic methods for alignment hence need to combine the two approaches. The actual strategy used in construction of an alignment and phylogeny varies with the biological problem, and the nature of the data available. Some of these are illustrated below :

1. Protein versus DNA - During our discussion of pairwise sequence comparisons, we mentioned that pairwise alignment of DNA sequences is far less reliable than protein alignment, due to the small alphabet size of 4 for DNA, compared to 20 for proteins. This problem is far more serious for multiple alignments, because there are $O(k2)$ pairwise comparisons, where k is the number of sequences. Therefore, alignments should be done with proteins, wherever possible. One exception might be tRNA or rRNA molecules where information on secondary structure can be used to guide an alignment.

2. Phylogeny construction depends on detecting mutational events.
   - The degeneracy of the genetic code can mask mutations, making it preferable to construct phylogenies using protein coding DNA sequences, rather than proteins.
   - DNA sequence may be under less selective pressure than the corresponding protein sequence.
   - For closely related sequences, little of no sequence divergence may have occurred at the amino acid level, while divergence can be detected at the DNA level.

3. Display of the alignment in various ways can yield important insights into an alignment.

4. A very small data set of only a few genes or proteins may give a misleading answer simply because there are too few examples.

5. Very large data sets may impose computational constraints on the choice of methods used. As data sets get larger, redun-dant sequences may creep into the data set.

13.8. STEPS IN CONSTRUCTING ALIGNMENTS AND PHYLOGENIES

There is no one protocol for constructing alignments and phylogenies. At each step, decisions must be made as to which approach to take. In some cases, it may be necessary to try several methods before choosing one. As well, results at one step often make it necessary to go back several steps and refine the data set. For example, a poor phylogeny may indicate the need to re-do the alignment, and then to retry the phylogeny.

The steps in constructing an alignment and a phylogeny are illustrated using programs from the BIRCH system (Fig. 13.5). Assume a set of GenBank entries has been retrieved, all of which represent homologous genes from several species. In GenBank entries, protein coding sequences are annotated as 'CDS' features. The FEATURES program can extract CDS sequences from a group of GenBank entries automatically. Next, the coding sequences must be translated. Two multiple alignment programs are available. CLUSTALX aligns by successive addition of sequences, using a phylogenetic tree as a guide. PIMA uses a clustering method based on hierarchical groupings of amino acids according to chemical structure. To display the alignment for evaluation or final publication, it is best to try several of the programs listed to tailor the output to your needs. REFORM generates straight ASCII text, which can be easily imported into a word processor or drawing program. The other programs listed generate PostScript output for direct viewing or printing.

If an aligned DNA sequence is desired, MRTRANS from the FASTA package can read in an aligned protein sequence and the corresponding DNA sequence and generate a file containing the DNA alignment. The most complex part of the decision process involves choosing a strategy for phylogeny construction.

13.9. CONSIDERATIONS IN CHOICE OF THE METHOD

The distance and character based methods use different approaches as discussed above. These methods may find that more than one tree meets the criterion chosen for being the most likely tree. The branching patterns in these trees may be compared to find which branches are shared and hence are more strongly supported. PAUP program can be used for finding consensus trees. PHYLIP package also has the CONSENSE program for this purpose.

Different programs and program options are different for DNA and protein sequences. The alignment of the sequence pairs should not have a large number of gaps that are obviously necessary to align identical or related characters. The phylogenetic analysis should only be performed on parts of sequences that can be reasonably aligned. In general, phylogenetic methods analyze conserved regions that are represented in all the sequences. The simplest evolutionary models assume that the variations in each column of the multiple sequence alignment represents single-step changes and that no reversals have occurred. With the increase in observed variations, more multiple-step changes and reversions are likely to happen. One may apply corrections for such variation, which increases the observed amount of change to a more reasonable value. These corrections assume a uniform rate of change at all sequence positions over time. Gaps in the multiple sequence alignments are not scored.

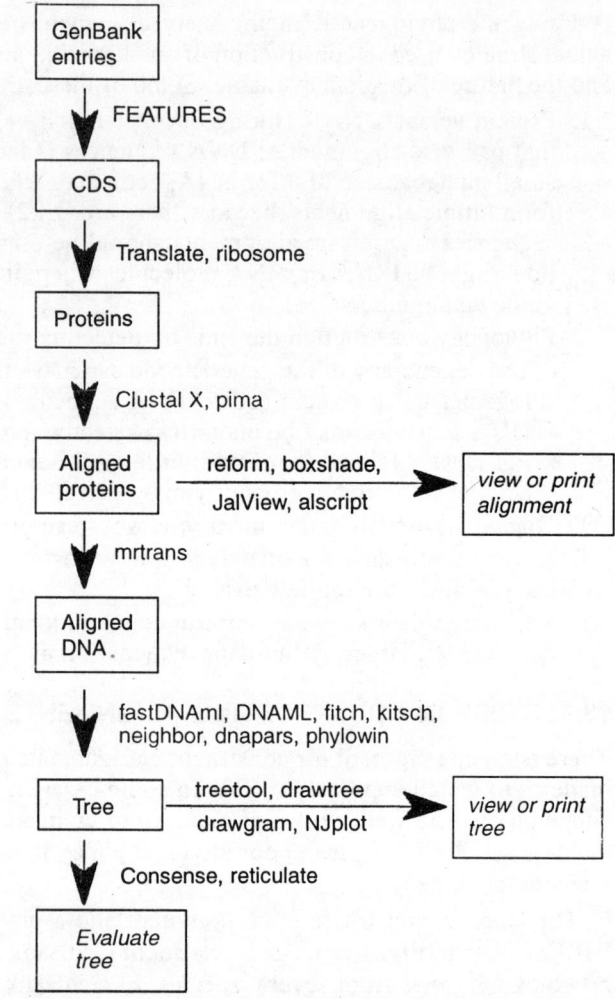

Fig. 13.5. Steps in constructing an alignment form the BIRCH system

For parsimony analysis, the best results are obtained when the amount of variation among all pairs of sequences is similar and when the amount of variation is small. The MP method attempts to fit all possible trees to the data, the method is hence not suitable for more than 11 or 12 sequences because there are too many trees to test. More than one tree may be found to be equally parsimonious. A consensus tree representing the conserved features of the different trees may then be produced.

Distance methods are able to predict an evolutionary tree when variation among the sequences is present and when the amount of variation is intermediate. The number of changed positions in an alignment between two sequences divided by the total number of matched positions is the distance between the sequences. As distances increase, corrections are necessary for deviations from single-step changes between sequences. The uncertainty of alignments also increases with the increase in distances. Distance methods may be used with a large number of sequences.

Maximum likelihood methods are used for any set of related sequences, but they are particularly useful when the sequences are more variable. These methods are computationally intense and the complexity increases with the number of sequences since the probability of every possible tree must be calculated. An advantage of these methods is that they provide evolutionary models to account for the variation in the sequences.

13.10 WORKING WITH PHYLOGENETIC TREES - AN ILLUSTRATION

Reconstruction of additive trees (Fig. 13.6)

The following algorithm for the reconstruction of an additive tree from a given distance matrix was introduced by Beyer, Singh, Smith and Waterman. (There are others also). We need to :

- Verify that the distance matrix constitutes an additive metric
- Choose a pair of objects, which results in the first path in the tree.
- Choose a third object and establish the linear equations to let the object branch off the path.
- Choose a pair of leaves in the tree constructed so far and compute the point a newly chosen object is inserted at.
  1. The new path branches off an existing branch in the tree: do the insertion step once more in the branching path.
  2. The new path branches off an edge in the tree: This insertion is finished.

An alternative algorithm inserts a new object into the tree by trying to solve the linear equations which result from trying to let the new edge branch off each edge in the tree, whereat there exists a solution for one edge only:

Given a distance matrix constituting an additive metric, the topology of the corresponding additive tree is unique.

Approximating additive metrics

Let a distance matrix on the species be given. In practice, the distance matrix between molecular sequences will not be additive. A tree T is searched whose distance matrix approximates the given one. Although the true difficulty lies in finding the best topology, one may formulate two alternative formalizations of the approximation task when the topology is given.

Let A be the path-edge incidence matrix of the given tree topology where by a path a leaf-to-leaf path is meant. Each row of matrix A corresponds to a path between two species and each column corresponds to an edge (Fig. 13.7). If an edge lies on a certain path the corresponding matrix entry is 1 and otherwise it is 0. The vector of edge-lengths of an edge-weighted tree shall be denoted by a column-vector e.

Here the above example again:

Heuristics

1. Heuristics for tree construction

The methods for exact tree reconstruction provide an inventory for heuristics for tree construction based on approximating additive metrics. Heuristics give exact results when operating on additive metrics, but the performance of solutions gets unclear when biased additive metrics are handled.

- *Insertion heuristics* : Step by step new objects are inserted into the tree. Each edge is tested for insertion, and for each edge an objective function is minimized. Finally the object is inserted at the edge, which minimizes the objective function best.

	A	B	C	D	E
A	0	2	7	4	7
B		0	7	4	7
C			0	7	6
D				0	7
E					0

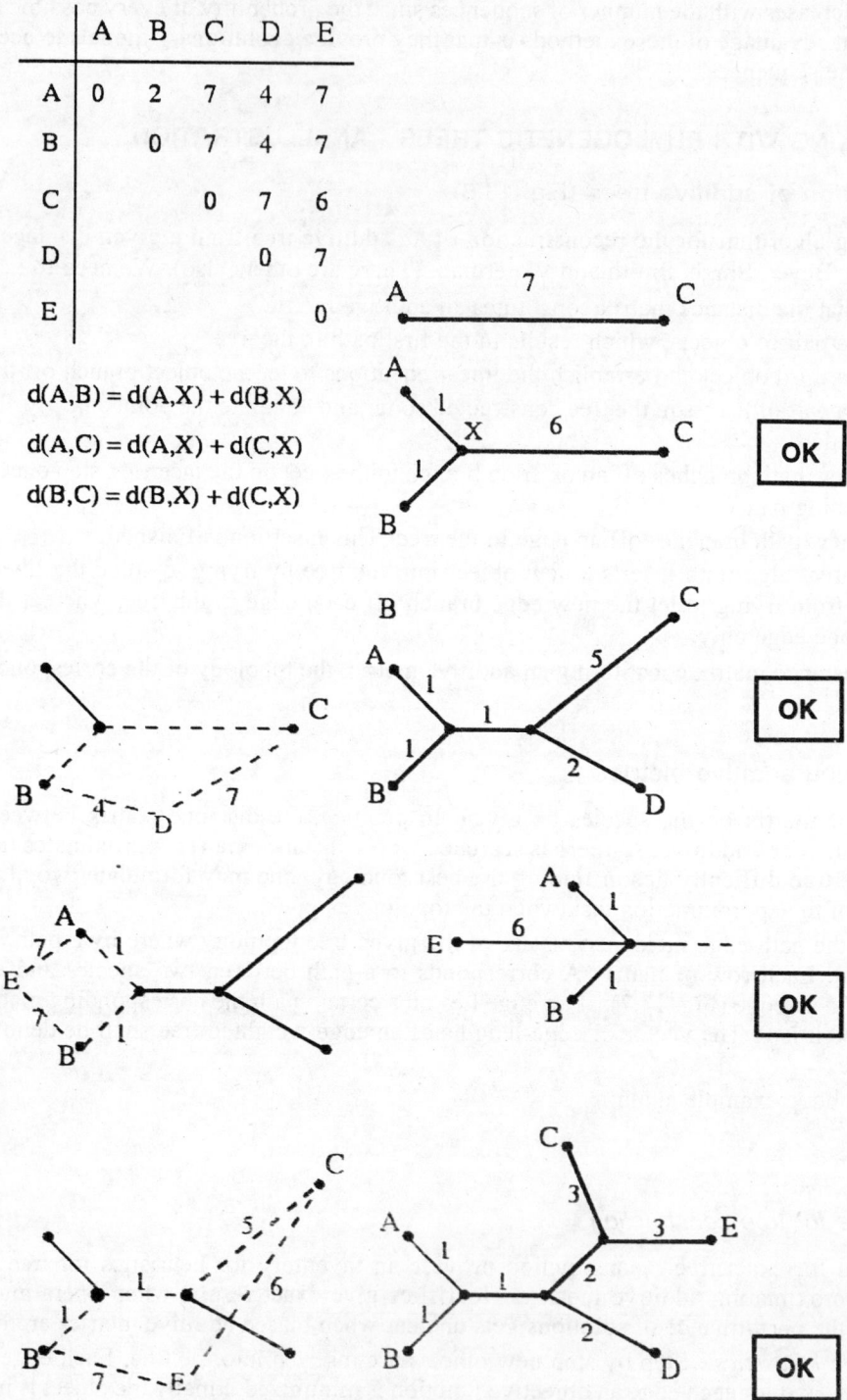

$$d(A,B) = d(A,X) + d(B,X)$$
$$d(A,C) = d(A,X) + d(C,X)$$
$$d(B,C) = d(B,X) + d(C,X)$$

Fig. 13.6. Additive tree construction

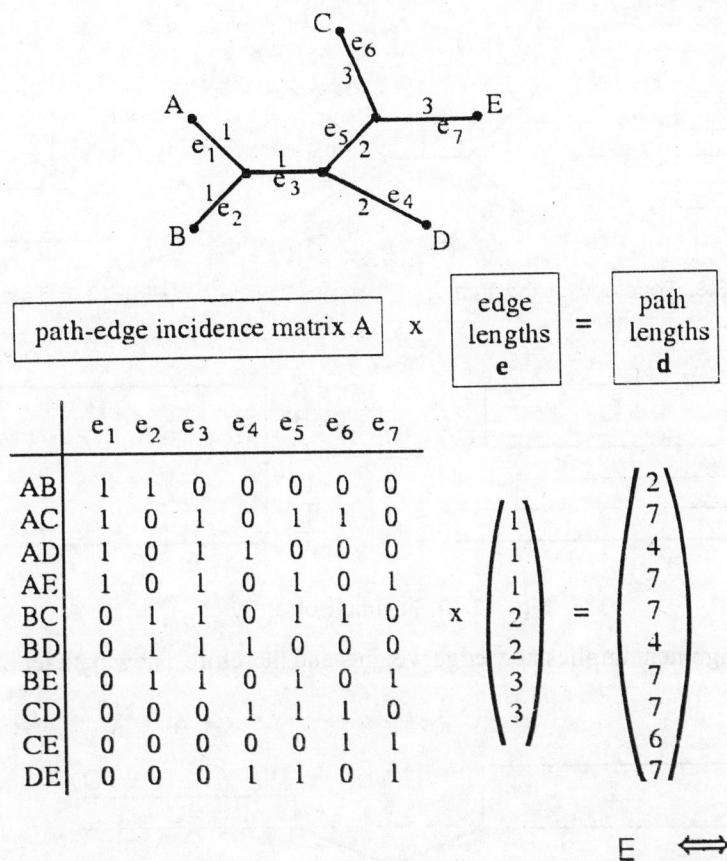

Fig. 13.7. The distance matrix on a set of objects constitutes an additive metric

- Rearrangement : In addition to inserting objects, objects are taken out, the tree is rearranged and new insertions of objects are tested.
- Nearest Neighbor Interchange : The tree topology is changed by exchanging two nearest leaves, and for each topology, an objective function is minimized.

2. The Three-Way-Alignment

The principle of the Three-Way-Alignment is to build up a multiple alignment by constructing a tree and aligning sequences and pre-aligned groups of sequences simultaneously:

Given N sequences and assume, that there is a tree topology for n (n<N), sequences and a multiple alignment for n sequences coupled to the tree, i.e $n=5$ (Fig. 13.8):

Each edge of the tree is tested for an insertion of a new sequence, i.e. test edge e (Fig. 13.9):

For an insertion of a sequence in edge e, a three-way-alignment between the following groups of sequences is computed (Fig. 13.10)

- The aligned sequences on the left of e
- The aligned sequences on the right of e
- The new sequence

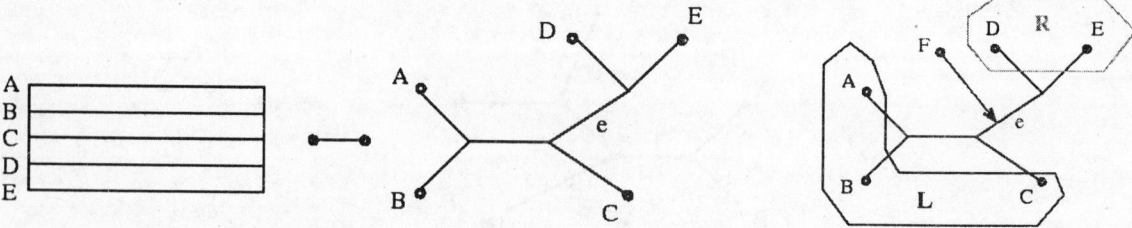

Fig. 13.8. Topology of the tree.

Fig. 13.9. Tree showing the edge

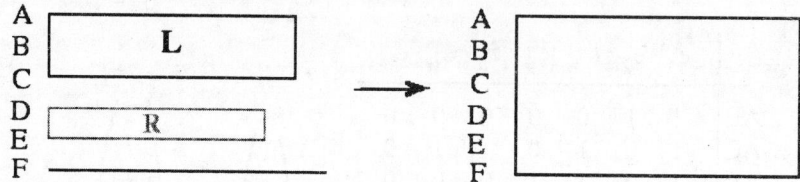

Fig. 13.10. Insertion of an edge.

The three-way alignment implies new edge weights and therefore a new path length for the complete tree (Fig. 13.11):

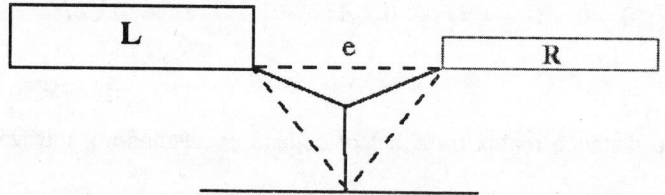

Fig. 13.11. Three-way alignment for the complete tree.

In order to keep the amount of evolution as small as possible, one chooses the topology resulting in the smallest path length. In the example an alignment of $n+1$ sequences now is coupled with a tree topology for six sequences and a new sequence may be inserted. When constructing a multiple alignment iteratively in this way, a correction of positions in the profile alignments is possible (Fig. 13.12).

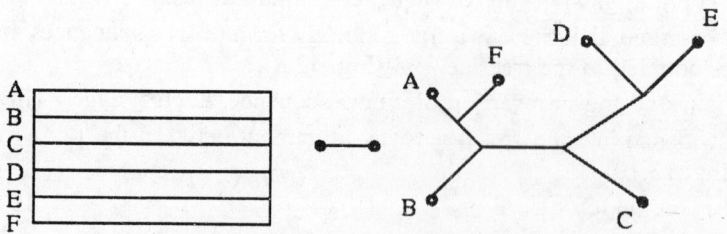

Fig. 13.12. Extension of the tree topology for 6 sequences.

14

Gene Prediction Methods

14.1. INTRODUCTION

We have discussed the structure and function of gene in an earlier chapter. The objective of gene prediction is to identify regions of genomic DNA that encodes proteins. The genomic DNA sequence may be that of an insert of genomic DNA in a bacterial artificial chromosome (BAC) or similar vector or that of an assembled chromosome or chromosomal fragment. Gene prediction programs are used to search through new sequences and then annotate the sequence database entry with this information. The annotation includes gene structure, gene location and any matches of the translated exons with the protein sequence databases. The amino acid sequence of the predicted gene may also be entered in the annotated information. The standards of gene prediction are not uniform and also they may not be entirely correct. Confirmation can be done by cDNA sequencing. If EST sequences are available in a sufficient coverage of the genome, these are also useful for confirmation of predicted gene sequences.

There are a number of gene prediction programs. They all have in common to varying degrees the ability to differentiate between gene sequences characteristic of exons, introns, splicing sites, and other regulatory sites in expressed genes from other non-gene sequences that lack these patterns. However, a program trained on one organism may not work as efficiently for the other.

Just to refresh and provide the context for gene prediction, this is a brief discussion on gene structure and function.

Gene Structure

Transcription is the process of copying the portion of the DNA containing a gene into RNA. Something has to happen to instigate transcription at genes and not at non-coding regions. Thus there must be signals in the DNA sequence, which tell where to start the transcription. Enzyme RNA polymerase binds to specific patterns at approximately 10 and 35 bases before the gene to start transcription. Other binding sites upstream from before the gene called promoters help signal when to express or inhibit the gene from expressing as RNA. Transcription stops when it encounters a DNA palindrome flanking repeated *A*s, forming a 'knot'.

Translation is the process of building proteins according to the template RNA. Ribosome works its way along an RNA molecule, grabbing the appropriate amino acid for the next codon and adding to the end of the given protein.

The appropriate bases get to the right places by essentially random motion, guided by electrostatic forces. Binding sites ensure that the right things stick together when they bang into each other. The coding regions of genes are called exons. Gene recognition in eukaryotes is complicated by the presence of *introns*, or non-coding regions. DNA in eukaryotes resides in the cell's nucleus, but proteins are translated outside the nucleus. Issues of how proteins/RNA cross membrane boundaries are critical in understanding their function, and designing drugs.

Basis of Gene Prediction

In general, introns are flanked by *donor* and *acceptor* sites GT and AG - however, such pairs should each happen by chance every $4^2 = 16$ bases. Genes start with ATG and end with a stop codon (TAA, TAG, or TGA) - however, such codons should happen every codons. The length of all coding regions must be a multiple of three - however coding regions can be split over multiple exons. The distribution of base triples and heximers differs between coding and non-coding regions - but one needs a sufficiently long enough region to trust statistical variations.

Problems Which Complicate Gene Prediction

- Gene transfer mechanisms often introduce extra copies of genes into genomes, which then diverge through evolution. Distinguishing broken pseudo-genes from working genes is a difficult problem.
- Sequencing errors can step on donor/acceptor sites and cause apparent frame shifts.
- Exons can be separated by several thousand bases.
- Genes can overlap each other, appear in different reading frames and on different strands.
- Exons can be assembled in multiple ways through alternative splicing (Fig. 14.1).

The objective of gene prediction is to locate a particular gene in the nucleotide sequence. Then locate exons and introns with in the gene. One simple method of doing this is to do pattern searches. This is discussed below.

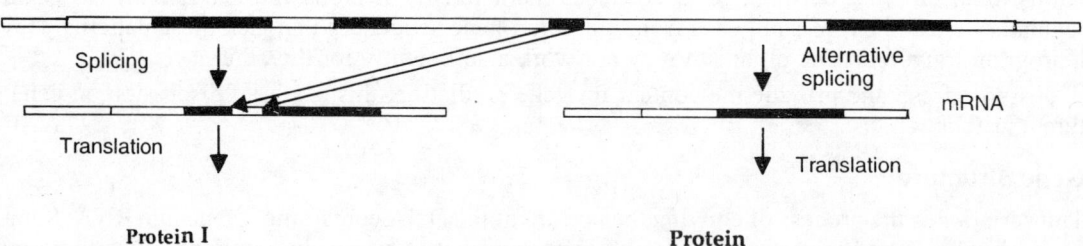

Fig. 14.1. Alternative splicing

14.2 USING PATTERNS TO PREDICT GENES

Pattern Searching

Pattern finding is the procedure of scanning a nucleic acid or protein sequence for matches to short sequence patterns. These short patterns are usually known to be important indicators of some biological function. The presence of the matching pattern in the target nucleic acid or protein sequence is a signal of the same function for the target gene or protein sequence.

Patterns most often examined in DNA sequences are:
- Recognition sites of restriction endonucleases
- Codons specifying the amino acid sequence of a protein
- Intron splice sites
- Promoter
- Binding sites for regulatory proteins which activate or repress transcription

Patterns in protein sequences (motifs), can be used to predict:
- Presence of active sites
- Prediction of protein secondary structure
- Presence of signals used to localize the protein in the cell.

Types of Matches

Computer programs search for one of two types of matches in a target sequence:
- Exact matches to a large number of possible patterns such as the presence of sites recognized by certain restriction endonucleases
- Approximate matches to a given pattern such as DNA binding site for a protein or the structural motif in a protein, which vary from one sequence to another. A simple example of approximate pattern searching might be looking for a DNA pattern that is one base different from a restriction endonuclease cleavage site.

In general, pattern searching programs should allow several options including:
- Presence of ambiguous symbols in the specified patterns
- Variable spacing between matched positions
- Choice of alternative matches to particular positions
- Matches that include gaps in the pattern or target sequence

Sequences of related protein families sometimes also have multiple consensus patterns that increase the prediction of function (for example, using the BLOCKS database). Pattern searching in sequences is the basis for performing rapid searches through a sequence database for the closest matches to a given sequence by the BLAST and FASTA programs. The program FASTA has been used successfully to locate previously unidentified DNA binding sites for *E.coli* LexA protein. Function predictions based on pattern searching can often be greatly improved if several patterns are present in a row or if the patterns are in the usual expected order for that type of function.

14.3. METHODS OF GENE PREDICTION

The major methods of gene prediction are as follows:
1. Laboratory-based approaches
2. Feature-based approach
3. Homology-based approach
4. Statistical and HMM-based approaches

Laboratory-Based Approaches to Gene Prediction

This is the traditional way to find a gene was to do it in the laboratory. Experimental procedures for locating genes in new DNA are basically of three types:

1. Identification via hybridization to mRNA or cDNA.
2. Identification of the 5'-end and intron-exon junctions of the gene.
3. Exon trapping

1. Identification via hybridization to mRNA or cDNA

Northern blots

Northerns are the same as Southerns except that mRNA is run out on the Gel. Thus, transcripts resulting from expression of a gene can be detected and isolated to any given new DNA sequence by using a labeled probe of the same sequence as this new DNA sequence. This methodology can also be used to distinguish exons from introns by appropriate probe construction, although a more complete experimental approach is to sequence the mRNA via the cognate cDNA and compare the sequence directly with the genomic DNA sequence.

Zoo blots

Zoo blots are simply Southern blots of a labeled probe from the new DNA sequence against genomic DNA R.fragments from different organisms (the Zoo). The point is to determine if DNA sequences that are highly similar, and hence possibly homologous, to the new DNA sequence are present in one or more of these other organisms. An observed hybridization signal argues strongly that:

- The DNA probe comes from an intragenic region
- Both organisms encode homologous proteins that probably execute similar functions.

Zoo blots thus provide both gene location information as well as predictive gene function information.

2. Identification of the 5'-end and Intron-Exon Junctions of the Gene

S1 Nuclease mapping and Primer Extension (Fig. 14.2)

In S1 nuclease mapping, a DNA probe labeled at its 5'-end and which overlaps the gene 5'-end or the 5'-end of an exon is hybridized to the gene DNA. S1 nuclease, which is specific for either ssDNA or RNA, is used to digest the single-stranded DNA. The resulting 5'-labeled DNA probe is then "sized" via a Southern blot. Its size pinpoints the 5'-end of the gene or exon.

In primer extension, a DNA probe labled at its 5'-end and which is contained within the gene is hybridized to mRNA from the gene. The probe DNA is used as a primer for a Reverse Transcriptase which will extend this primer, using the mRNA as Template, synthesizing DNA to the end of the mRNA. The resulting 5'-labled DNA probe, identical to the one produced in the S1 nuclease mapping approach, is then "sized" via a Southern blot, to pinpoint the 5-end of the gene.

3. Exon Trapping

This method is used most often to isolate exons from new DNA, rather than simply to identify exon-intron boundaries. In exon trapping, an R.fragment from a new DNA sequence is cloned into a cognate R.site in an intron of a cloned Gene; Cloning Vehicles have been constructed that make this relatively easy to do. This chimeric DNA is introduced into an appropriate eukaryotic host, usually *Yeast*, and the cloned gene is expressed. During processing of the initial transcript, introns are spliced out, leaving only the exon from the cloned R.fragment behind. DNA from this mRNA is obtained via RT-PCR, and its sequence determined. Comparison of this sequence, containing only the exon from

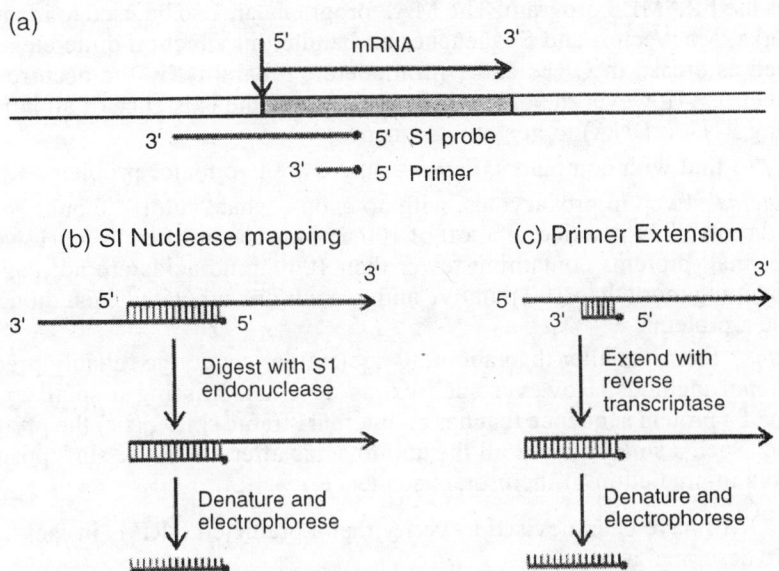

Fig. 14.2. S1 Nuclease mapping and Primer Extension.

the cloned R.fragment, with the sequence of the R.fragment itself shows where the intron-exon boundaries are located.

RT-PCR is a variation on PCR in which the first polymerization step of the PCR reaction is executed by a reverse transcriptase, thereby converting the mRNA into a cDNA. This cDNA is then amplified further using a thermostable DNA polymerase such as Taq polymerase. A problem with many laboratory methods is that relatively few genes tend to dominate the population of expressed sequences, and hence one discovers duplicates instead of new genes.

Feature-Based Approaches to Gene Prediction

Web-based gene recognition systems such as *Grail*, *GeneID*, and *GeneParser* work by searching for various ad hoc features of genes, and then identifying regions which score high enough. Typical features include codon bias, donor / acceptor sites, and coding frame length.

Since stop codons should occur every 20 codons or so, long *open reading frames* or ORFs without stop codons are strongly suggestive of genes. The key to the analysis of an unknown DNA sequence is the identification of ORFs. ORF has the presence of a long series of codons in a DNA sequence without the series being interrupted by a termination codon. An ORF signal is enhanced even further by the presence of sequence patterns for starting and stopping transcription before and after the ORF. Dynamic programming can be used to identify the highest scoring regions. The best gene recognition systems tend to be species-specific, trained on examples of known genes in the given organism.

Scanning DNA for ORFs : The transcription initiation site is always an ATG codon and it is always about 30 base pairs downstream from a TAATAA sequence. This is enough information to specify a pattern for the GCG program FINDPATTERNS . It may be even easier to just produce a map of ORFs in all 6 reading frames and look for a long one. Simple software that maps an ORF starting at every ATG and stops it at every stop codon is available in a wide variety of forms.

GCG provides the FRAMES program. The MAP program can also be used to identify open reading frames. GeneWorks, MacVector, and Sequencher all handle this function quite elegantly. Introns can often be identified as breaks in ORFs and with moderate reliability by the occurrence of consensus splice signal sequences. However the only way to truly prove the existence of an intron is experimentally by comparing RNA (cDNA) to genomic sequences.

ORFs are easy to find with computers, however there are two major problems:

(i) *Small Proteins* : Even in prokaryotes, with no exons, what "cutoff" should be used for a minimum sized protein? In practice, a cutoff of 100 amino acids is often used. However, in so doing, some true small proteins containing fewer than 100 amino acids are not annotated and some ORFs containing more than 100 putative amino acids are annotated even though they in fact do not encode a protein.

(ii) *Small Exons* : Exons smaller than about 30 nucleotides cannot be reliably predicted by normal computational methods. However such exons do exist. Missing a small exon can result in prediction of a protein sequence that has an internal "frame shift", (i.e) the protein coding frame has shifted. Such a shift changes all the amino acids after the frame shift position, resulting in major errors in prediction of the protein sequence.

Three tests of ORFs have been devised to verify that a predicted ORF is in fact likely to encode a protein. These are described below:

1. This is based on an unusual type of sequence variation that is found in ORFs - every third base tends to be the same one much more often than by chance alone. This property is due to non-random use of codons in ORFs and is true for any ORF, independent of the species. The program TESTCODE (from GCG) provides a plot of the non-randomness of every third base in the sequence.

2. This is based on the analysis to determine whether the codons in the ORF correspond to those used in other genes of the same organism. For this test, information on codon use for an organism is necessary, averaged over all genes.

3. The ORF may be translated into an amino acid sequence and the resulting sequence then compared to the databases of existing sequences. If one or more sequences of significant similarity are found, there will be much more confidence in the predicted ORFs.

Homology-Based Approaches to Gene Prediction

Searching for a known homolog is the most widely understood means of identifying new protein-coding genes. Such searches depend only on evolutionary relatedness, and so are widely applicable. A major advantage of finding homologous product is that some of the biology of the gene may be already elucidated. Usually databases are searched for ACRs (Ancient Conserved Region) and ESTs (Expressed Sequence Tags).

Hence evidence for genes can consist of matches to

• Known proteins
• Protein motifs (e.g. zinc finger, ATP and GTP-binding motifs, etc.)
• ESTs and ACRs

Homology-based gene prediction systems such as *Procrustes* scan databases find similarities to previously identified coding regions. Such homology-based approaches can only identify previously known genes, of course, but the fraction of known genes is growing rapidly. A different homology-based approach to identify totally unknown genes is to compare two whole genomes and look for conserved regions, on the theory that sequence is only conserved if it is important.

*Finding coding regions by similarity searching :*An approach to this problem is to translate the sequence in all six reading frames (3 forward and three reverse) and do a similarity search against the protein databanks. There is a variant of the BLAST program (BLASTX) that automatically translates a DNA query sequence and performs a similarity search against protein databanks. If a protein sequence matches, get its DNA sequence and align it with your unknown sequence. The start and stop codons should line up nicely. If the query sequence is genomic, then the introns should also be obvious.

Statistical and HMM Approaches to Gene Prediction (Fig. 14.3)

There are other statistical methods for identifying ORFs in DNA sequences. GCG provides several tools that help to identify protein coding sequences by statistics that measure codon usage (CODON-PREPERENCE) and the non-random use of particular nucleotides in the third position of each codon (ESTCODE). These statistical methods are imprecise, but can help identify possible coding regions in large chunks of genomic DNA sequence.

An alternate approach to building prediction programs based on ad hoc features is to train a learning program on positive and negative examples and have the program select the most important features. Such learning-based approaches can work surprisingly well, often better than hand-crafted programs if the task is sufficiently fuzzy. Standard learning approaches for pattern recognition include *neural networks* and *hidden Markov models* (HMMs). *HMM gene* and *GeneMark* are popular gene recognition programs based on HMMs. Building good training sets are complicated by sequencing errors and duplications in Genbank.

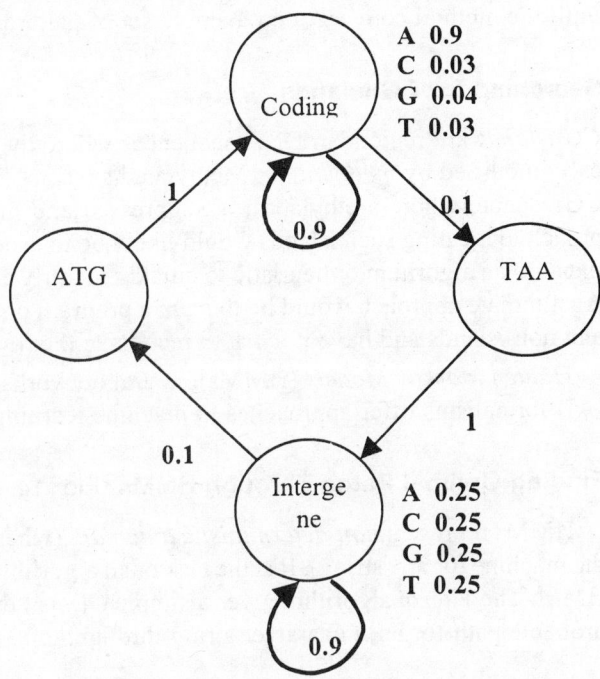

Fig. 14.3. HMM approach for gene prediction

Searching for Protein Binding Sites in DNA Sequences

DNA and protein sequences, which have a related function, may share consensus patterns that can be found by sequence analysis methods. An example is a set of DNA sequences that contains signals for transcriptional promoters. Sequences of proteins in families may also have conserved amino acid patterns or motifs. These patterns serve as a signature of function and may be used to identify other sequences that may have the same function. SIGNALSCAN is an example of a program that utilizes a database of transcription factor sequences to find potential transcription factor binding sites in DNA sequences.

If the members of a set of sequences are similar to each other, the simplest method of finding consensus patterns is to:

- Align the sequences by Multiple Sequence Alignment and make a profile
- Search for patterns with a statistical method such as the expectation maximization method

DNA binding sites for proteins may be composed of several such conserved patterns separated by variable spaces between the patterns. A computer algorithm called the Expectation Maximization Algorithm has been devised for finding such regions in unaligned sequence fragments (Cardon and Stormo in 1992). In this method, a best scoring comparison matrix is obtained. In a second step, this matrix is then used to find the approximate locations of the binding sites in the original sequences. In the third step, the predicted binding sites are then used to make a new matrix, which in a fourth step is again used to define even better the locations of the binding sites in the sequences. This process is repeated until the method converges on a single set of patterns in the sequences.

Searching for CG Islands

CG islands are regions in DNA sequences where the dimer CG repeatedly occurs. CG sites are typically modified by *methylation*. Methylated sites are likely to mutate to TG sites, so concentrations of CGs denote where methylation is suppressed and thus have biological significance. A possible approach to locating such islands would likely be to produce a list of all positions where CG's occur, and then use an algorithm or heuristic to quickly identify all sufficiently long, sufficiently dense sequences. An alternate approach would be to *train* a program on appropriately identified examples of CG islands and non-islands and have it *learn* to recognize them.

Hidden Markov Models (HMMs), neural networks, decision trees, and other Artificial Intelligence (AI) formalisms offer approaches to machine learning.

Finding Optimal Paths Through HMMs (Fig. 14.4)

HMMs represent *non-deterministic automata* (where there can be exponentially many ways through the machine for any string). It is the task of an algorithm like Viterbi to find the optimal path through the HMM. The *Viterbi* algorithm gives a simple $O(nm^2)$ dynamic programming algorithm to find the most probable path for an n character string through an m state automata.

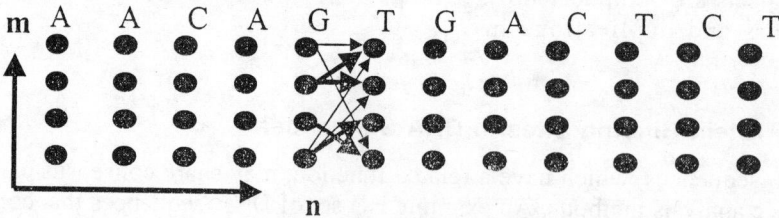

Fig. 14.4. Viterbi algorithm

Training HMMs

If the fine structure of the training examples is properly annotated in accord with the states of the model, the state transition probabilities can be easily determined. If not, parameters can be found through *iterative* algorithms, where each training sequence is run through the model and weights adjusted to increase the probability that training examples are correctly classified. In one such algorithm, the *Baum-Welch* algorithm, we calculate the forward and backward probabilities for each sequence/each state, and adjust accordingly. In the *Viterbi* algorithm, we only reinforce the strongest path for an input sequence.

The overall training method used is as follows :

1. The model is initialised with estimates of transition probabilities and amino acid composition for each match and insert date. If an initial alignment of the sequences is known, or some other kinds of data suggest which sequence positions are the same, then these data may be used in the model. For other cases, the initial distribution of amino acids to be used in each state is described below. The initial transition probabilities generally favour transitions from one match state to the next rather than favouring insert and delete states, which build more uncertainty into a sequence motif.

2. All possible paths through the model for generating each sequence are examined. As there are many possible such paths for each sequence, it would normally take a long time for such computations. The algorithm - Forward-backward algorithm, is used to reduce the number of computations to the number of steps in the model times the total length of the training sequences. This computational approach provides a probability of the sequence, given all possible paths through the model, and, from this value, the probability of any particular path may be found. The Baum-Welch algorithm is now used to count the number of times a particular state-to-state transition is used and a particular amino acid is required by a particular match state to generate the corresponding sequence position.

3. A new version of the HMM is produced that uses the results in step 2 to generate new transition probabilities and match-insert state compositions.

4. State 3 and 4 are repeated up to 10 more times until the parameters do not change significantly.

5. The trained model is used to provide the most likely path for each sequence by using the Viterbi algorithm. The alignment can be done by using the dynamic programming technique instead of going though all the possible alignments. The collection of paths for the sequences provides a MSA of the sequences with the corresponding match, insert and delete states for each sequence. The columns in the MSA are defined by the match states in the HMM such that amino acids from a particular match state are placed in the same column. For columns that do not correspond to a match state, a gap is added.

6. The HMM is then used to search a sequence database for additional sequences that share the same sequence variation. In this case, the sum of probabilities of all possible sequence alignments to the model is obtained. This probability is computed by the forward component of the forward-backward algorithm. This gives a type of distance score of the sequence from the model, thus providing an indication of how well a new sequence fits the model and whether the sequence may be related to the sequences used to train the model.

To reduce the number of parameters the model must learn, it is often a good idea to initialize, force, or combine certain parameters in light of a priori knowledge. Forcing certain transition probabilities to zero imparts a non-complete *topology* to the network. Multistage recognition problems such as prokaryotic genes (promoter sites, start codon, coding sequences, stop codon) are best modeled as progressing sequent

14.4 : GENE PREDICTION TOOLS

GRAIL

GRAIL (Gene Recognition and Analysis Internet Link) is perhaps the most widely used ORF identification tool. (It was also one of the first to be made available). It provides analysis of protein coding potential of a DNA sequence. GRAIL uses variable-length windows tailored to each potential exon candidate defined as an open reading frame bounded by a pair of start/donor, acceptor/donor or acceptor/stop sites. This scheme facilitates the use of more genomic context information (splice junctions, translation starts, non-coding scores of 60-base regions on either side of a putative exon) in the exon recognition process. GRAIL finds about 91% of all coding regions with an apparent false positive rate of 8.6%. Three further refinements of the program - GRAIL 1a, GRAIL II and GRAIL-EXP have made the appearance after the original program.

Grail II provides analysis of protein-coding regions, poly (A) sites, and promoters; constructs gene models; predicts encoded protein sequences; and provides database searching capabilities. A list of most likely exon candidates is first established, and these are evaluated further using a neural network approach. The algorithm makes its final prediction by selecting the best candidates. A DP approach is then used to define the most probable gene models.

GenLang

GenLang is a syntactic pattern recognition system, which uses the tools and techniques of computational linguistics to find genes and other higher-order features in biological sequence data. Patterns are specified by means of rule sets called grammars, and a general purpose parser, implemented in the logic programming language Prolog, then performs the search.

BCM GeneFinder

GeneFinder offers some unusual custom algorithms. The algorithm first predicts all possible potential internal exons, and potential 5' and 3'-exon for each internal by linear discriminant functions combining characteristics describing various contextual features of these exons. Then by method of dynamic programming it searches for optimal combination of these exons and construct gene model.

Procrustes

Procrustes is a homology-based tool. The input for Procrustes is a genomic DNA sequence. It then scans databases to find similarities to previously identified coding regions. The algorithm is unusual - it does not use a DNA sequence by itself to look for the signal. The user provides the DNA sequence.

GeneParser

This program predicts the most likely combination of exons and introns in a genomic sequence by a DP approach. GeneParser uses a likelihood score for each sequence position being in an intron and exon. The intron and exon positions are then aligned with the constraint that they must alternate within a gene structure. In this manner, a combination of the most likely intron and exon regions that comprise a gene structure are found. GeneParser uses a scheme for adjusting the weights used for several types of sequence patterns that make up the intron and exons.

14.5 SUMMARY OF TOOLS FOR DNA/RNA STRUCTURE AND FUNCTION ANALYSIS

1. Poly-A Site Prediction

HCpolyA - Poly-A Site Prediction (Hamming Clustering Method) - WebGene
Server POLYA - Recognition of 3'-end Cleavage & Poly-A Signals - BCM

Summary of estimated performance measures for some of the tools

Tool	Prediction type	Sensitivity (%) nucl.	Specificity (%) nucl.	Sensitivity exact exon	Specificity exact exon	Missed exons	Wrong exons
FGENES	Gene structure	83	93	73	78	15	11
GeneID	Gene structure	69	77	42	46	28	24
Gene Parser	Gene structure	66	79	35	40	29	17
GENSCAN	Gene structure	93	93	78	81	9	5
GRAIL II	Gene structure	83	87	-	52	25	10
MZEF	Internal exons	87	95	78	86	14	7

2. TATA Signaling, Promoter & Trans-Factor Bind Site Prediction

HCtata - TATA Signaling Prediction (Hamming Clustering Method) -WebGene
Server MatInspector - Search Sequence for Transcription Factor
Binding Sites - GSF
McPromoter - Prediction of Transcription Start Sites in Eukaryotic DNA -Erlangen
NNPP - Promoter Prediction - LBNL Human Genome Center
Recognition of PolII Promoter Region & Transcription Start Signals Using
Signal Scan - Search Search for Eukaryotic Transcriptional Elements - BIMAS
Target Finder - Search for target genes of DNA-binding proteins - TigemNet
TESS - Transcription Factor Binding Site Sequence Search - U Penn
Tfsitescan - Promoter analysis - MIRAGE -IFTI

3. Exon (ORF) Prediction

Cassandra - Recognition of Protein-Coding Segments - CCEG-USC
CDSB - Search for Protein Coding Regions in E.coli - BCM
DNA Sequence Translation - Analysis of ORF in Gene Sequence -FramePlot
- Protein Coding Region Prediction in Bacterial DNA - NIH-NET
Gene Finder - Gene Structural Analysis, Exon and Splice Site Prediction - BCM
GENEID - Prediction of Exons and Gene Structure in Query Sequences
GenHunt - Search for Exons in Query Sequence - Weisman Institute
GENIE - Gene (Prediction) Finder
GenView - Protein-Coding Gene Prediction - WebGene Server (Italy)
GRAIL - Exon Prediction/Analysis
HEXON - Search for Prediction of Internal Exons in Human DNA - BCM
ORF Finder - Open Reading Frame Finder at - NCBI
ORFGene - Gene Structure Prediction - WebGene Server
PROCRUSTES - Gene Recognition via Spliced Alignment - USC

4. Splice Site Prediction

Gene Finder - Gene Structural Analysis, Exon and Splice Site Prediction - BCM
NetGene - Splice Site Location Prediction Email-Server Information
NNSSP - Splice Site Prediction by Neural Network - LBNL Human Genome Center
Search/Prediction of Potential Splice Sites in DNA
Splice Site - Splice Site Prediction by Neural Network - LBNL
SpliceView - Splicing Signals Prediction - WebGene Server
YSPL (BCM Gene Finder) - Search for Exon-Exon Junction Positions in cDNA -BCM

5. Repetitive DNA & CpG Isles Analyses

CENSOR - Query Sequence Comparison against Human/Rodent
Repeats Database - GIRI
GRAIL - CpG Isle, Repetitive DNA prediction/Analysis
PYTHIA - Identification of Human Repetitive DNA
RepEater - Search for Sequence Repeats in Query Sequence
RepeatMasker2 - Analysis of Repetitive Elements in DNA Sequences

6. tRNA Gene Prediction

Pol3Scan - Analysis of tRNA Genes & Related Elements
tRNAscan - Genomic tRNA Gene Identification

Some of the important programs and their electronic addresses

Program	Electronic address
GeneID	www.imim.es/GeneIdentification/Geneid/geneid_input.html
GeneParser	beagle.colorado.edu/~eesnyder/GeneParser.html
Genie	www-hgc.lbl.gov/inf/genie.html
GenLang	www.cbil.upenn.edu/~sdong/genlang_home.html
GENSCAN	genomic.stanford.edu/GENSCANW.html
GENVIEW	www.itba.mi.cnr.it/webgene
GRAIL	avalon.epm.ornl.gov
HEXON/FGENEH	dot.imgen.bcm.tmc.edu:9331/gene-finder/gf.html
MORGAN	www.cs.jhu.edu/labs/compbio/morgan.html
MZEF	clio.cshl.org/genefinder
ORFgene	www.itba.mi.cnr.it/webgene
PROCRUSTES	www-hto.usc.edu/software/procrustes/index.html
SorFind	www.rabbithutch.com
VEIL	www.cs.jhu.edu/labs/compbio/veil.html
Xpound	ftp://igs-server.cnrs-mrs.fr/pub/Banbury/xpound
Banbury	Cross igs-server.cnrs-mrs.fr

RNA Structure Prediction

15.1 INTRODUCTION

One of the guiding principles in molecular biology is that structure is much more conserved than sequence. RNA molecules are involved in important biochemical functions, including translation, RNA splicing, processing and editing, cellular localization, and catalysis. RNA sequence analysis needs to be treated differently than DNA sequence analysis because RNA structures fold and base pair with themselves to form secondary structures. Hence, it is not necessarily the sequence but the *structure conservation* that is most important in RNA sequence analysis.

Variations in RNA sequence maintain base-pairing patterns that give rise to these secondary structures. Therefore, to maintain the secondary structure, when a nucleotide in one base changes, the base with which it pairs must also change to maintain the same structure. For instance, if you have the base pair G-C, and the G mutates to an A, then the C should mutate to a U to maintain a base pairing at this location, which promotes the same secondary structure. Such a variation is referred to as *covariation*.

In RNA, sequence conservation among functional homologues is usually limited to short (<10 nucleotide) segments, making homology searching even more difficult than for proteins. RNA secondary structures are amenable to phylogenetic covariation analysis, giving RNA biologists an advantage in determining the functional family to which a molecule belongs. Frequently, sequence conservation within these RNA families becomes apparent in the context of the secondary structure. In group I introns, for example, the conserved positions of functionally critical residues within the RNA secondary structure revealed the location of the catalytic core (Fig. 15.1). The representation shows features typical of RNA

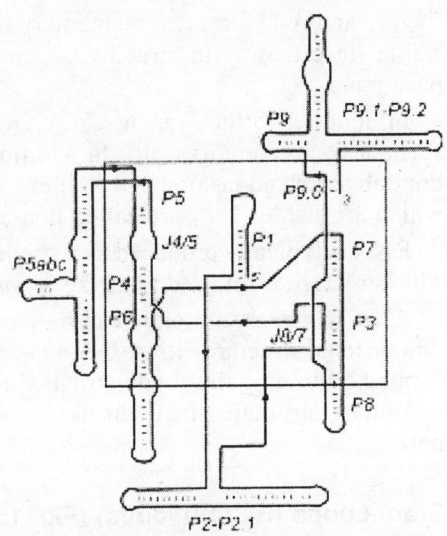

Fig. 15.1. Secondary structure of the group I class of self-splicing introns.

235

secondary structures, including base-paired segments (P) connected by joining regions (J). The boxed region is the catalytic core, identified by conservation of functionally critical residues.

Some of the characteristics of RNA structure are as follows :

1. RNA structure is dynamic in solution, i.e. constantly fluctuating between different folded states;
2. There are many alternative structures that are nearly identical in energy (both predicted and actual);
3. RNA molecules are highly sensitive to solution conditions, e.g. salt and temperature. They are also highly sensitive to protein binding;
4. Biologically important structure may not have lowest predicted free energy, but it should be one of the lower ones. Hence, we need to look at sub-optimal structures also;
5. Three dimensional structure of RNA is difficult to determine due to flexibility of molecule;
6. Most analysis of correctness is based on phylogenetically determined models. Phylogenetic models look for invariant base pairs, but may not identify all unique structures;
7. Structural information can also be obtained from nuclease digestion studies and sometimes cross-linking.

In order to determine the secondary structure of the RNA molecule, all possible choices of complementary sequences are considered, and the sets that provide the most energetically stable molecules are chosen. Another method to predict secondary structure in RNA takes into account conserved patterns of base-pairing. Positions of covariance are studied, and are taken to be conserved matches, since they maintain the secondary structure. Locating regions of covariance in sequence data is a computationally challenging tasks.

15.2 OVERVIEW OF RNA SECONDARY STRUCTURE

RNA is a polymer composed of a combination of four nucleotides: adenine (A), cytosine (C), guanine (G), and uracil (U).

G-C and A-U form complementary hydrogen bonded base pairs, with the GC base pairs being more stable since they form three hydrogen bonds as opposed to the two hydrogen bonds formed by AU base pairs.

In addition to the Watson-Crick GC and AU base pairs, non-canonical pairs can occur in RNA secondary structure as well. In addition, we consider the weaker G-U wobble pair, where the bases bond in a skewed fashion. All of these are called canonical base pairs. Other base pairs occur, some of which are stable. They are called non-canonical base pairs.

RNA is typically produced as a single stranded molecule, which folds upon itself to form base pairs. This structure is referred to as the *secondary structure* of the RNA.

RNA secondary structure can be viewed as an intermediary between a linear molecule and a three-dimensional structure. RNA secondary structure is mainly composed of double-stranded RNA regions formed by folding the single-stranded RNA molecule back on itself. There are a number of different secondary structures that can be formed from this base-pairing. These structures are summarized here.

Stem Loops (Hairpin loops) (Fig. 15.2)

Stem loop is a lollipop-shaped structure formed when a single-stranded nucleic acid molecule loops back on itself to form a complementary double helix (stem) topped by a loop. Stem loops are generally at least 4 bases long.

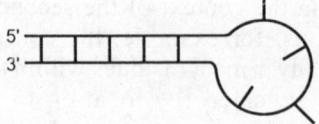

Fig. 15.2. Structure of stem loops.

Bulge Loops (Fig. 15.3)

Bulge loops are commonly found in helical segments of cellular RNAs. Bulge Loops occur when bases on one side of the structure cannot form base pairs and they cause bends in the helix.

Interior Loops (Fig. 15.4)

Interior loops occur when bases on both sides of the structure cannot form base pairs.

Junctions or Multiloops (Fig. 15.5)

Junctions include two or more double-stranded regions converging to form a closed structure.

15.3 OVERVIEW OF RNA TERTIARY STRUCTURE

In addition to the above secondary structures, tertiary interactions can be present as well. The three-dimensional structure of yeast tRNA(Phe) was determined by Kim and Rich in 1974 and it turned out not to have an extended cloverleaf structure but rather folded into an L shape in which each of the arms of the L was made up of two of the stem-loops of the cloverleaf. Each arm of the molecule is around 60Å long and the distance from the acceptor end to the anticodon loop is about 67Å. Such tertiary interactions are located using covariance analysis. The types of tertiary interactions present in RNA molecules include kissing hairpins, pseudoknots and hairpin-bulge interactions.

Kissing Hairpins (Fig. 15.6)

In kissing hairpins, the unpaired bases of two separate hairpin loops base pair with one another.

Pseudoknots (Fig. 15.7)

When the parts of the RNA sequence spanned by two base pairs are neither disjoint, nor have one contained in the other, the two base pairs form a *pseudoknot*. Almost all RNA structures contain one or more pseudoknots.

Hairpin-Bulge Interactions (Fig. 15.8)

15.4 ASSUMPTIONS IN RNA STRUCTURE PREDICTION

Most of the methods for RNA structure prediction are based on a set of three assumptions. These assumptions are :

1. The most likely structure is similar to the energetically most stable structure.

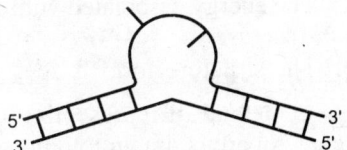

Fig. 15.3. Bulge loops.

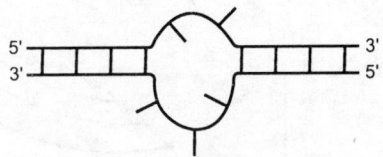

Fig. 15.4. Interior loops.

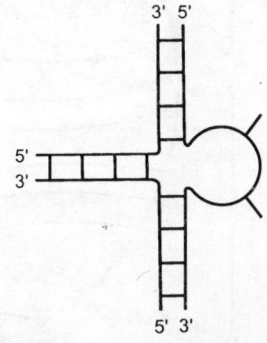

Fig. 15.5. Junctions or multiloops.

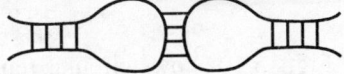

Fig. 15.6. Kissing hairpins.

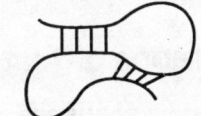

Fig. 15.7. Pseudoknots.

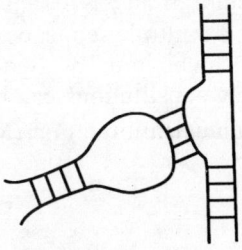

Fig. 15.8. Hairpin-bulge interaction.

2. The energy associated with any position in the structure is only influenced by local sequence and structure.

3. The structure formed does not produce pseudoknots.

One method of representing the base pairs of a secondary structure is to draw the structure in a circle. An arc is drawn to represent each base pairing found in the structure. If any of the arcs cross, then a pseudoknot is present. An example of the representation of RNA in a circular form is shown in Fig. 15.9.

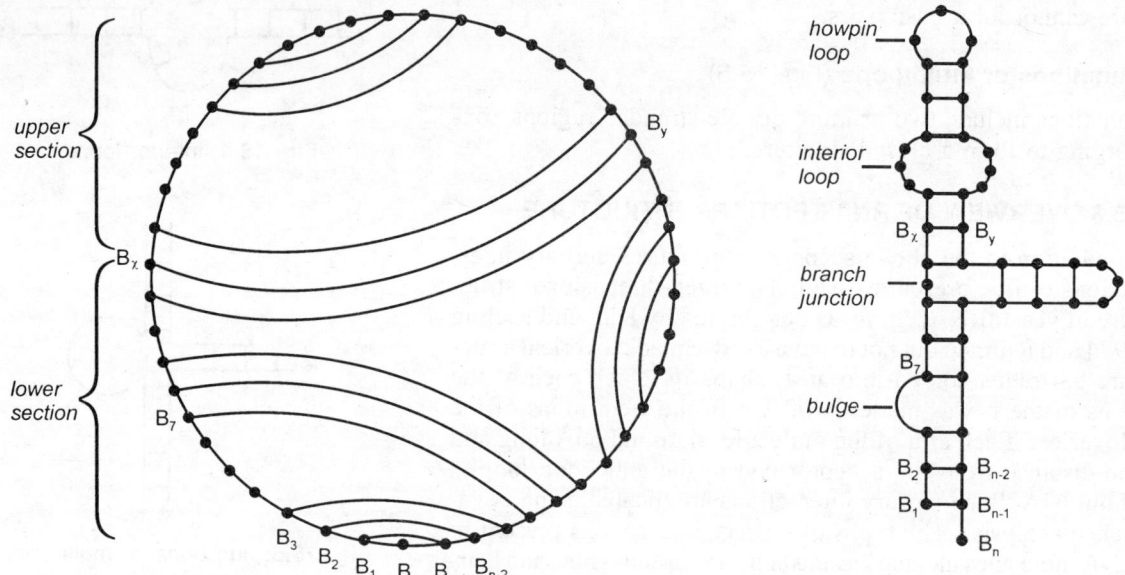

Fig. 15.9. RNA representation using the circular method.

Fig. 15.10 shows circular representation of *B.subtilis* RNA. The nucleotides are stretched out uniformly along the circumference of a circle and circular arcs that link paired bases and meet the circle at right angles represent the base pairs.

15.5 METHODS OF RNA STRUCTURE PREDICTION

Comparative sequence analysis

Comparative sequence analysis is the most reliable computational method for prediction of the secondary structure of an RNA sequence. In order to use comparative sequence analysis, the first step is to calculate a multiple sequence alignment. The pre-condition is that the sequences be similar enough so that they can be initially aligned. At the same time, the sequences should be dissimilar enough so that co-varying substitutions can be detected.

The mutual information (M_{ij}) gained by aligning two columns that co-vary is determined by the function:

$$M_{ij} = \sum_{x_i, x_j} f_{x_i x_j} \log_2 \frac{f_{x_i x_j}}{f_{x_i} f_{x_j}}$$

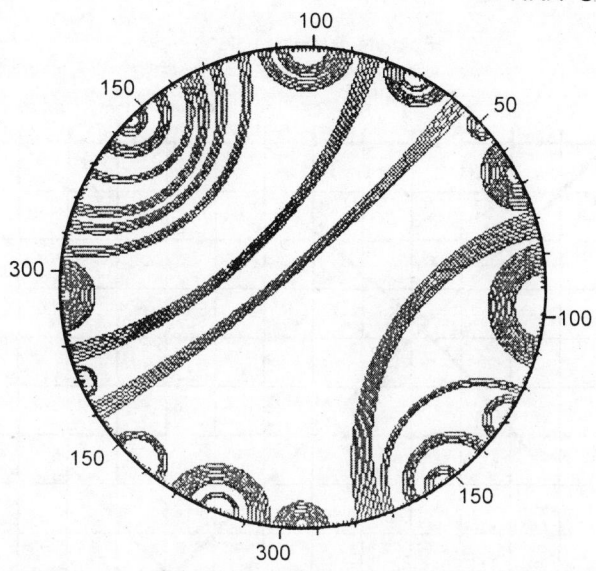

Fig. 15.10. Circular representation of *B.subtilis* RNA folding.

Here f_{x_i} is the frequency of a base in column i; $f_{x_i x_j}$ is the joint (pairwise) frequency of a base pair between columns i and j. For RNA, the information ranges from 0 and 2 bits. If columns i and j are uncorrelated, the mutual information is 0.

Self-complementary regions in RNA sequences

There are a number of possible secondary structures that can be determined from a single sequence. For example, an RNA molecule only 200 bases long has 10^{50} possible secondary structures, many of which are not plausible. A method to detect the correct structure is needed.

Dot-matrix method can be used to find self-complementary regions in an RNA sequence. The dot-plot of the sequence is performed against its complement. The repeat regions that are found can potentially base pair with each other to form secondary structures. More advanced dot-plot techniques incorporate free energy measures as well. For the following sequence S, using MFOLD (http://bioweb.pasteur.fr/seqanal/interfaces/mfold-simple.html), we get the dotplot shown in Fig. 15.11.

GCUUACGACCAUAUCACGUUGAAUGCACGCCAUCCCGUCCGAUCUGGCAAGUUAAGCAA
CGUUGAGUCCAGUUAGUACUUGGAUCGGAGACGGCCUGGGAAUCCUGGAUGUUGUAAGCU

The *energy dot plot* gives an overall visual impression of how "well-defined" the folding is. A cluttered plot, or cluttered regions, indicate either structural plasticity (the lack of well-defined structure) or else the inability of the algorithm to predict a structure with confidence.

Base Pair Maximization

This method is also called *Nussinov Folding Algorithm*. The approach is to find the configuration with the greatest number of paired bases. Testing and scoring each possible structure is numerically impossible. This method uses dynamic programming for finding an efficient solution.

According to the Nussinov algorithms, there are four ways to get the best structure from I to j from the best structures of the smaller subsequences:

  1. Add i,j pair onto best structure found for subsequence i+1, j-1

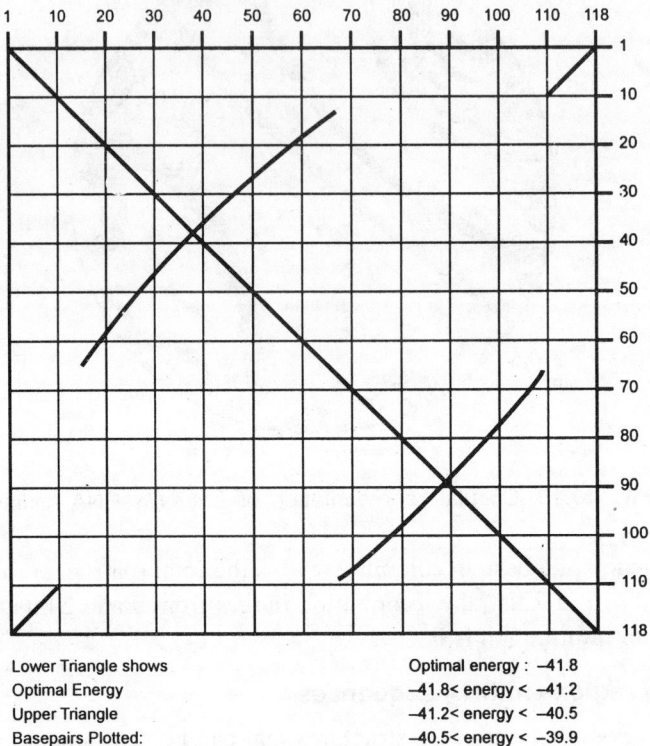

Fig. 15.11. Sample dotplot from MFOLD.

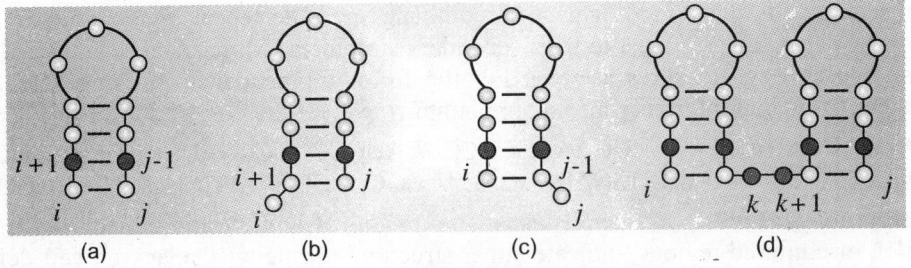

Fig. 15.12. (a) i,j pair , (b), i unpaired, (c) j unpaired and (d) bifurcation.

2. Add unpaired position i onto best structure for subsequence i+1, j
3. Add unpaired position j onto best structure for subsequence i, j-1
4. Combine two optimal structures i,k and k+1, j

The possible structures are shown in Fig. 15.12.

The Nussinov RNA folding prediction program works by comparing a sequence against itself in a dynamic programming matrix with the above rules for scoring the structure at a particular point. Since the structure is folding upon itself, it is only necessary to calculate half of the matrix.

Initialization step

In the matrix fill step, the score for the matches along the main diagonal and the diagonal just below it are set to zero. Formally, the scoring matrix, M, is initialized as follows:

M[i][i] = 0   for i = 1 to L (where L is the length of the sequence)

M[i][i-1] = 0 for i = 2 to L

Consider the RNA sequence T = GGGAAAUCC, the matrix looks like Fig. 15.13 (a), such that sequences of length 1 will score 0:

	G	G	G	A	A	A	U	C	C
G	0								
G	0	0							
G		0	0						
A			0	0					
A				0	0				
A					0	0			
U						0	0		
C							0	0	
C								0	0

Fig. 15.13(a). Initialisation step.

Now the matrix is filled in, starting with subsequences of length 2, and ending at subsequences of length L. The four rules for filling in the matrix are used:

M[i][j] = max of the following four:

   M[i+1][j] (Ith residue is hanging off by itself)

   M[i][j-1] (jth residue is hanging off by itself)

   M[i+1][j-1] + S(x_i, x_j) (ith and jth residue are paired; if x_i = complement of x_j,

then S(x_i, x_j) = 1; otherwise it is 0.

   M[i][j] = MAX$_{i<k<j}$ (M[i][k] + M[k+1][j]) (merging two substructures)

When looking for subsequences of length 2, the matrix is filled as Fig.15.13(b), since A-U is the only base-pair found.

	G	G	G	A	A	A	U	C	C
G	0	0							
G	0	0	0						
G		0	0	0					
A			0	0	0				
A				0	0	0			
A					0	0	1		
U						0	0	0	
C							0	0	0
C								0	0

Fig. 15.13 (b). Filling the matrix.

Filling in for subsequences of length 3, the matrix becomes as in Fig. 15.13 (c)

	G	G	G	A	A	A	U	C	C
G	0	0	0						
G	0	0	0	0					
G		0	0	0	0				
A			0	0	0	0			
A				0	0	0	1		
A					0	0	1	1	
U						0	0	0	0
C							0	0	0
C								0	0

Fig. 15.13 (c). Filling the matrix for subsequences of length 3.

The final filled matrix is as given in Fig. 15.13(d).

	G	G	G	A	A	A	U	C	C
G	0	0	0	0	0	0	1	2	3
G	0	0	0	0	0	0	1	2	3
G		0	0	0	0	0	1	2	2
A			0	0	0	0	1	1	1
A				0	0	0	1	1	1
A					0	0	1	1	1
U						0	0	0	0
C							0	0	0
C								0	0

Fig. 15.13 (d). The final filled matrix.

Nussinov has been implemented at (http://ludwig-sun2.unil.ch/~bsondere/nussinov/form.html). Using this program, for the above sequence T, the structure obtained is given in Fig. 15.14.

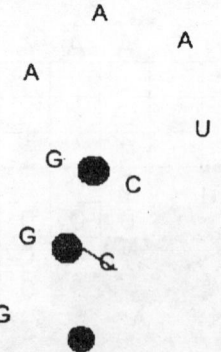

Fig. 15.14. Structure for sequence T using Nussinov algorithm.

Sequence S, which was more complex purports to the structure as given in the Fig. 15.15.

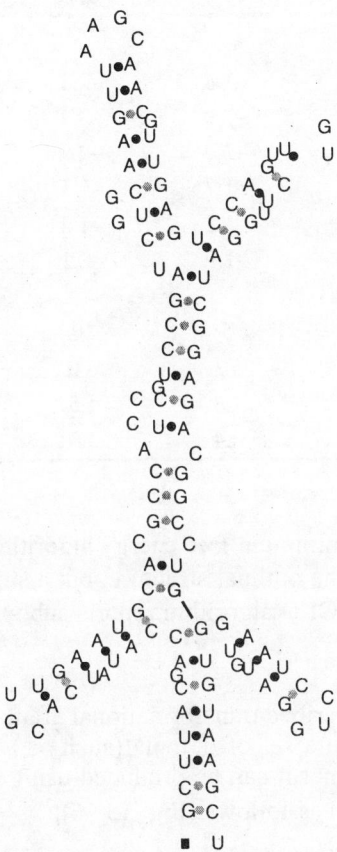

Fig. 15.15. Structure for sequence S using Nussinov algorithm.

Energy Minimization Methods

Since RNA folding is determined by biophysical properties, methods that take into account these properties are more likely to yield accurate predictions. One method that is widely used is the energy minimization algorithm that predicts the correct secondary structure is the one that minimizes the free energy (DG). The free energy of an RNA secondary structure is calculated as the sum of the individual contributions of loops, base pairs, and other secondary structure elements. Energies of stems are calculated as the stacking contributions between neighboring base pairs.

The predicted free-energy values (kcal/mole at 37°C) are calculated as shown in Table 15.1.

In order to find the structure for which the minimum free energy is found, the sequence is compared against itself using a dynamic programming approach similar to the maximum base-paired structure approach previously described. However, instead of using a scoring scheme for the base pairs present, the score is based upon the free energies described above. Gaps between matches represent some form of a loop, so the gap score is calculated using the above tables as well. The most widely

Table 15.1. Predicted free-energy values

	A/U	C/G	G/C	U/A	G/U	U/G
Stacking Energies for base pairs						
A/U	−0.9	−1.8	−2.3	−1.1	−.1	-0.8
C/G	−1.7	−2.9	−3.4	−2.3	−2.1	-1.4
G/C	−2.1	−2.0	−2.9	−1.8	−1.9	-1.2
U/A	−0.9	−1.7	−2.1	−0.9	−1.0	-0.5
G/U	−0.5	−1.2	−1.4	−0.8	−0.4	-0.2
U/G	−1.0	−1.9	−2.1	−1.1	−1.5	-0.4
Destabilizing Energies for Loops						
Number of Bases	1	5	10	20	30	
Internal	—	5.3	6.6	7.0	7.4	
Bulge	3.9	4.8	5.5	6.3	6.7	
Hairpin	—	4.4	5.3	6.1	6.5	

used software that incorporates this minimum free energy algorithm is MFOLD. The correct structure is not necessarily the structure with the optimal structure, but a structure within a certain threshold of the calculated minimum energy. MFOLD algorithm reports suboptimal foldings as well.

Tranformational Grammars

The linguist Noam Chomsky first described transformational grammars in the 1950's. The idea behind transformational grammars is to take a set of outputs (such as a sentence, or in our case, an RNA structure) and determine whether or not it can be produced using a set of rules for the language.

The Chomsky hierarchy is defined as follows (Fig. 15.16):

1. Regular grammars
   $$u \longrightarrow Xv \quad u \longrightarrow X$$
2. Context free grammars
   $$u \longrightarrow \beta$$
3. Context sensitive grammars
   $$\alpha_1 u \alpha_2 \longrightarrow \alpha_1 \beta \alpha_2$$
4. Unrestricted grammars
   $$\alpha_1 u \alpha_2 \longrightarrow \gamma$$

where μ is a non-terminal, X a terminal, α, γ any sequence of terminals/non-terminals except the null string, and b any sequence of terminals/non-terminals.

Transformational grammars consist of a set of symbols and production rules on which the symbols can be put together. The grammar consists of a set of abstract *non-terminal* symbols, a set of *terminal* symbols (those that actually appear in strings) and a set of *productions*.

Stochastic Context Free Grammars

Stochastic Context Free Grammars (SCFGs) have been used to model RNA secondary structure. Context free grammars are well suited to modeling RNA secondary structure because they can represent base pairing preferences.

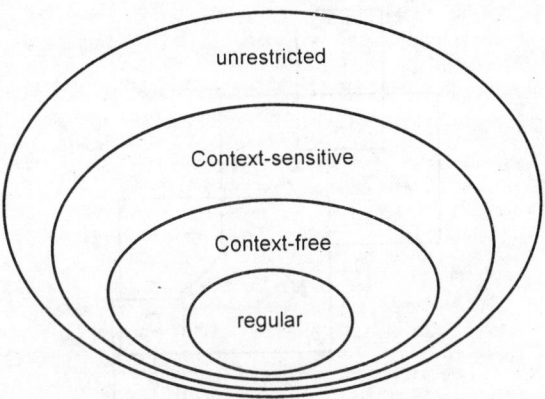

Fig. 15.16. Chomsky hierarchy of grammars.

Example of this is tRNAScan-SE (http://www.genetics.wustl.edu/eddy/tRNAscan-SE/). Typically, with SCFG approaches, using a training set of data creates the grammars, and then the grammars are applied to potential sequences to see if they fit into the language. SCFGs allow the detection of sequences belonging to a family, such as tRNAs, group I introns, snoRNAs, snRNAs, etc.

Grammar for Palindromic sequences

First, consider the case of palindromic DNA sequences. There are a total of five possible terminal symbols: {A, C, G, T, e) where e represents the blank terminal symbol. The production rules for creating a palindromic sequence are as follows, where S and W are non-terminal symbols:

$$S \rightarrow W$$
$$W \rightarrow aWa \mid cWc \mid gWg \mid tWt$$
$$W \rightarrow a \mid c \mid g \mid t \mid \varepsilon$$

Using these production rules, we can create a derivation of the palindromic sequence acttgttca as follows:

$$S \Rightarrow W \Rightarrow aWa \Rightarrow acWca \Rightarrow actWtca \Rightarrow acttWttca \Rightarrow acttgttca$$

Creating a parse tree

The parse tree for UAG can be created as follows.

$$s \rightarrow C_1 \qquad c_1 \rightarrow Uc_2 \qquad c_2 \rightarrow Ac_3 \qquad c_3 \rightarrow A$$
$$c_2 \rightarrow Gc_4 \qquad c_3 \rightarrow G$$
$$c_4 \rightarrow A$$

Parse tree is given in Fig. 15.17.

The root of the tree is the non-terminal start symbol, S. Leaves of the parse tree are the terminal symbols in the sequence, and internal nodes are the non-terminals. The leaves can be parsed from left to right to view the results of the production.

A parse tree for the example sequence acttgttca in the above section is shown in Fig. 15.18.

A SCFG for RNA secondary structure can be constructed as follows:

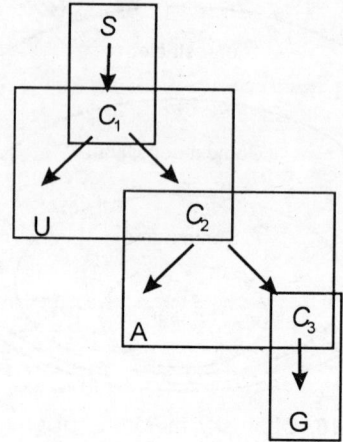

Fig. 15.17. A sample parse tree.

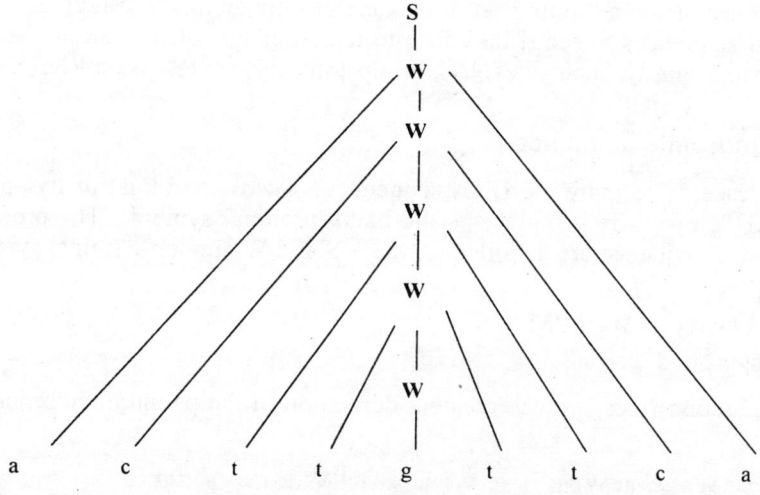

Fig. 15.18. Parse tree for acttgttca.

$S \rightarrow W$

$W \rightarrow WW$ (bifurcation)

$W \rightarrow aWu \mid cWg \mid gWc \mid uWa$ (loops)

$W \rightarrow gWu \mid uWg$

$W \rightarrow aW \mid cW \mid gW \mid uW$ (bulges on one side)

$W \rightarrow Wa \mid Wc \mid Wg \mid Wu$ (bulges on opposite side)

$W \rightarrow a \mid c \mid g \mid t \mid \varepsilon$

Using this grammar, the structure for the RNA structure for the sequence, can be constructed using the following productions (5' to 3') as follows:

GCUUACGACCAUAUCACGUUGAAUGCACGCCAUCCCGUCCGAUCUGGCAAGUUA
AGCAACGUUGAGUCCAGUUAGUACUUGGAUCGGAGACGGCCUGGGAAUCCUGGAU
GUUGUAAGCU

$S \Rightarrow W \Rightarrow Wu \Rightarrow gWcu \Rightarrow gcWgcu \Rightarrow gcuWagcu \Rightarrow gcuuWaagcu \Rightarrow$

$gcuuaWuaagcu \Rightarrow gcuuacWguaagcu \Rightarrow$

$gcuuacgWuguaagcu \Rightarrow gcuuacgaWuuguaagcu \Rightarrow$

$gcuuacgacWguuguaagcu \Rightarrow gcuuacgaccWguuguaagcu \Rightarrow gcuuacgaccaWguuguaagcu \Rightarrow$

The structure is shown in Fig. 15.19.

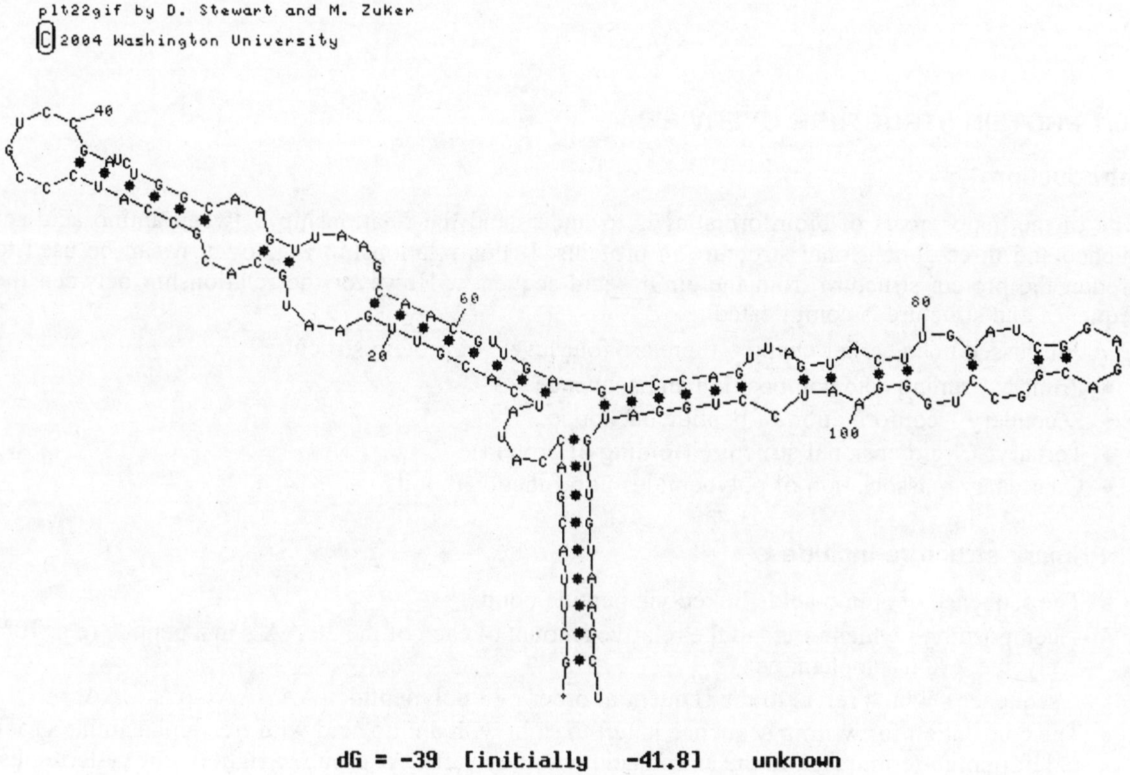

```
plt22gif by D. Stewart and M. Zuker
[C] 2004 Washington University
```

dG = -39 [initially   -41.8]   unknown

Fig. 15.19. RNA structure using MFOLD.

16

Visualization and Prediction of Protein Structure

16.1 PROTEIN STRUCTURE OVERVIEW

Introduction

One of the major goals of bioinformatics is to understand the relationship between amino acid sequence and three-dimensional structure in proteins. If this relationship is known, it can be used to predict the protein structure from the amino acid sequence. However the relationship between the sequence and structure is complicated.

As discussed in an earlier chapter, there are four levels of protein structure :

- Primary – amino acid composition and sequence
- Secondary – conformation of peptide backbone
- Tertiary – 3-dimensional structure (folding of protein)
- Quartenary – association of polypeptides into functional units

1. Primary structure includes

- The sequence of amino acids linked via peptide bonds
  - composition - which refers to the relative amount of each of the 20 AA's in a peptide (e.g, 10% glycine, 6% tryptophan, etc.)
  - sequence - which refers to the sequential order of a polypeptide (AA_1-AA_2-AA_3...AA_n)
- The convention for writing sequence is left to right with amino acid with free alpha amine group to left (amino-terminus) and the amino acid with free carboxyl group to right (carboxy-terminus)

2. Secondary structure includes

- Conformation of peptide backbone
  - Spatial arrangement of amino acid residues that are near one another in the linear sequence which can give rise to a periodic structure — typically intramolecular and intermolecular hydrogen bonding.
    - Alpha-helix

248

- Beta-pleated sheet
- Turns
- Collagen triple helix
   – Supersecondary structure, which includes clusters of secondary structure

Alpha-helix

Alpha helix, the right-handed helix is most common arrangement. Alpha-helix results from the conformation of peptide bonds and particular R-groups seeking the most stable arrangement which consists of. There are 3.6 residues/turn in right-handed helix. The periodicity or distance that the helix rises per turn is 0.54 nm. The rise per amino acid is 0.15 nm. H-bonding between every 4th peptide bond (amide and carboxyl) stabilizes alpha-helix. In helical region of a protein, every peptide bond therefore participates in H-bonding which leads to a very stable structure. A consequence of the structure of the alpha-helix is that amino acids which are three to four amino acids apart in primary structure are spatially close to each other in the helix. Hydrogen-bonding is the strongest when groups are in straight line which is the configuration in alpha-helix. Tight packing within the core of the helix also stabilizes the helix.

Molecular Visualization of Alpha-helix

One method of visualization is using Kinemages. (C2motif.kin). Kinemage 1 is amphipathic. The other method is using Chemscape Chime Molecular Visualization.

Beta-pleated sheet

Beta- strands are typically 5-8 amino acid residues which form an extended, chain - silk/spider webs. They form a fully extended structure - adjacent amino acids are 3.5 angstroms away (compared to only 1.5 for alpha helix). These strands can form sheets when two strands are grouped and hydrogen bonded. Kinemage anti-parallel beta-sheet can be used to visualize beta sheets. Arrangements of β-sheets can be :

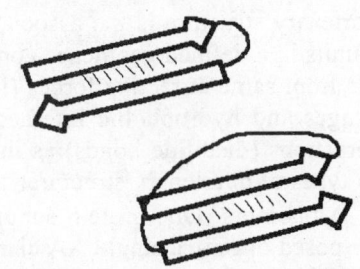

- Anti-parallel, which have amino-terminal end at one end of the polypeptide oriented toward carboxy-terminus of polypeptide. Anti-parallel is the most common arrangement (Fig. 16.1).

Fig. 16.1. Parallel and anti-parallel arrangements

- Parallel, which have amino and carboxy-termini of peptide chains are oriented in the same direction. They are often grouped into structural units of 2-5 sheets. Beta sheets can have a mix of parallel and antiparallel components.

Turns or Loop Regions

Loop regions typically connect different combinations of secondary structures and they may be flexible allowing conformational changes in the protein. They are often on the protein surface. They can form hydrogen bonds with water molecules. Loops that connect two adjacent antiparallel beta-strands (thus forming a beta-sheet) are called hairpin loops or reverse turns. Such loops lead to reversal of the direction of the polypeptide chain. The short loops or turns typically have 3-5 residues. Often glycine residues are present in one type of hairpin turn (Type II - second of two residues in turn). The small R-group of glycine allows in to fit inside the turn. Other R-groups would be too bulky, lead to steric problems, and prevent a structural turn. Another type of typical bend, loop, or turn results from gly-pro-ser. Proline's angle is fixed and forces the bend, while glycine is the least sterically hindering and thus does not get in way inside the turn. Turns facilitate the folding of a protein into a compact structure by reversing chain direction into a central region.

Random Coil

Coils comprise of amino acid residues in chains that do not lead to a consistent secondary structure or disrupt alpha-helix or beta-sheet. Coils may form due to electrostatic repulsion or bulkiness of R-groups that disrupt structure. This may happen due to amino acids such as proline in which the N is part of a rigid ring that prevents rotation of the ring carbons and leads to a "kink".

3. Tertiary Structure

Tertiary structure represents spatial arrangement of amino acids that are far apart in the linear sequence. It results from interactions between R-groups via van der Waals, ionic, hydrophobic and hydrogen bonding. Groupings or arrangements of secondary structures into combinations that are present in a variety of proteins are often described as motifs or domains. Examples include :
- Parallel and antiparallel β-sheets (also known as the Hairpin Beta-motif)
- Greek Key motif - four adjacent antiparallel beta strands
- Beta–alpha–beta motif (can be either two parallel or two anti-parallel β)

4. Quartenary

Quartenary structure is the association of polypeptide subunits in a defined geometric configuration. This results from same attractive forces (i.e., H-bonding, salt linkages and hydrophobic interactions) and covalent interactions (disulfide bonds) as in tertiary. There are two types of quartenary structures :
- Monomers (One protein subunit) – protein composed of only a single AA chain
- Oligomers – proteins composed of more than one AA chain (Fig. 16.2)

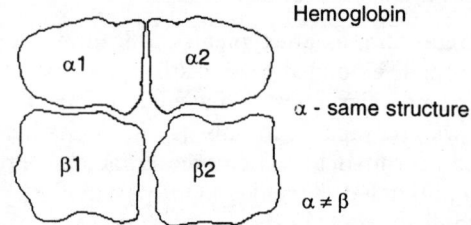

Fig. 16.2. Different structural proteins.

4° structure is not required for all proteins to be functional - many proteins may have only 2° or 3° structure.

16.2. DIFFERENT STRUCTURAL PROTEINS (Fig. 16.3)

Proteins and their structures are built from domains (motifs) and polypeptides. A motif is a short conserved region in a protein sequence. A domain is a discrete portion of a protein assumed to fold independently of the rest of the protein and possessing its own function. Motifs are frequently highly conserved parts of domains. Several motifs, groups or individual tertiary structures which combine to form a compact globular structure that acts as an independent region of a protein. Thus domains are different combinations of secondary structure elements and motifs. Simple motifs combine to form complex motifs. Proteins may have different domains that serve different functions (catalysis versus regulation) and which may be made of several different general types of domains in terms of general organization (i.e., globular versus fibrous domains).

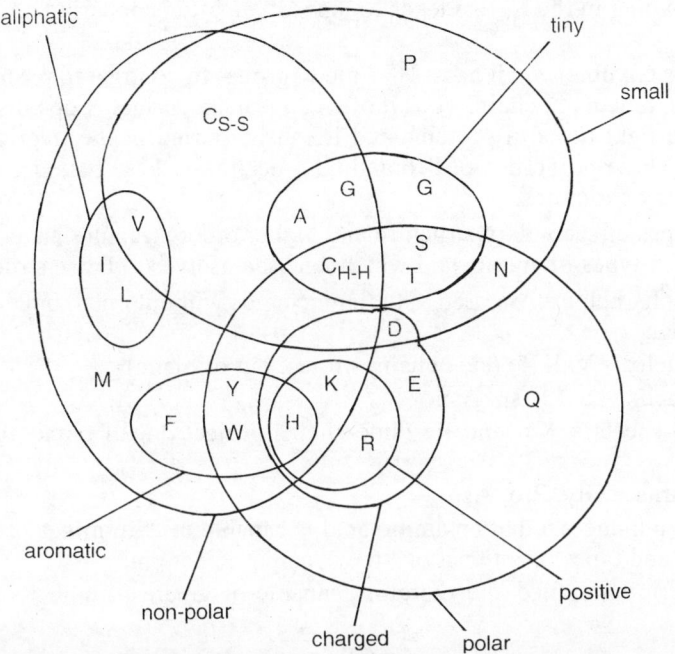

Fig 16.3. A Venn diagram showing the relationship of the 20 naturally occurring amino acids to a selection of physio-chemical properties thought to be important in the determination of protein structure.

There are four types of protein structure classifications :

- **Alpha or a/a** = Predominantly or core exclusively alpha helices
  - General types of mainly alpha
    - Bundle
    - Non-bundle
- **Beta or b/b** = Predominantly or core primarily beta strand
  - General types beta
    - Single sheet
    - Roll
    - Barrel
    - Sandwich
- **Alpha/Beta or a/b** = Predominantly alternating alpha-helix and beta-strand
  - For example, BaB motifs and combinations of this motif (usually parallel β sheets)
  - Note that typically β-sheets are found in the interior of proteins while alpha-helixes are found on the exterior of proteins
- **Alpha and beta or a + b** = alpha helices and beta strand regions as separate groupings
  - Anti-parallel β sheets, segregated a and B regions
  - Helices typically on one side of the sheet

Steric properties of amino acids can greatly affect the local structures that a protein adopts. The best example of this is perhaps proline. Proline exhibits reduced torsional freedom with the main chain phi angle fixed). This leads to the conformation of the peptide backbone being locked in a turn and with the loss of a hydrogen bonding in the N, this leads to the residue often appearing on the surface loops of a protein.

Another example is Glycine which has a H as the R-group. In contrast to proline, Gly has complete torsional freedom about the main chain. Thus it often appears in surface loops. Its small size lends it to being associated with tight turns in proteins and it can be buried in the interior of the protein in a hydrophobic pocket. These properties of Pro and Gly mean that these residues do not typically lend themselves to secondary structures.

Other particular types of secondary structure and higher order structure have reasonable probabilities of having particular types of amino acid which lend themselves to those structural configurations.

- Propensity for alpha-helix = Ala, Leu, Glu (amino acids without much bulk, or polar atoms, close to the alpha carbon)
  - Disrupt alpha-helix = Val, Ile (side chains project out of plane)
  - Disrupt alpha-helix = Ser, Asp, Asn
- Propensity for β-sheets = Val and Ile (side chains project out of plane and thus conducive to sheets)
- Propensity for turns = Gly, Pro, Asp
- Conformation in phi and psi that an amino acid is capable of determines propensity to form secondary structure and types of interactions they can participate in.
- Gly has least steric hindrance and therefore capable of greatest number of conformations in a protein

One of the difficulties in protein structure prediction is that the context in which amino acids find themselves in a protein has a large affect on their conformation (phi and psi rotation) and thus their propensity to form particular secondary structures.

16.3 PROTEIN STRUCTURE DATABASES AND VISUALIZATION TOOLS

PROWL

This is a site that provides information on properties of amino acids, bond geometry they allow, probability for being interior vs. exterior residues and which amino acid substitutions are likely to maintain structure and function. It also provides other information that is used to make predictions about protein structure based on primary amino acid sequence.

Cn3D

"See in 3-D," a structure and sequence alignment viewer for NCBI databases. It allows viewing of 3-D structures and sequence-structure or structure-structure alignments. Cn3D works as a helper application to the browser. Files are downloaded to the computer and the helper application is launched.

Chemscape Chime, Rasmol, and Protein Explorer

Chemscape Chime works as a plug-in to allow visualization of structures with the browser. Protein Explorer also works as a plug-in to allow visualization of structures with your browser. Rasmol is an external application on which both of these browser-based applications are primarily derived

RasMol is one of the most popular tools for protein structure visualization. It reads molecular structure files from the Protein Data Bank (PDB).

Mage and Kinemages

A "kinemage" (kinetic image) is a scientific illustration presented as an interactive computer display. Operations on the displayed kinemage respond immediately: the entire image can be rotated in real time, parts of the display can be turned on or off, points can be identified by selecting them, and the change between different forms can be animated. A kinemage is prepared in order to better communicate ideas that depend on 3-dimensional information. The kinemages are distributed as plain text files of commented display lists and accompanying explanations. They are viewed and explored in an open-ended way by the reader using a simple graphics program called MAGE. A utility called PREKIN makes a starting kinemage from a PDB-format coordinate file which can then be modified on-screen in MAGE or off-line in any text editor.

Protein Data Bank

PDB is a very large global repository for the processing and distribution of 3-D macromolecular structure data primarily determined experimentally. Depositors to the PDB have derived the structures using a variety of tools and techniques like X-ray crystal structure determination, NMR, cryoelectron microscopy and theoretical modeling. The database provides access to the structural data as well as methods to visualize the structures and to download structural information.

NCBI Structure Database (MMDB)

NCBI's Entrez includes a database of experimentally determined three-dimensional biomolecular structures. Most 3D-structure data are obtained from X-ray crystallography and NMR-spectroscopy. They provide a wealth of information on the biological function, on mechanisms linked to the function, and on the evolutionary history of and relationships between macromolecules. The addition of structure data to Entrez makes this information easily accessible to biologists, and to facilitate comparative analysis involving 3-D structure.

The NCBI Structure Database is called MMDB, Molecular Modeling Database, and contains macromolecular 3D structures, as well as tools for their visualization and comparative analysis. The majority of data files for MMDB are experimentally determined biopolymer structures which are primarily obtained from the Protein Data Bank (PDB). The Molecular Modelling Database (MMDB) contains both proteins and polynucleotides with over 10,000 structures which are linked to the rest of the NCBI databases, including sequences, bibliographic citations, taxonomic classifications, and sequence and structure neighbours.

MMDB reorganizes and validates the information in a way that enables cross-referencing between the chemistry and the three-dimensional structure of macromolecules. Its data specification includes a description of a biopolymer's spatial structure, a description of how it is organized chemically, and a set of pointers linking the two. By integrating chemical, sequence, and structure information, MMDB is designed to serve as a resource for structure-based homology modeling and protein structure prediction. MMDB records are stored in ASN.1 format and can be displayed with the Cn3D, Rasmol, or Kinemage viewers. In addition, similar structures within the database have been identified using VAST, and new structures can be compared against the database using VAST search.

Protein sequences from MMDB are extracted and available in the Entrez protein sequence database. They are linked to the 3-D structures, therefore it is possible to determine whether a protein sequence in Entrez has homologs amongst known structures by examining its Related Sequences or Protein Neighbors and checking whether this set has any structure links. Text searches in MMDB will yield

"Structure Query pages", providing access to entries that matched the keywords. "Structure Summary pages" for one/several/all of these may be retrieved.

From the "Structure Summary pages" one may:

- access amino acid and nucleic acid sequences
- retrieve MedLine documents
- get taxonomy information
- view sequence neighbors
- view structure neighbors

VAST

VAST - Vector Alignment Search Tool - is a computer algorithm developed at NCBI and used to identify similar protein 3-dimensional structures. The "structure neighbours" for every structure in MMDB are pre-computed and accessible via links on the MMDB Structure Summary pages. These neighbors can be used to identify distant homologs that cannot be recognized by sequence comparison alone. VAST generates a domain division based on the compactness of adjacent secondary structure elements in space.

VAST Search

VAST Search is NCBI's structure-structure similarity search service. It compares 3D coordinates of a newly determined protein structure to those in the MMDB/PDB database. VAST Search computes a list of structure neighbors that you may browse interactively, viewing superpositions and alignments by molecular graphics. Protein structure neighbors in Entrez are determined by direct comparison of 3-dimensional protein structures with the VAST algorithm. Each of the more than 18,000 domains in MMDB is compared to every other one. From the MMDB structure summary pages, retrieved via Entrez, structure neighbors are available for protein chains and individual structural domains.

On the structure summary page, use "Structure Neighbors" to retrieve a list of similar structures. For example, select a chain identifier such as "B", or a domain identifier such as "B.4", to get a list of neighbors. The results of the precompiled VAST search will then present a table of structural neighbours. Using the checkboxes in the left most column of this table, select those structures you would like to see superimposed, and click on "View/Save Alignments" to view these with the mime-typed helper application you have installed (e.g. Cn3D or MAGE).

VAST Search is a service that allows searching for structural neighbors starting with a set of 3D-coordinates specified by the user. This service is meant to be used with newly determined protein structures which are not yet part of MMDB. Structure neighbors for proteins already in MMDB have been pre-computed and can simply be looked up from MMDB's structure summary pages.

CDD

Conserved Domain Database (CDD) is a collection of sequence alignments and profiles, representing protein domains conserved in molecular evolution, is now available via the CD-search service. Proteins often contain several modules or domains, each with a distinct evolutionary origin and function. The CD-Search service may be used to identify the conserved domains present in a protein sequence.

It uses the following domain definition:

- A compact substructure of a protein based on the 3-D fold

- Defined without regard to the sequence conservation shared with other members of protein families.
- Defined without regard to sequence continuity (i.e., topology)

Conserved domains are defined based on recurring sequence patterns or motifs. CDD currently contains domains derived from two popular collections: Smart and Pfam. The source databases also provide descriptions and links to citations. Since conserved domains correspond to compact structural units, CDs contain links to 3D-structure via Cn3D whenever possible.

To identify conserved domains in a protein sequence, the CD-Search service employs the reverse position-specific BLAST algorithm. The query sequence is compared to a position-specific score matrix prepared from the underlying conserved domain alignment. Hits may be displayed as a pairwise alignment of the query sequence with a representative domain sequence, or as a multiple alignment. CD-Search now is run by default in parallel with protein BLAST searches. While the user waits for the BLAST queue to further process the request, the domain architecture of the query may already be studied.

DART

DART is the Domain Architecture Retrieval Tool that can be used to search for proteins with similar domain architectures. DART uses precomputed CD-search results to quickly identify proteins with a set of domains similar to that of the query.

PDBsum

PDBsum is a web-based database providing a largely pictorial summary of the key information on each macromolecular structure deposited at the Protein Data Bank (PDB). It includes images of the structure, annotated plots of each protein chain's secondary structure, detailed structural analyses generated by the PROMOTIF program, summary PROCHECK results and schematic diagrams of protein; ligand and protein; and DNA interactions.

RasMol scripts highlight key aspects of the structure, such as the protein's domains, PROSITE patterns and protein; ligand interactions, for interactive viewing in 3D. Numerous links take the user to related sites.

The PDB structures can be displayed and manipulated in 3D using RasMol and/or a VRML browser. The former is also used for focusing on specific aspects of the structure, such as protein-ligand interactions and residues belonging to PROSITE patterns.

Each PDBsum entry contains the following information and analyses:

- Name, date and description of macromolecule(s) in the PDB entry.
- Thumbnail image, rendered using Raster3D, of the structure in the given entry. Protein secondary structure is depicted as cylinders for helices, arrows for beta strands and threads for random coil; ligands and metals are shown in spacefill. For DNA structures, and elongated proteins/multimers, three orthogonal views are given.
- Authors, resolution and *R*-factor.
- Links to Related entries, as defined in the header records of the PDB file.
- Enzyme Classification number
- Summary PROMOTIF information.
- Protein Motif Fingerprints and link to the PRINTS database and multiple alignments in CINEMA.

Several databases attempt to use structural similarities of proteins for their classification. One of these is "A Structural Classification of Proteins" (SCOP). The SCOP database, was created by manual inspection and abetted by a battery of automated methods, aims to provide a detailed and comprehensive description of the structural and evolutionary relationships between all proteins whose structure is known. As such, it provides a broad survey of all known protein folds, detailed information about the close relatives of any particular protein, and a framework for future research and classification. The SCOP database aims to provide a detailed and comprehensive description of the structural and evolutionary relationships between all proteins whose structure is known, including all entries in the Protein Data Bank. It is available as a set of tightly linked hypertext documents which make the large database comprehensible and accessible

16.4. PROTEIN CLASSIFICATION

Protein classification methodology

Proteins are classified to reflect both structural and evolutionary relatedness. Many levels exist in the hierarchy, but the principal levels are family, superfamily and fold, described below. The exact position of boundaries between these levels is to some degree subjective. Our evolutionary classification is generally conservative: where any doubt about relatedness exists, we made new divisions at the family and superfamily levels. Thus, some researchers may prefer to focus on the higher levels of the classification tree, where proteins with structural similarity are clustered.

The different major levels in the hierarchy are:

Family : *Clear evolutionarily relationship*

Proteins clustered together into families are clearly evolutionarily related. Generally, this means that pairwise residue identities between the proteins are 30% and greater. However, in some cases similar functions and structures provide definitive evidence of common descent in the absence of high sequence identity; for example, many globins form a family though some members have sequence identities of only 15%.

Superfamily: *Probable common evolutionary origin*

Proteins that have low sequence identities, but whose structural and functional features suggest that a common evolutionary origin is probable are placed together in superfamilies. For example, actin, the ATPase domain of the heat shock protein, and hexakinase together form a superfamily.

Fold: *Major structural similarity*

Proteins are defined as having a common fold if they have the same major secondary structures in the same arrangement and with the same topological connections. Different proteins with the same fold often have peripheral elements of secondary structure and turn regions that differ in size and conformation. In some cases, these differing peripheral regions may comprise half the structure. Proteins placed together in the same fold category may not have a common evolutionary origin: the structural similarities could arise just from the physics and chemistry of proteins favoring certain packing arrangements and chain topologies.

Protein classification tools

CATH (Class, Architecture, Topology, and Homologous superfamily)

CATH is a novel hierarchical classification of protein domain structures, which clusters proteins at four major levels, Class(C), Architecture(A), Topology(T) and Homologous superfamily (H). Class, derived from secondary structure content, is assigned for more than 90% of protein structures automatically. Architecture, which describes the gross orientation of secondary structures, independent of connectivity, is currently assigned manually. The topology level clusters structures according to their toplogical connections and numbers of secondary structures. The homologous superfamilies cluster proteins with highly similar structures and functions. The assignments of structures to topology families and homologous superfamilies are made by sequence and structure comparisons. CATH includes the following :

- Class : Similar secondary structure content and all alpha, all beta , alpha/beta etc.
- Architecture (Fold) : Major structural similarity and secondary structure elements in similar arrangement
- Topology (Superfamily) : Probable common ancestry
- Family : Clear evolutionary relationship and sequence similarity usually >25%

16.5. PROTEIN STRUCTURE PREDICTION

Introduction

The problem of predicting protein structure from sequence remains fundamentally unsolved despite a high focus by researchers on this problem.

- Mean-force-potentials derived from the protein databases can distinguish between correct and incorrect models.
- Inter-residue contacts can be detected by analysis of correlated mutations, although with low accuracy.
- Secondary structure, solvent accessibility, and transmembrane helices can be predicted with significantly improved accuracy using multiple sequence alignments.

Multiple sequence alignments tailored to particular protein families intrude into the twilight zone of sequence similarity. Combination of advanced sequence alignment, and threading techniques with expertise permits to intrude into the midnight zone of extremely low sequence identity, even. Some of these new prediction methods have proven accurate and reliable enough to be useful in genome analysis, and in experimental structure determination.

The Protein Folding Problem

Its 3D shape (fold, conformation), determines the function of a protein. The three-dimensional (3D) structure of proteins is determined by the amino acid sequence. Can we predict the 3D shape of a protein given only its amino-acid sequence?

It is difficult, in general, to predict structure from sequence. However, from the growing database of experimentally determined protein structures, some rules are emerging :

- The number of unique protein folds is quite limited.
- There are many proteins with the same fold, but no similarity of sequence.
- 'Neutral' mutations altering the protein structure are likely.

These rules suggest that a key to understanding protein structure lie in the patterns of neutral amino acid exchange.

How to solve the protein folding problem?

The protein folding problem is one of the key problems in molecular biology. The classical methods for structure analysis of proteins are X-ray crystallography and nuclear magnetic resonance (NMR). Unfortunately, these techniques are expensive and can take a long time. On the other hand, the sequencing of proteins is relatively fast, simple, and inexpensive. As a result, there is a large gap between the number of known protein sequences and the number of known three-dimensional protein structures. This gap has grown over the past decade (and is expected to keep growing) as a result of the various genome projects worldwide. Thus, computational methods that may give some indication of structure and/or function of proteins are becoming increasingly important.

Overview of methods of protein structure prediction

Sequence with significant similarity to a protein of known structure: In this case, homology modelling can be used to construct a 3D model with correct fold, but it does not give accurate loop regions. Homology modelling effectively increases the number of 'known' 3D structures to a great extent.

Sequence with insignificant sequence identity: Threading techniques can potentially detect remote homologies.

When homologies modelling and threading are inapplicable: In such cases, the prediction problem has to be simplified. There are some generic methods for prediction at three different levels of simplification, namely one, two, and three dimensions.

Comparative modelling exploits the fact that evolutionarily related proteins with similar sequences as measured by the percentage of identical residues at each position based on an optimal structural superposition often have similar structures. For example, two sequences that have just 25% sequence identity usually have the same overall fold. Threading methods compare a target sequence against a library of structural templates, producing a list of scores. The scores are then ranked and the fold with the best score is assumed to be the one adopted by the sequence. The ab initio prediction methods consist in modelling all the energetics involved in the process of folding, and then in finding the structure with lowest free energy. This approach is based on the 'thermodynamic hypothesis', which states that the native structure of a protein is the one for which the free energy achieves the global minimum. While ab initio prediction is clearly the most difficult, it is arguably the most useful approach.

There are two components to ab initio prediction: devising a scoring (i.e, energy) function that can distinguish between correct (native or native-like) structures from incorrect ones, and a search method to explore the conformational space. In many methods, the two components are coupled together such that a search function drives, and is driven by, the scoring function to find native-like structures. Unfortunately, this direct approach is not really useful in practice, both due to the difficulty of formulating an adequate scoring function and to the formidable computational effort required to solve it. To see why this is so, note that any fully-descriptive energy function must consider interactions between all pairs of atoms in the polypeptide chain, and the number of such pairs grows exponentially with the number of amino acids in the protein. To make matters worse, a full model would also have to contend with vitally important interactions between the protein's atoms and the environment, the so-called 'hydrophobic effect'. Thus, in order to make the computation practical, simplifying assumptions must necessarily be made.

Prediction in 1D (secondary structure, solvent accessibility and transmembrane helices) : use of evolutionary information.

Prediction in 2D (inter-residue contacts, inter-strand contacts, disulphide bonds): use of evolutionary information. However the effectiveness is limited.

Prediction in 3D: (1) particular protein structures (coiled-coil proteins) can be predicted from sequence, (2) incorrect structures can be detected with remarkable accuracy (mean-force potentials).

Determinants of protein structure

Hierarchy of protein structure terminology. To reiterate, primary structure denotes the amino acid sequence and secondary structure denotes regular patterns of the main chain atoms (like α-helices or β-strands). Tertiary structure is the representation of all atoms in a protein chain in three dimensions and quaternary structure denotes the arrangement of all atoms of the whole protein, consisting of multiple chains.

Sequence determines structure. A fully unfolded amino acid sequence diluted in the appropriate solvent (under proper conditions in terms of pH value and temperature) folds into a unique tertiary (3D) structure. This process is usually reversible. Consequently, it is hypothesized that folding is determined exclusively by the information contained in the amino acid sequence. It is also thought that the formation of some secondary structure precedes tertiary organisation. Possible exceptions to this hypothesis (Anfinsen-hypothesis) constitute molecular chaperones, i.e., proteins which assist or hinder folding.

Secondary structure facilitates dense packing. Pauling and Corey first proposed the existence of secondary structure elements on theoretical grounds prior to their discovery in protein structures. The main driving force for folding water-soluble globular protein molecules is the need to pack hydrophobic side chains into the interior of the molecule. This creates a hydrophobic core and a hydrophilic surface. But how can that be realised with the main chain being highly polar (with NH as hydrogen donor and C=O as hydrogen acceptor? The solution is to neutralise the NH and CO groups by a formation of hydrogen bonds. These bonds affect the formation of the regular patterns of secondary structure like α-helix and β-strand. Any region of the protein that is not in either helix or strand is termed 'loop'. Helices and strands form dipoles.

Function-specific motifs of secondary structure. Combinations of a few secondary structure segments with a specific geometric arrangement occur frequently in protein structures (3D structure). Such combinations are termed super-secondary structure or motifs. Some of these motifs are associated with particular functions. Examples are the helix-loop-helix DNA binding motif, the calcium binding motif, or the Greek key or β-meander motif.

Classification of proteins into structural classes. Motifs can be used to classify proteins. Three widely used databases of structure classifications are SCOP, FSSP, and CATH. A more simple classification is based purely on the content of secondary structure. A protein can be classified as, e.g., all-α, if it contains almost no strand structure and a high content of helix.

Variety of protein structures. Protein structures show a fascinating variety. Structure is more conserved by evolution than sequence. 3D structure is closely related to the function of the protein. Although the mutation of a few residues in a protein is likely to destabilise the fold, evolution has created a record of sequence variation by not changing the 3D structure. Two natural protein sequences can differ by 75% of their residues and, yet, have the same 3D structure.

3D structure is encrypted in the sequence. Solving the protein folding problem means deciphering the code according to which the 3D structure is encrypted in the amino acid sequence. Prediction methods can be distinguished according to the principle they start from: physics or statistics. The prediction success of methods based on physical principles is still very limited.

What determines protein stability? It is the marginal entropy differences that determine protein stability. According to the Anfinsen hypothesis, the folded state of a globular protein is characterised by a minimum in free energy. The folding transition is largely a two-state process: unfolded non-native chain (U) -> folded native structure (N). As a first approximation, usually intermediate states can be neglected. The difference in free energy between unfolded and native state can be approximated by :

$$Æ\ G\ α\ -\ RT\ \ln\ K$$

with R being the gas constant, T the absolute temperature, and the equilibrium constant K = number of chains in U / number of chains in N. Typical values for ÆG are −5 to −15 kcal/mol

Why do proteins fold? Hydrophobic forces drive folding stability. The driving force for folding is the reduction of solvent accessible surface. Folding is driven by the attempt for dense packing. Globular proteins are known to have a very high packing density. This density can possibly be explained by the complementarity between interior side chains, fitting tightly together.

What determines the specific conformation of a fold? The dense packing determines the conformational specificity. One explanation could again be the density of packing, i.e. only very specific conformations allow the residues to pack into the jigsaw puzzle. However, there is evidence that such a grouping can readily be done, i.e. does not require one particular conformation. This suggests that dense packing is not the primary source of conformational specificity. What then determines the fold? One candidate is the stereo-chemical code.

A single mutation can destabilise a protein. The mutation of a single residue typically causes an approximate reduction of the free energy difference between native and unfolded state of about 1 kcal/mol. Thus, the exchange of a few residues can destabilise a protein of more than 100 residues. Does this imply that two proteins with some different residues have a different 3D structure? And if yes, are all potential 3D structures expressed in nature, i.e. are there some 20N different folds for proteins with N residues realised in nature? The fact that a single mutation can destabilise a protein implies only that the majority of the 20N possible sequences adopt different structures. It does not mean that all of them exist in natural form.

Only mutations not altering the structure survive through the evolutionary chain. Random errors in the DNA lead to the wrong translation of the information coded in the genes into sequences of amino acids. These errors are the basis for evolution. As the structure and the environment of the protein determine the function, mutations resulting in a structural change are not likely to survive, since the protein cannot perform its task. Thus, only those errors are likely to be accepted which do not alter the structure. However, it is also to be noted that usually proteins consist of functional modules, which are combined in various ways to yield different properties for the proteins.

How much variation in sequence is possible? Mutations of amino acids survive if they do not change the 3D structure of the folded protein. The known proteins are a record of exploration for variation of sequence with no effect to structure. A protein sequence folds into a unique three-dimensional protein structure. Different sequences, though, can fold into similar structures. Structure is more conserved than sequence. But, how much variation of the sequence can exactly be accepted without changing the structure? How stable is a protein structure with respect to sequence changes? What percentage of the sequence are 'anchor' residues, i.e., are crucial for protein structure and function? Evolution has realised pairs of proteins that have the same 3D structure, although they have only 25 of their 100 residues alike. Not any two residues can be exchanged anywhere in the sequence. Instead, the possible exchanges depend on the details of the structure and on the physico-chemical properties of the amino acids involved. Thus, the pattern of residue substitution - the record of the unlikely - carries information rather specific for a particular protein structure.

How many different protein folds exist? The number of different protein folds realised by nature is fairly limited. However, the concept of 'similarity' between folds is not clear-cut. The number of unique structures is about 300. Based on this number and recent analyses of entire chromosomes the estimate for the number of folds appears to confirm the notion of 1,000 folds (factor of 3 possible).

Goal of structure prediction. For over 30 years, there has been an ardent search for methods to predict 3D structure from the sequence. Many methods were found which looked initially very promising - but always the hope has been dashed. The search has been driven by the belief that the 3D structure of a protein is determined by its amino acid sequence. While it is now known that chaperones often play a role in the folding pathway, and in correcting misfolds, it is believed that the final structure is at the free-energy minimum. Thus, all information needed to predict the native structure of a protein is contained in the amino acid sequence.

Limitations of ab initio prediction of protein structure from sequence. Given only the amino acid sequence, it should be possible in principle to directly predict protein structure from physico-chemical principles using, for example, molecular dynamics methods. In practice, however, such approaches are frustrated by the enormous complexity of the calculation (requiring many orders of magnitude more computing time than is currently feasible) and by inaccuracies in the experimental determination of basic parameters. Thus, the most successful structure prediction tools are knowledge-based, using a combination of statistical theory and empirical rules.

16.6 METHODS OF STRUCTURE PREDICTION FOR KNOWN FOLDS

Sequence alignments

Any sequence analysis starts with database searches for homologous proteins by sequence alignment procedures. When pairwise sequence identity is over 40%, alignment procedures are usually straightforward. For less similar protein sequences, alignments may fail. Multiple alignments improve as data banks grow. The most advanced sequence alignment tools base the alignment on profiles derived from databases or particular sequence families. New methods like HMM may be more successful in the twilight zone of sequence alignments.

Homology modelling

The basic assumption of homology modelling is that unknown structure (U) and the homologous template protein of known structure (T) have nearly identical backbone structure in the aligned regions. The basic action is to correctly place the side chains of U into the backbone of T. For levels of above 70-90% sequence identity, the resulting models are quite accurate. However, the limiting factor is the computation time required. For sequence identities down to about 30% sequence identity, U and T will still have the same fold, but the number of loops inserted grows and the divergence between U and T becomes considerable. For lower levels of pairwise sequence identity, the accuracy of the sequence alignment becomes an additional problem. However, even down to levels of 25-30% sequence identity, homology modelling produces coarse-grained models for the overall fold of proteins of unknown structure.

Remote homology modelling (threading)

Threading is used for cases with <25% pairwise sequence identity. Threading has to go through three steps :

1. The remote homology between U and T has to be detected
2. U and T have to be aligned correctly
3. The homology modelling procedure has to be tailored to the harder problem of extremely low sequence identity.

Although automatic threading methods still are fairly inaccurate, both in recognising the correct fold and in getting the alignment correct, it is clearly superior to traditional sequence alignments at this low level (<25%) of sequence identity.

Sequence alignments

1. Database search

The most common tools for starting a database search are BLAST and FASTA. Some of the search tools automatically check regions that are composition biased (e.g., Gly-Arg-Ala in DNA binding proteins).

Selecting the putative homologues from the hit list. Given a list of proteins aligned (hit list) to U, which ones are likely to be homologues? Where to set the threshold in terms of the score reported by the alignment program (e.g. the BLAST score)? Few programs help with that decision (e.g. MAXHOM) or the consistent alignment parser CAP in BLAST. The best strategy may be to select a large number of proteins from the hit list (>100) and repeat a more accurate full dynamic programming alignment of U against this list (rather than against the entire database).

Finding sequence motifs. Complements to alignment programs are tools that search for motifs, blocks or patterns. Examples are PROSITE , PFSCAN, or the tools associated with databases of block alignments (BLOCKS, PRINTS, PRODOM). Motifs can be used to detect more distantly related homologues (<30% sequence identity) and to refine the alignment (e.g. by defining a family specific profile that can be given as input to, e.g., CLUSTALW.

Refining the alignment. There are four major approaches to automatically refine alignments:

1. A more accurate dynamic programming algorithm (BIOACCELERATOR or SSEARCH, or MAXHOM).
2. Build a profile and to thus generate a more family-specific alignment (e.g. by ClustalW).
3. Use Hidden Markov models.
4. Expert tool that enables to investigate the final alignment (e.g.) TopAlign.

2. Alignment

Finding the best match for two strings. At the level of protein molecules, selective pressure results from the need to maintain function, which in turn requires maintenance of the specific 3D structure. This evolutionary history is the basis for attempts to align protein sequences, i.e., to optimally detect equivalent positions in strings of amino-acid letters. Sequence alignments unravel information about structural and functional relations between residues in different proteins. It is not trivial to map the complexity of factors determining protein structure and function onto 1D relations between letters. The objective is to find the best match between two strings of letters (amino acids or nucleotide acids). Once the time demanding task of scanning the entire database is accomplished, more refined dynamic programming-based or HMM-based alignment programs can be applied to refine the alignment for the hits found.

Task for high levels of sequence identity. Any sequence analysis starts with database searches: all known databases are scanned by sequence alignment procedures for proteins homologous to the search sequence U. When the pairwise sequence identity between U and a putative homologue H is over 25-30% (for more than 80 residues), alignment procedures are usually straightforward. For less similar protein pairs, alignments may fail. One of the difficulties in comparing different alignment procedures is the lack of well-defined criteria for measuring the quality of an alignment. The second problem is that most methods do not supply a cut-off criterion for distinguishing between homologous and non-homologous sequences (i.e., false positives). For some large sequence families remote homologues can be aligned correctly, but for most cases sequences with less than 25% sequence identity will be false positives, i.e., will have no structural or functional similarity to the guide sequence.

3. Multiple alignments

Merging pairwise alignments into a multiple alignment. MSA is implemented by the program MAXHOM (implemented for the PredictProtein prediction service) or the generation of the HSSP database. The usual process is as follows :

1. A fast algorithm (BLAST) is used to scan the database for possible homologues.
2. A length-dependent cut-off threshold for structural homology filters the list of putative homologues.
3. All sequences that fall above the threshold are aligned consecutively to the guide sequence (U) by a standard dynamic programming algorithm
4. After each sequence has been added to the alignment an alignment profile is compiled and used to align the next sequence.
5. After all the sequences have been aligned the profile is recompiled and the dynamic programming algorithm starts once again to align consecutively the sequences, this time using the conservation profile as derived after completion of the first sweep.
6. A slightly different method is to additionally sort the aligned sequences according to evolutionary trees. In general the power of multiple alignment methods grows with the databases.

Hidden Markov models and genetic algorithms. The principal idea is to deduce a family specific model reflecting evolutionary processes and to align new sequences according to the model derived. The idea is the same as for traditional family specific profiles used with dynamic programming. Hidden Markov-based alignments appear to be particularly sensitive to detecting less obvious homologues. Another interesting method is the application of genetic algorithms to the multiple alignment problems; the particular advantage being that any objective function can be optimised by the genetic algorithm.

Homology Modelling

If the database search with U picked a homologue that has known 3D structure one can predict 3D structure for U by homology modelling. Homology modelling can be done by using Modeller and SWISS-MODEL.

An analysis of sequence alignments for proteins of known structure reveals that all protein pairs with more than 30% pairwise sequence identity (for alignment length > 80), have homologous 3D structures. This is the basis for homology modelling. The principal idea is to model the structure of U (protein of unknown structure) based on the template of a sequence homologue of known structure (T). The accuracy of homology modelling depends on the level of similarity between U and T.

As discussed earlier, the basic assumption of homology modelling is that U and T have identical backbones (main chain C). The task is to correctly place the side chains of U into the backbone of T. For very high levels of sequence identity between U and T (ideally differing by one residue only), side chains can be 'grown' during molecular dynamics simulations. For slightly lower levels (still of high sequence similarity), side chains are built based on similar environments in known structures.

Rotamer libraries (libraries containing all side-chain orientations observed in known structures) are used in the following way:

1. Rotamer distributions are extracted from a database of non-redundant sequences.
2. Fragments of seven (helix, strand) or five residues (other) are compiled.
3. Fragments of the same length are successively shifted through the backbone of U.
4. For modelling the side chains of U only those fragments from the rotamer library are accepted which have the same amino acid in the centre as U, and for which the local backbone is similar to that around the evaluated position). Over the whole range of sequence identity between U and T for which homology modelling is applicable, the accuracy of the model drops with decreasing similarity.
5. For levels of at least 60% sequence identity, the resulting models are quite accurate. For even higher values, the models are as accurate as is experimental structure determination.

Homology modelling Tools

Name	Comments
Modeller : *http://guitar.rockefeller.edu/modeller/* *modeller.html*	Takes the inputs - alignment file and a Modeller script and calculates multiple models for the inputs
Swiss-Model : http://expasy.hcuge.ch/swissmod/ SWISS-MODEL.html	An automated knowledge-based protein modelling server; first approach and optimise

Remote homology modelling (threading)

Naturally evolved sequences with more than 30% pairwise sequence identity have homologous 3D structures. Does that mean that all others are non-homologous? Not necessarily - in the PDB database there are thousands of pairs of structurally homologous pairs of proteins that are remote homologues. Actually, most similar protein structures are such remote homologues.

If a correct alignment between U and a remote homologue T is given, one could build the 3D structure of U by (remote) homology modelling based on the template of T. A successful remote homology modelling must solve three different tasks:

1. The remote homologue (T) has to be detected.
2. U and T have to be correctly aligned.
3. The homology modelling procedure has to be tailored to the harder problem of extremely low sequence identity (with many loop regions to be modelled).

There are two basic algorithms for threading:

1. Profile Method
2. Core threading model

Profile method is the one in which the structure of the template is coded into a vector. This vector contains fingerprint of the structural environment of each residue inside the template protein. The main idea of this threading model is that the target protein reproduces the structural features of the template protein. However, the profile method fails when the structural profiles change from the template protein to the target.

So a second model is introduced to overcome this problem. It is based on analyzing pairwise interactions between structurally adjacent residues in the protein. Thus the threading problem optimizes a kind of pseudopotential based on the relative attraction of the residue pairs. It is also called core threading model, in which branch-and bound method is used. The problem of this model is that it concentrates only on the core regions and overlooks the loop regions which are also very important for some proteins.

A very recent model is a recursive dynamic programming (RDP) method for protein threading which can overcome the above problem. RDP is based on the divide-and-conquer paradigm and maps the target onto the template in a stepwise fashion.

The following are the some of the variations in threading techniques:

1. Use of structural propensities of amino acids (such as preferences for secondary structure formation, hydrophobicity, and polarity), and then to assess whether or not a given sequence with its structural preferences fits into the structural environment of a given structure.

2. A different approach is to use the rich knowledge deposited in the database of protein structures (PDB) by extracting mean-force potentials. Such potentials monitor the observed distances between residue pairs of particular amino acids, with a particular sequence separation (number of residues between the two).

3. Another threading method is based on 1D predictions: first 1D structure (secondary structure and solvent accessibility) is predicted for a sequence of unknown structure, then the 1D structure is extracted for a library of known structures, and finally the observed and the predicted 1D structure strings are aligned by typical dynamic programming algorithms

Since the different mean-force-potentials that have been proposed capture different aspects of protein structure, the correct remote homologue is likely to be found by at least one of them. However, so far, no single method has been able to detect the correct remote homologue for more than half of all test cases. This is still clearly superior to that of traditional sequence alignments at this low level (<25%) of sequence identity.

Threading tools

Name	Accuracy	Comments
PHDthreader: http://www.embl-heidelberg.de/predict protein/	< 30%, less than 30% of the predicted first hits are true remote homologues. Evaluated by cross-validation on 89 unique protein structures.	Prediction-based threading detecting the fold type and aligning a protein of unknown structure and a protein of known structure for low levels of sequence identity (< 25%).
T3P2: http://www.mbi.ucla.edu/people/frsvr/frsvr.html		Prediction-based threading detecting the fold type and aligning a protein of unknown structure and a protein of known structure for low levels of sequence identity (< 25%).

16.7. METHODS OF STRUCTURE PREDICTION FOR UNKNOWN FOLDS

Prediction in 1D

Prediction of 1D aspects of 3D structure (e.g. secondary structure, solvent accessibility, transmembrane helices, coiled-coils) is a much simpler task than homology modelling. In general, prediction accuracy is significantly superior if predictions are based on multiple alignments.

The basic idea underlying most secondary structure prediction methods is the fact that segments of consecutive residues have preferences for certain secondary structure states. Thus, the prediction problem becomes a pattern-classification problem tractable by pattern recognition algorithms. The goal is to predict whether the residue at the centre of a segment of typically 13-21 adjacent residues is in a helix, strand or in none of the two (no regular secondary structure, often referred to as the 'coil' or 'loop' state.

Many different algorithms have been applied to tackle the protein structure prediction problem: physico-chemical principles, rule-based devices, expert systems, graph theory, linear and multi-linear statistics, nearest-neighbour algorithms, molecular dynamics, and neural networks. The later techniques have been centred around the evolutionary information and has become a key to significantly improved predictions.

On the one hand, about 75 out of 100 residues can be exchanged in a protein without changing structure. On the other hand, exchanges of 1-5 residues can readily destabilise a protein structure. These statements may appear contradictory. However, the explanation is simple: evolution has explored exactly the unlikely exchanges of particular amino acids at particular positions that do not change structure, as a change of structure usually results in a loss of function (and thus would not survive). Thus, the residue exchange patterns extracted from a protein family (i.e. alignments of similar sequences) are highly indicative of the specific structural details for that family.

1. Solvent accessibility prediction

It has long been hypothesized that if the segments of secondary structure could be accurately predicted, the 3D structure could be predicted by simply trying different arrangements of the segments in space. One criterion for assessing each arrangement could be to use predictions of residue solvent accessibility. The principal goal is to predict the extent to which a residue embedded in a protein structure is accessible to solvent. Solvent accessibility can be described in several ways. The simplest is a two-state description distinguishing between residues that are buried (relative solvent accessibility < 16%) and exposed (relative solvent accessibility 16%). The classical method to predict accessibility is to assign either of the two states, buried or exposed, according to residue hydrophobicity. However, a neural network prediction of accessibility has been shown to be superior to simple hydrophobicity analyses.

Solvent accessibility at each position of the protein structure is evolutionarily conserved within sequence families. This fact has been used to develop methods for predicting accessibility using multiple alignment information. Prediction accuracy is about 75±7%, four percentage points higher than for methods not using alignment information. Predictions of solvent accessibility have also been used successfully for prediction-based threading, as a second criterion towards 3D prediction by packing secondary structure segments according to upper and lower bounds provided by accessibility predictions, and as basis for predicting functional. More recently, predictions of accessibility were also used successfully to predict sub-cellular location.

Solvent accessibility prediction tools

Name	Accuracy	Comments
PHDacc: http://www.embl-heidelberg.de/predictprotein/	> 75% (+/-10%, one standard deviation)	Multiple alignment-based neural network system

2. Predicting transmembrane helices

Very little structural data is available for proteins that do not stay solvent in water. Transmembrane proteins exemplify this property. The major obstacle with these proteins is that they do not crystallise, and are hardly tractable by NMR spectroscopy. Consequently, for this class of proteins structure prediction methods are even more needed than for globular water-soluble proteins. Computational methods can be used to predict which proteins in a genome will be transmembrane proteins.

The prediction task is simplified by strong environmental constraints on transmembrane proteins: the lipid bilayer of the membrane reduces the degrees of freedom to such an extent that 3D structure formation becomes almost a 2D problem. Two major classes of membrane proteins are known:

1. Proteins which insert helices into the lipid bilayer. Once the location of transmembrane segments is known for helical transmembrane proteins, 3D structure can be predicted by exploring all possible conformations. Additionally, predicting the locations of these transmembrane helices is a much simpler problem than is the prediction of secondary structure for soluble proteins. Elaborated combinations of expert-rules, hydrophobicity analyses and statistics yields a two-state per-residue accuracy of about 90% (residues predicted correctly as either transmembrane helix, or other)

2. Proteins that form pores by a barrel of 16 strands (the only known cases of this type are porins. Since there is not much experimental information available on different porin-like membrane proteins, we can hardly estimate prediction accuracy for this class.

The best current prediction methods have a similar high accuracy around 95%. One such method uses a system of neural networks. In order to predict the orientation of the helices (i.e. the topology) a simple rule is applied: positively charged residues occur more often in intra-cytoplasmic than in extra-cytoplasmic regions. The advanced neural network system has been improved significantly by adding a dynamic programming algorithm to the neural network output. The basic idea is to use the neural network output as an energy landscape and to find the optimal path through this landscape. As reliable data for the locations of transmembrane helices exists only for a few proteins, data used for deriving these methods originate predominantly from experiments in cell biology and gene-fusion techniques. Different experimental groups often report different locations for transmembrane regions. Thus, the level of 95% accuracy is not verifiable. Despite this uncertainty in detail, the prediction of transmembrane helices is a valuable tool to quickly scan entire chromosomes.

The classification into membrane/not-membrane proteins has an expected error rate of less than two percent, i.e., about two percent of the proteins predicted to contain transmembrane regions will probably be false positives. The predictions of transmembrane helices has provided a lower bound to approach the question of how many proteins organisms need for, e.g., communication: the percentage of proteins with transmembrane helices has been estimated to be about 25% for yeast and haemophilus influenzae, and around 10-15% for mycoplasma genitalium and methanococcus jannaschii.

Transmembrane helix and signal peptide prediction tools

Name	Accuracy	Comments
PHDhtm: http://www.embl-heidelberg.de/predictprotein/	> 95% (+/-10%, one standard deviation)	Multiple alignment-based neural network system predicting the locations of transmembrane helices
TMAP: http://www.embl-heidelberg.de/tmap/tmap_sin.html	> 95%.	Single sequence-based statistical prediction of the locations of transmembrane helices.
PHDtopology: http://www.embl-heidelberg.de/predictprotein/	> 85% of all proteins all helices and topology are predicted correctly	Refinement of PHDhtm by dynamic programming and prediction of topology (orientation of N-term with respect to membrane).
TMpred: http://ulrec3.unil.ch/software/TMPRED_form.html		Single sequence-based prediction of location and topology for helical transmembrane proteins using statistics and similarity metrices.
Signalp : http://www.cbs.dtu.dk/services/SignalP/		Neural network prediction of presence and location of signal peptide cleavage sites in amino acid sequences from different organisms: Gram-positive and Gram-negative prokaryotes, and eukaryotes.
DAS - Dense Alignment Surface prediction of transmembrane regions in proteins		

3. Identification and characterization-composition using ExPASy

AACompIdent is an important tool to identify a protein by its amino acid composition. It uses the amino acid composition of an unknown protein to identify known proteins of the same composition. Some of the other tools are summarised below :

- AACompSim - Compare the amino acid composition of a SWISS-PROT entry with all other entries

- MultiIdent - Identify proteins with pI, Mw, amino acid composition, sequence tag and peptide mass fingerprinting data

- PeptIdent - Identify proteins with peptide mass fingerprinting data, pI and Mw Experimentally measured, user-specified peptide masses are compared with the theoretical peptides calculated for all proteins in SWISS-PROT, making extensive use of database annotations

- TagIdent - Identify proteins with pI, Mw and sequence tag, or generate a list of proteins close to a given pI and Mw

- FindMod - Predict potential protein post-translational modifications and potential single amino acid substitutions in peptides. Experimentally measured peptide masses are compared with the theoretical peptides calculated from a specified SWISS-PROT entry or from a user-entered sequence, and mass differences are used to better characterize the protein of interest.

- GlycoMod - Predict possible oligosaccharide structures that occur on proteins from their experimentally determined masses (can be used for free or derivatized oligosaccharides and for glyco-peptides)

- GlycanMass - Calculate the mass of an oligosaccharide structure
- FindPept - Identify peptides that result from unspecific cleavage of proteins from their experimental masses, taking into account artefactual chemical modifications, post-translational modifications (PTM) and protease autolytic cleavage
- PeptideMass - Calculate masses of peptides and their post-translational modifications for a SWISS-PROT or TrEMBL entry or for a user sequence

4. Some of the other identification and characterization tolls are as follows :

- PepMAPPER - Peptide mass fingerprinting tool from UMIST
- Mascot - Peptide mass fingerprint, sequence query and MS/MS ion search from Matrix Science Ltd., London
- PepSea - Protein identification by peptide mapping or peptide sequencing from Protana, Denmark
- PeptideSearch - Peptide mass fingerprint tool from EMBL
- ProteinProspector - A variety of tools from UCSF (MS-Fit,MS-Tag, MS-Digest, etc.) for mining sequence databases in conjunction with mass spectrometry experiments
- PROWL - Protein chemistry and mass spectrometry resource from Rockefeller and NY Universities
- CombSearch - An experimental unified interface to query several protein identification tools accessible on the web

5. Primary structure analysis

Compute pI/Mw is a tool that calculates the isoelectric point and molecular weight of an input sequence. The sequence can be input in the FASTA format, the output is the pI and molecular weight for the entire length of the sequence.

pI/Mw example

Theoretical pI/Mw for the protein sequence
MNIAEEPSDE ... FSSGDYSMDY :
Theoretical pI/Mw: 5.19 / 89512.78

MNIAEEPSDEVISSGPEDTDICSQQTSASAEAGDQSIKIERKTSTGLQLEQLANTNLLTIRIKWQLQEEE
DDHCNSRITDQIMDTIQHYKGISVNNSDTETYEFLPDTRRLQVLEQNKDIYLYEHGSQEYEKSYKDNEEE
DDWRYDTVLQAQFKYPKSLENACTDISELLKSEPIGQHIDKWSIGVNKHALTYPGNIFVGGIAKSLSIGE
LSFLFSKYGPILSMKLIYDKTKGEPNGYGFISYPLGSQASLCIKELNGRTVNGSTLFINYHVERKERERI
HWDHVKENNNDDNFRCLFIGNLPYHNPEKVETLITPKEVIEVIKKELSKKFPDFDIISYYFPKRSNTRSS
SSVSFNEEGSVESNKSSNNTNGNAQDEDMLKGYGFIKLINHEQALAAIETFNGFMWHGNRLVVNKAVQHK
VYNNHNSHDRHPSISNHNDMEVLEFANNPMYDYNNYTYDRYYFNNNKNGNSNDTSNVRYFDSVRSTPVAE
KMDLFYPQRESFSEGRGQRVPRFMGNKFDMYQYPSTSYSLPIPMSNQQESNLYVKHIPLSWTDEDLYDFY
KSFGEIISVKVITVGGSKNKYRQQSNDSSSDNDLPVGSSRGYGFVSFESPLDAAKAILNTDGYQVSKDQV
LSVSFAQKRGNLSSSDDDDQSQTDNSSKFQNFQPHNDYHKAYPTKYNKKFINALMTQNQSQQQVSRENYF
IPLQYPNTNTKPVNSYNLISANQNNANWMMPMFPSFGFIPQVPPVPYIIPPQNPAANHIPIMANGSNEEE
EFSSGDYSMDY

SAPS

SAPS (Statistical Analysis of Protein Sequences) algorithm provides extensive statistical information for any given sequence. The output begins with a composition analysis - amino acids, with their counts. It is followed by a charge distribution analysis, including the locations of positively and negatively charged clusters.

COMPOSITIONAL ANALYSIS

```
A-  : 28 (3.6%);   C : 5 (0.6%);   D : 50 (6.4%); E : 54 (6.9%); F  : 36 (4.6%)

G   : 40 (5.1%);   H : 20 (2.6%); I : 49 (6.3%); K : 49 (6.3%); L  : 46 (5.9%)

M   : 17 (2.2%);   N+: 75 (9.6%); P : 40 (5.1%); Q : 42 (5.4%); R  : 2 6 (3.3%)

S   : 82 (10.5%);  T : 34 (4.4%); V : 36 (4.6%); W : 7 (0.9%);  Y +: 4 5 (5.8%)

KR :75 (9.6%);    ED       : 104 (13.3%);AGP : 108 (13.8%);

KRED : 179 (22.9%); KR-ED : -29 (-3.7%); FIKMNY : 271 (34.7%);

LVIFM : 184 (23.6%); ST : 116 (14.9%).

CHARGE

DISTRIBUTIONAL ANALYSIS

DISTRIBUTION OF OTHER AMINO ACID TYPES

High scoring trans me mbrane seg ments:

SPACINGS OF C.

REPETITIVE STRUCTURES.

A. SEPARATED, TANDEM, AND PERIODIC REPEATS: amino acid alphabet

B. SEPARATED AND TANDEM REPEATS
```

6. Tools for physical properties

Some of the other tools for determining the physical properties based on the amino acid sequence are as follows :

- ProtParam - Physico-chemical parameters of a protein sequence (amino acid and atomic compositions, pI, extinction coefficient, etc.)
- MW, pI, Titration curve - Computes pI, composition and allows to see a titration curve
- REP - Searches a protein sequence for a repeats
- Coils - Prediction of coiled coil regions in proteins
- Paircoil - Prediction of coiled coil regions in proteins
- Multicoil - Prediction of two- and three-stranded coiled coils
- PEST - Identification of PEST regions
- PESTfind - Identification of PEST regions at EMBnet Austria
- ProtScale - Amino acid scale representation (Hydrophobicity, other conformational parameters, etc.)

- Drawhca - Draw an HCA (Hydrophobic Cluster Analysis) plot of a protein sequence
- Protein Colourer - Tool for coloring amino acid sequence
- Colorseq - Tool to highlight (in red) a selected set of residues in a protein sequence
- HelixWheel / HelixDraw - Representations of a protein fragment as a helical wheel
- RandSeq - Random protein sequence generator

7. Profiles, Patterns, Motifs and Fingerprints

Profiles

Profiles are a numerical representation of a multiple sequence alignment. Within the multiple sequence alignment is the intrinsic sequence information that represents the common characteristics of that particular collection of sequences. Profiles help find the similarities between these sequences and help in identification and analysis of distant related proteins. Profiles are constructed by taking a multiple sequence alignment representing a protein family. A position-specific scoring table (PSSM) is constructed on the lines of PAM or BLOSUM.

Profile searching has four steps:

1. Assembly of a family of related sequences into a multiple sequence alignment with PILEUP
2. Construction of a profile from the alignment with the program PROFILEMAKE
3. Comparison of the profile to a database of sequences with PROFILESEARCH
4. Display of the best similarities found with PROFILEGAP or PROFILESEGMENTS

A single sequence can be searched with a library of different profiles using the PROFILESCAN program.

Patterns

Patterns also represent the common characteristics of a protein family, but it does not contain any weighting information.

FINDPATTERNS uses a text string of DNA or amino acids such as TAATAATG as a pattern.

FINDPATTERNS allows for ambiguity in pattern matching by enclosing different choices in parenthesis and separating the choices with commas. For instance, RGF(Q,A)S means RGF followed by either Q or A followed by S. Variable numbers of N characters (which match any base) or X (which match any amino acid) may also be included.

FINDPATTERNS works best with short patterns (less than about 50 characters). A number of patterns can be searched simultaneously by creating a pattern list file (see the GCG documentation for the format of this file). The GCG program MOTIFS is essentially an implementation of FINDPATTERNS that uses the entire PROSITE database as a large pattern file.

Patterns vs. Profiles

In some cases, you may wish to reverse the pattern searching process. Rather than search your sequence for the known patterns found in a database, you might wish to search a database with a new pattern of your own creation.

GCG has two different types of pattern searching tools, FINDPATTERNS and MOTIFS work with simple text patterns, while PROFILESEARCH and PROFILESCAN use mathematical profiles that are created from multiple alignments of a number of sequences that share a conserved domain.

Motif search

The best starting point for motif search is in the PROSITE database: PROSITE contains a comprehensive list of documented protein domains constructed by expert molecular biologists. Several tools have been developed to compare an amino acid sequence to the patterns in PROSITE. GCG provides the programs MOTIFS and FINDPATTERNS.

In addition, each of the motifs in PROSITE have been exhaustively searched against the SwissProt database (which contains all well-annotated protein sequences) and the results correlated into several derived databases:

BLOCKS from the Henikoff group at the Fred Hutchinson Cancer Research Center in Seattle, WA (USA)

ProDom : Protein Domain Database from Daniel Kahn at the INRA in Toulouse (France)

Fingerprints

Fingerprints are groups of conserved motifs or elements that together form a diagnostic signature for particular protein families.

Profiles search methodology

An illustrative flow of studying profiles is as follows:
1. **blast** to locate members of an extended family
2. **pileup** to make an automated alignment
3. **lineup** to optimise that alignment
4. **profilemake** to generate a .prf (profile) file.
5. **profilesearch to** search a databases
6. **profilesegments** to look at identified hits.

Note that profilesearch can only search a 'like' database; a DNA database with a DNA profile and vice versa. The EGCG program tprofilesearch can search a DNA database with a protein query. A number of pre-generated profiles, from the PROSITE motifs database, can be found in /usr/software/gcg/gcgcore/data/profile. These can be used with the profilescan program to make a more sensitive version of the motifs program.

Pattern identification by the profile method.

Multiple sequence alignment with GCG PILEUP.

```
1  50Hsp70 ........ MASNKILGI DLGTTNSAFA VMEGGDPEII VNGEGERTTP
   Hsp70-2 ........ MAKVIGI DLGTTNSCVA VMDGKNAKVI ENAEGARTTP
   Hsp70-3 ......... MSGKGPAIGI DLGTTYSCVG VFQHGKVEII ANDQGNRTTP
   Hsp70-4 ......... MSKGPAVGI DLGTTYSCVG VFQHGKVEII ANDQGNRTTP
   Hsp70-5 ........ MAKAAAIGI DLGTTYSCVG VFQHGKVEII ANDQGNRTTP
   Hsp70-6 ........ MAKSVAIGI DLGTTYSCVG VFQHGKVEII ANDQGNRTTP
   Hsp70-7 ........ MATKGVAVGI DLGTTYSCVG VFQHGKVEII ANDQGNRTTP
   Hsp70-8 ........ M SAPKGVAFGI DLGTTYSCVG VFQHGKVEII ANNQGNRTTP
   Hsp70-9 ........ MPNAIGI DLGTTYSCVG VFQHGKVEII ANDQGNRTTP
```

Hsp70-10 .... MASAKGSKPN LPESNIAIGI DLGTTYSCVG VWRNENVDII ANDQGNRTTP
Hsp70-11 .... M SKYTGPAVGI DLGTTYSCVG IWQNDRVEII ANDQGNRTTP
Hsp70-12 .... MTYEGAIGI DLGTTYSCVG VWQNERVEII ANDQGNRTTP
Hsp70-13 .... MTYEGAIGI DLGTTYSCVG VWQNERVEII ANDQGNRTTP
consensus ..... m.kg.aiGI DLGTTyScvg vfqhgkveiI aNdqGnRTTP

Scoring matrix for HSP70 proteins based on the above alignment usingGCG program PROFILEMAKE.

Cons	A	B	C	D	E	F	G	H	I	K
	L	M	N	P	Q	R	S	T	V	W
	Y	Z	Gap	LenI						
	8	3	-2	5	4	5	5	-4	24	0
	15	13	1	1	1	-7	2	22	21	-18
	-6	4	100	100T						
	13	19	-5	24	18	-18	19	7	1	7
	-7	-4	14	11	10	-1	9	29	3	-28
	-14	15	100	100L						
	5	5	-5	3	4	13	4	2	8	-4
	14	12	8	-5	0	-10	0	10	10	-1
	5	2	100	100S						
	17	14	17	13	10	-12	29	-5	-5	6
	-14	-9	12	10	0	-2	34	19	1	-8
	-15	4	100	100T						
	15	3	22	0	-1	-5	12	-2	7	-3
	-8	-6	5	7	-8	-7	16	29	9	-22
	6	-4	100	100T						
	8	-1	12	-2	0	5	6	-4	19	-4
	8	5	-1	2	-8	-8	7	22	19	-15
	4	-3	100	100C						
	17	0	24	-1	-3	11	8	-1	7	-10
	1	-2	1	-3	-8	-14	8	5	9	-5
	14	-7	100	100V						
	11	0	18	-1	-2	2	14	-10	26	-4
	9	7	-3	7	-7	-7	21	10	31	-19
	-5	-5	100	100C						
	10	-8	15	-11	-11	6	8	-7	11	-10
	4	3	-7	0	-11	-4	11	5	15	-22
	14	-11	100	100V						
	7	7	-3	8	8	-3	11	1	20	-1
	14	10	4	2	8	-5	0	5	26	-24
	-6	8	100	100						

To find motifs in proteins first requires alignments of the sequences. Most methods of multiple sequence alignments rely on first producing a phylogenetic tree predicting evolutionary relationships of the organisms from which the sequences were derived to each other. Pairs of sequences that are most closely related are then aligned. These alignments are then used to align the other sequences according to their order in the tree. This procedure has the effect of basing alignments of several sequences on alignments of the most closely related sequences, a procedure that is called a greedy algorithm by computer scientists. The resulting motifs will also be biased by the most alike sequences. The filtered dot matrix is an alternative method for aligning several sequences which weights the sequences more equally. The method performs a dot matrix analysis on all pairs of sequences and then compares these dot matrices to find motifs in the sequences. An advantage of this algorithm is in providing a reliable method to find common regions in distantly related protein sequences. However, using this method requires the assistance of an experienced computer programmer.

Two powerful methods for detecting subtle patterns in two or more protein sequences have recently been described. The first, Aligned Segment Statistical Evaluation (ASSET), can locate patterns, combine related patterns and provide a measure of statistical significance of the patterns without any prior information that the patterns are actually present (Neuwald and Green 1994).The second method GIBBS (Lawrence et al. 1993) searches for previously identified patterns that may be weakly conserved in a given sequence. The Blocks and Meme servers provide such an analysis.

Some of the tools for patterns and profiles are listed below :

- InterPro Scan - Integrated search in PROSITE, Pfam, PRINTS and other family and domain databases
- ScanProsite - Scans a sequence against PROSITE or a pattern against SWISS-PROT and TrEMBL
- ProfileScan - Scans a sequence against protein profile databases
- Frame-ProfileScan - Scans a short DNA sequence against protein profile databases
- Pfam HMM search; scans a sequence against the Pfam protein families db [At Washington University or at Sanger Centre]
- FPAT - Regular expression searches in protein databases
- PRATT - Interactively generates conserved patterns from a series of unaligned proteins.
- PPSEARCH - Scans a sequence against PROSITE (allows a graphical output)
- PROSITE scan - Scans a sequence against PROSITE (allows mismatches); at PBIL
- PATTINPROT - Scans a protein sequence or a protein database for one or several pattern(s); at PBIL
- SMART - Simple Modular Architecture Research Tool; at EMBL
- TEIRESIAS - Generate patterns from a collection of unaligned protein or DNA sequences; at IBM
- Hits - Relationships between protein sequences and motifs

ProfileScan

It uses a method called pfscan to find similarities between a protein or a nucleic acid query sequence and a profile library. It uses profile libraries like Pfam and PROSITE.

Pfam HMM search results

MNIAEEPSDEVISSGPEDTDICSQQTSASAEAGDQSIKIERKTSTGLQLEQLANTNLLTIRIKWQLQEEE
DDHCNSRITDQIMDTIQHYKGISVNNSDTETYEFLPDTRRLQVLEQNKDIYLYEHGSQEYEKSYKDNEEE
DDWRYDTVLQAQFKYPKSLENACTDISELLKSEPIGQHIDKWSIGVNKHALTYPGNIFVGGIAKSLSIGE
LSFLFSKYGPILSMKLIYDKTKGEPNGYGFISYPLGSQASLCIKELNGRTVNGSTLFINYHVERKERERI
HWDHVKENNNDDNFRCLFIGNLPYHNPEKVETLITPKEVIEVIKKELSKKFPDFDIISYYFPKRSNTRSS
SSVSFNEEGSVESNKSSNNTNGNAQDEDMLKGYGFIKLINHEQALAAIETFNGFM WHGNRLVVNKAVQHK
VYNNHNSHDRHPSISNHNDMEVLEFANNPMYDYNNYTYDRYYFNNNKNGNSNDTSNVRYFDSVRSTPVAE
KMDLFYPQRESFSEGRGQRVPRFMGNKFDMYQYPSTSYSLPIPMSNQQESNLYVKHIPLSWTDEDLYDFY
KSFGEIISVKVITVGGSKNKYRQQSNDSSSDNDLPVGSSRGYGFVSFESPLDAAKAILNTDGYQVSKDQV
LSVSFAQKRGNLSSSDDDDQSQTDNSSKFQNFQPHNDYHKAYPTKYNKKFINALMTQNQSQQQVSRENYF
IPLQYPNTNTKPVNSYNLISANQNNANWMMPMFPSFGFIPQVPPVPYIIPPQNPAANHIPIMANGSNEEE
EFSSGDYSMDY

rrm 197-268 RNA recognition motif. (a.k.a. RRM, RBD, or RNP domain)
rrm 297- 413 RNA recognition motif. (a.k.a. RRM, RBD, or RNP domain)
rrm 542-633 RNA recognition motif. (a.k.a. RRM, RBD, or RNP domain)
Align ments of top-scoring do m ains:
rrm: do m ain 1 of 3, from 197 to 268: score 69.1, E = 4.9e-18
*->lfVgNLppdvteedLkdlFskfGpivsikivrDiiekpketgkskGf
+fVg++ ++ + +L lFsk+Gpi+s+k+++D k +g ++G+
query 197 IFVGGIAKSLSIGELSFLFSKYGPILSMKLIYD——KTK G E P N G Y 238 .
aFVeFeseedAekAlealnGkelggrklrv<-*
+F+ + ++A ++++lnG++++g +l +
query 239 GFISYPLGSQASLCIKELNGRTVNGSTLFI 268

Prosite

MNIAEEPSDEVISSGPEDTDICSQQTSASAEAGDQSIKIERKTSTGLQLEQLANTNLLTIRIKWQLQEEEDDHCNSRITD
QIMDTIQHYKGISVNNSDTETYEFLPDTRRLQVLEQNKDIYLYEHGSQEYEKSYKDNEEEDDWRYDTVLQAQFKYPKSLE
NACTDISELLKSEPIGQHIDKWSIGVNKHALTYPGNIFVGGIAKSLSIGELSFLFSKYGPILSMKLIYDKTKGEPNGYGF
ISYPLGSQASLCIKELNGRTVNGSTLFINYHVERKERERIHWDHVKENNNDDNFRCLFIGNLPYHNPEKVETLITPKEVI
EVIKKELSKKFPDFDIISYYFPKRSNTRSSSSVSFNEEGSVESNKSSNNTNGNAQDEDMLKGYGFIKLINHEQALAAIET
FNGFMWHGNRLVVNKAVQHKVYNNHNSHDRHPSISNHNDMEVLEFANNPMYDYNNYTYDRYYFNNNKNGNSNDTSNVRYF
DSVRSTPVAEKMDLFYPQRESFSEGRGQRVPRFMGNKFDMYQYPSTSYSLPIPMSNQQESNLYVKHIPLSWTDEDLYDFY
KSFGEIISVKVITVGGSKNKYRQQSNDSSSDNDLPVGSSRGYGFVSFESPLDAAKAILNTDGYQVSKDQVLSVSFAQKRG
NLSSSDDDDQSQTDNSSKFQNFQPHNDYHKAYPTKYNKKFINALMTQNQSQQQVSRENYFIPLQYPNTNTKPVNSYNLIS
ANQNNANW MMPMFPSFGFIPQVPPVPYIIPPQNPAANHIPIMANGSNEEEEFSSGDYSMDY
Si milarity percentage 100
---N-
glycosylation site.
Prosite access number: PS00001
Prosite docu mentation access num ber: PDOC00001
N-{P}-[ST]-{P}.
Randomized probability: 5.138e-03 .
Site : 95 to 98 NN S D. Identity.
Site : 262 to 265 NGST. Identity.

```
Site : 364 to 367 NKSS. Identity.
Site : 368 to 371 NNT N. Identity.
Site : 455 to 458 NYTY. Identity.
Site : 472 to 475 NDT S. Identity.
Site : 586 to 589 ND S S. Identity.
Site : 641 to 644 NLSS. Identity.
Site : 655 to 658 NSSK. Identity.
Site : 688 to 691 NQSQ. Identity.
Site : 764 to 767 NGSN. Identity.
```

cA MP- and cG MP-dependent protein kinase phosphorylation site.

[RK](2)-x-[ST].

Protein kinase C phosphorylation site. (12)

[ST]-x-[RK].

Casein kinase II phosphorylation site. (20)

[ST]-x(2)-[DE].

Tyrosine kinase phosphorylation site. (1)

[RK]-x(2,3)-[D E]-x(2,3)-Y.

N- myristoylation site.(7)

G-{EDRKHPFY W}-x(2)-[STAGCN]-{P}.

Eukaryotic RNA Recognition Motif (R R M) R N P-1 region signature.(2)

[RK]- G-{E D R K H P C G}-[A G S CI]-[FY]-[LIV A]-x-[FYLM].

Site : 381 to 388 KGYGFIKL. Identity.

Site : 600 to 607 RGYGFVSF. Identity.

BLOCKS

The BLOCKS database used the concept of blocks to identify a family of proteins.

```
Poly-adenylate binding protein, unique do main
Block Fra m e Location (aa) Block E-value
IPB002004C 0 235-277 1.2e-05
IPB002004C <->C (108,208):234
Q9H361   137 SKGYGFVHFETHEAAERAIKKMNGMLLNGRKVFVGQFKSRKER
|||  ||| || || | |  |    | | |
Unknown  235   pnG Y G FisYplgsqAslcIKeLN GrtVN GstlFinyHVeRKER
IPB002004E C<->E (157,215):113
PABX_ARATH|Q9ZQA8 354 PEEAIDAVKTFHGQMFHGKPLYVAIAQKKEDRKMQL
| | | || | | | || | | |
Unknown   391   hEqALAAIeTFN GfM w H GnrLvVnkAvqhkVynnHn
Block IPB002004A
ID PABP; BLOCK
AC IPB002004A; distance fro m previo u s block =(-1 4,8 0)
DE Poly-adenylate binding protein, unique do m ain
```

```
BL LRC; width=48; seqs=33; 99.5%=1997; strength=1575
PAB2_HU MA N|Q15097 (-13) XXXXXXXXXXXXXXXMLYEKFSPAGPILSIRVCRDMITRRSLGYAYVNF    13
PABP_SCHP O|P31209 (81) SLYVGELDPSVTEAMLFELFNSIGPVASIRVCRDAVTRRSLGYAYVNF      30
PAB2_ARATH|P42731 (37) SLYVGDLDFNVTDSQLFDAFGQMGTVVTVRVCRDLVTRRSLGYGYVNF      47
PAB3_ARATH|O64380 (50) SLYAGDLDPKVTEAHLFDLFKHVANVVSVRVCRDQNRRSLGYAYINFS      61
PAB5_ARATH|Q05196 (46) SLYVGDLDPSVNESHLLDLFNQVAPVHNLRVCRDLTHRSLGYAYVNFA      62
PABX_ARATH|Q9ZQA8 (25) SLYVGDLHPSVTEGILYDAFAEFKSLTSVRLCKDASSGRSLCYGYANF     100
PABP_YEAST|P04147 (38) SLYVGDLEPSVSEAHLYDIFSPIGSVSSIRVCRDAITKTSLGYAYVNF      39
```

Pscan

Pscan is a tool for searching fingerprint matches. Pscan is a program of the EMBOSS package. It requires a protein sequence but will accept most formats. Pscan scans a protein using the PRINTS database. (PRINTS is a database of diagnostic protein signatures, or fingerprints.) An uncharacterised sequence matching all motifs or elements can then be readily diagnosed as a true match to a particular family fingerprint.

Interproscan

Interpro brings together information in participating protein family, domains and motif databases to make them easily searchable, and the results of those searches easy to compare.

Some of the databases participating in Interpro are:

- Prosite
- ProDom
- Prints
- Pfam
- Smart
- Swissprot

The search methods incorporated into Interproscan are:

ScanRegExp and Ppsearch for searching the PROSITE pattern database.

Pfscan for searching PROSITE profiles.

FingerPrintScan for searching the PRINTS database.

Hmmpfam for searching the Pfam and Smart databases.

BlastProDom.pl for searching the ProDom database.

8. DNA to Protein translation

Translate - Translates a nucleotide sequence to a protein sequence

Protein machine - Nucleotide to protein translation at EBI

MBS translator - Nucleotide to protein translation at MBS

Backtranslation - Translates a protein sequence back to a nucleotide sequence

Genewise - Compares a protein sequence to a genomic DNA sequence, allowing for introns and frameshifting errors

FSED - Frameshift error detection

LabOnWeb - Elongation, expression profiles and sequence analysis of ESTs using Compugen LEADS clusters

Translate a sequence

ATCTGCACCTGCGCTGCTTTCTGGATTTGGAGTTGGCGTGGCACTGATTTCTTCGTTCTG
GGCGGCGTCTTCTTCGAATTCCTCATCCCAGTAGTTCTGTTGGTTCTTTTTACTCTTTTT

5'3' Frame 1
I C T C A A F W I W S W R G T D F F V L G G V F F E F L I P V V L L V L F T L F
5'3' Frame 2
S A P A L L S G F G V G V A L I S S F W A A S S S N S S S Q Stop F C W F F L L F
5'3' Frame 3
L H L R C F L D L E L A W H Stop F L R S G R R L L R I P H P S S S V G S F Y S F
3'5' Frame 1
K K S K K N Q Q N Y W D E E F E E D A A Q N E E I S A T P T P N P E S S A G A D
3'5' Frame 2
K R V K R T N R T T G Met R N S K K T P P R T K K S V P R Q L Q I Q K A A Q V Q
3'5' Frame 3
K E Stop K E P T E L L G Stop G I R R R R R P E R R N Q C H A N S K S R K Q R R C R

Backtranslate

```
Back-translated
AT AT G CA CAT GT GC A GC A TTT T G G ATT T G G
A G T T G G A G A G G A A C A G A T TT C TT C G T T TT A
G G A GGA GTA TTT TTT GAA TTC CTC ATC CCA
GTG GTA CTG CTT GTC CTA TTC ACA TTG TTT

Starting sequence
A T C T G C A C C T G C G C T G C T TT C T G G ATT T G .G
AGT TGG CGT GGC ACT GAT TTC TTC GTT CTG
G G C G G C G T C T T C T T C G A A T T C C T C A T C C C A
G T A G TT CT G TT G G TT CTT TTT A C T CTT TTT

Protein
I C T C A A F W I W S W R G T D F F V L G G V F F E F L I P V V L L V L F T L F

Back-translate using S. cerevisiae
A T C T G C A C C T G T G C T G C A TTT T G G ATT T G G
AGT TGG AGA GGC ACT GAT TTT TTT GTT CTT
G G A G G T G T A TTT TT C G A A TT C TT G ATA C C A
G T G G T C CT G TT G G TT TTA TTT A C A CT A TT C
```

2D prediction

1. Predicting inter-residue contacts

Given all inter-residue contacts or distances, 3D structure can be reconstructed by distance geometry or molecular dynamics. This is used for the determination of 3D structures by nuclear magnetic resonance (NMR) spectroscopy which produces experimental data of distances between protons. Can inter-residue contacts be predicted? Some fraction of these contacts can be - helices and strands can be assigned based on hydrogen-bonding pattern between residues. Thus, a successful prediction of secondary structure implies a successful prediction of some fraction of all the contacts. However, contacts predicted from secondary structure assignment are short-ranged, i.e., between residues nearby in sequence. For successful applications of distance geometry, long-range contacts have to be predicted, i.e., contacts between residues far apart in sequence.

In sequence alignments, some pairs of positions appear to vary in a physico-chemically plausible manner, i.e., a 'loss of function' point mutation is often rescued by an additional mutation that compensates for the change. One hypothesis is that compensations would be most effective in maintaining a structural motif if the mutated residues were spatial neighbours. In general, prediction accuracy is rather poor, with a direct trade-off between predicting enough contacts, and predicting only correct ones, e.g., taking 5% of the best-predicted long-range contacts (sequence separation above 10 residues) the accuracy prediction is about 50%.

Analysing correlated mutations is only one way to predict long-range inter-residue contacts. Other methods use statistics, mean-force potentials, or neural networks. So far none of the methods appears to balance predicting too many false contacts and missing out on too many true contacts. However, some of the methods provide sufficient information to distinguish between alternative models of 3D structure.

2. Predicting inter-strand contacts

One simplification of the problem to predict inter-residue contacts focuses on predicting the contacts between residues in adjacent strands. Such an attempt is motivated by the hope that such interactions are more specific than are sequence-distant (long-range) contacts in general, and hence are easier to predict.

How to identify the correct β-strand alignment? The method for predicting inter-strand contacts is based on potentials of mean-force similar to those used in the evaluation of strand-strand threading. Propensities are compiled by database counts for $2 \infty 2 \infty 2$ classes (parallel/anti-parallel, H-bonded/not H-bonded, N-/C-terminal). Each of the eight classes is divided further into five sub-classes in the following way. Suppose the two strand residues at positions i and j are in close in space. Then the following five residue pairs are counted in separate tables: *i/j-2, i/j-1, i/j, i/j+1, i/j+2* . Such pseudo-potentials identify the correct b-strand alignment in 35-45% of the cases.

Even if the locations of strands in the sequence are known exactly, the pseudo-potentials cannot predict the correct inter-strand contacts in most cases. However, when using multiple alignment information, the signal-to-noise ratio increases such that inter-strand contacts have been predicted correctly for most of the strands inspected in some test cases. For the purpose of reliable contact prediction, this result is inadequate, especially as the locations of the strands are not known precisely.

3. Algorithms used for secondary structure prediction

The three widely used methods of protein secondary structure prediction are :
  1. The Chou-Fasman and GOR methods
  2. Nearest neighbor methods
  3. Hidden Markov models

Chou-Fasman method

- Frequencies of amino acids i in each kind of secondary structure s are counted (ni,s/ni).
- ni,s/ni is divided by Ns / Nt, the frequency of all residues in structure s, to give 3 x 20 sets of structure prediction parameter (Pa, Pb and Pt)
- Each amino acid position in a query sequence is evaluated by these parameters, using an averaging window
- Rules are made to predict the secondary structure of a region e.g if a row of amino acids have a high chance of being in a helix, then predict a helix.

GOR (Garnier, Osguthorpe and Robson) method

- This method assumes that amino acids up to 8 residues on each side influence the secondary structure of the central residue
- The frequency of amino acids at the central position in the window, and at -1, ... -8 and +1,....+8 is determined for α, β and turns to give three 17×20 scoring matrices
- The GOR method uses information theory and the values in these tables to calculate the probabilities that the central residue is one type of secondary structure and not another
- Early versions of GOR assumed that the amino acids in the window influenced secondary structure independently, later versions that there are pairwise correlations between the flanking residue and the central one, and the most recent version (GOR4) that there are pairwise correlations in the window.
- Correctly predicts 64% of the residue conformations in known structures and quite drastically (36.5%) underpredicts the number of residues in β strands.

Nearest neighbor methods

- A list of short sequence fragments is made by sliding a window of length n (e.g. n =16) along a set of approximately 100-400 training sequences of known structure but minimal sequence similarity
- The secondary structure of the central amino acid in each training window is recorded
- A sliding window of the same size is then selected from the query sequence
- The sequence in the window at each position of the query sequence is compared to each of the above training fragments and the 50 best matching fragments are identified (scoring matrices, multiple sequence alignments, etc may be used at this step)
- The frequencies of the known secondary structure of the middle amino acid in each of these matching fragments are then used to predict the secondary structure of the middle amino acid in the query window
- Rules or a neural network is used to make a final prediction for each amino acid position.
- WWW programs PREDATOR AND NNSSP are used - accuracy about 75%

Hidden Markov models

- Models are made that predict the secondary structure of a protein of a given structural class (e.g. α + β) as shown in the structural classification databases
- Each model is trained with the sequences of the proteins in that structural class
- The models are used with a query sequence to predict both the class and the secondary structure of the protein.

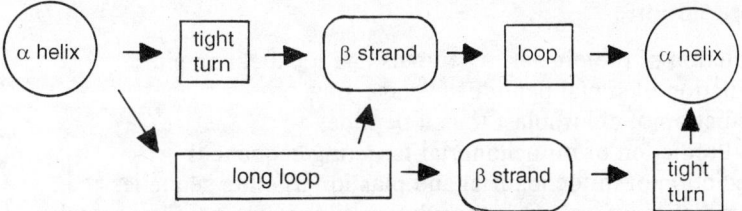

Hidden Markov model for hypothetical protein structure

Fig. 16.4. HMM for protein structure prediction

4. Secondary structure prediction tools

- AGADIR - An algorithm to predict the helical content of peptides
- BCM PSSP - Baylor College of Medicine
- Prof - Cascaded Mutiple Classifiers for Secondary Structure Prediction
- GOR I (Garnier et al, 1978)
- HNN - Hierarchical Neural Network method (Guermeur, 1997)
- Jpred - A consensus method for protein secondary structure prediction at EBI
- nnPredict - University of California at San Francisco (UCSF)
- PredictProtein - PHDsec, PHDacc, PHDhtm, PHDtopology,PHDthreader, MaxHom, EvalSec
- PREDATOR - Protein secondary structure prediction from single or multiple sequences at EMBL
- PSA - BioMolecular Engineering Research Center (BMERC)/PSIpred - Various protein structure prediction methods at Brunel University

nnPREDICT

```
Tertiary structure class: none
Sequence:
MNIAEEPSDEVISSGPEDTDICSQQTSASAEAGDQSIKIERKTSTGLQLEQLANTNLLTI
RIKWQLQEEEDDHCNSRITDQIMDTIQHYKGISVNNSDTETYEFLPDTRRLQVLEQNKDI
... etc ....
Secondary structure prediction (H = helix, E = strand, -= no prediction):
--------------EE--------------E---------------H--------HHH E E------------HHHHHHHH----HEE
EHH-------------------------HHH H H H-----------E E------------EE-----------HHE-----------------EEEE---------
HHH---------------------HHH   H H   H-------------------HHH H H----------------------
HH-H--------------EEE------------E-H-EHE   E   H-----------E-HEE E--------------------E
EE------------HEH H-------------------EEE   E-H-------HHH-EH---------------------EEEE------------------------
E--------HHHHHHHH---------------EE-E-------------...--------------EE----------------------------
HHHHH-EEEEHHHHHHHHHHHHHHHHH-HHHH--HHHH-HHHHH
E-------------------------------HHH H   H----------------EEE----------------------EEEE  E
------------------------------------------------H-------EE------------------------------------HHHEE--------------------
HHHHH——EEEEEEEEE————E-------------------
EEEE------HHHHHHEE-------E------EEEHHHH-------------------------------
HHHHHHH----------------------------------------------------EE-------------------------------------
EE--------------HHE-------------
```

5. Localization prediction

- PSORT - Prediction of protein sorting signals and localization sites
- SignalP - Prediction of signal peptide cleavage sites
- ChloroP - Prediction of chloroplast transit peptides
- MITOPROT -Prediction of mitochondrial targeting sequences
- Predotar - Prediction of mitochondrial and plastid targeting sequences
- NetOGlyc - Prediction of type O-glycosylation sites in mammalian proteins
- big-PI Predictor - GPI Modification Site Prediction
- DGPI -Prediction of GPI-anchor and cleavage sites
- NetPhos - Prediction of Ser, Thr and Tyr phosphorylation sites in eukaryotic protein

6. Transmembrane regions detection

- DAS - Prediction of transmembrane regions in prokaryotes using the Dense Alignment Surface method
- HMMTOP - Prediction of transmembrane helices and topology of proteins
- PredictProtein - Prediction of transmembrane helix location and topology
- SOSUI - Prediction of transmembrane regions Transmembrane detection based on multiple sequence alignment
- TMHMM - Prediction of transmembrane helices in proteins
- TMpred - Prediction of transmembrane regions and protein orientation
- TopPred 2 - Topology prediction of membrane proteins Hyrophobicity plot of EnvZ, a membrane-spanning protein

7. Secondary Structure Prediction comparison

Name	Accuracy	Comments
PHDsec: http://www.embl-heidelberg.de/predictprotein/	>72% (+/-10%, one standard deviation)	Multiple alignment-based neural network system
NSSP: http://dot.imgen.bcm.tmc.edu:9331/pssprediction/pssp.html	>71%. Evaluated on > 200 unique proteins	Multiple alignment-based nearest-neighbor method
SOPM: http://www.ibcp.fr/predict.html	> 70%	Multiple alignment-based method combining various other prediction programs
DSC: http://bonsai.lif.icnet.uk/bmm/dsc/dsc_read_align.html	70%	Multiple alignment-based program using statistics
SSPRED: http://www.embl-heidelberg.de/sspred/ssp_mul.html	> 70%	Multiple alignment-based program using statistics
MultiPredict: http://kestrel.ludwig.ucl.ac.uk/zpred.html	>65%	Multiple alignment-based method using physicochemical information from a set of aligned sequences and statistical secondary structure decision constants.
PSA: http://bmerc-www.bu.edu/psa/ classes		The PSA server analyzes amino acid sequences to predict secondary structures and folding
NNPREDICT: http://www.cmpharm.ucsf.edu/~nomi/nnpredict.html	>65%	Single-sequence based neural network prediction

Prediction in 3D

Introduction

In contrast to the above methods, the goal of *ab initio* prediction is to build a model for a given sequence without using a template by minimizing knowledge based energy functions and lattice models. How to accurately predict 3D structure for coiled-coil proteins. A particular class of proteins is coiled-coils. These are proteins that can be defined by the geometry of long helices, of which two or more wind around one another.

One of the important advances in 3D prediction in recent years has been the development of mean-force-potentials. Before these potentials, structure prediction was normally done with 'physical' potentials, i.e., bonds, angles, torsion angles, and van der Waals as well as electrostatic non-bonded terms which describe the internal energy of the molecule. In contrast, the mean-force-potentials, derived from databases of protein structure, attempt to describe the free-energy of the molecule. The physical potentials have been used very successfully to refine experimentally determined structures. In contrast, mean-force-potentials of pairwise residue distances are quite successful in fold recognition, as well as remote homology modelling.

Tertiary structure

- SWISS-MODEL - An automated knowledge-based protein modelling server
- Geno3d - Automatic modelling of protein three-dimensional structure
- CPHmodels - Automated neural-network based protein modelling server
- 3D-PSSM - Protein fold recognition using 1D and 3D sequence profiles coupled with secondary structure information (Foldfit)
- SWEET - Constructing 3D models of saccharides from their sequences
- Swiss-PdbViewer - A program to display, analyse and superimpose protein 3D structures

Protein Structure & Information Databases

- 3D-ALI - Protein Structural-Sequence Information Library - EMBL-Heidelberg
- BioMagResBank-Database of NMR-derived Protein Structures-BIMAS-NIH BMCD-Biological
- Macromolecule Crystallization Database - CARB
- CAMPASS - CAMbridge DB of Protein Alignments organized as Structural Superfamilies
- CATH - Protein Structure Classification at the - U College London
- Culled PDB - Unique/Representative Proteins in the PDB - Fox Chase Cancer Center
- DIP - Database of Interacting Proteins - UCLA-DOE
- DSMP - Database of Structural Motifs in Proteins - CDFD
- DSSP - Definitions of the Secondary Structures of Proteins Database - EMBL-Heidelberg
- ENTREZ Structure - Biomolecule 3D Structure Search - NCBI
- Enzyme Structure Database - UCL
- FSSP - Families of Structurally Similar Proteins Database - EBI
- MMDB - ENTREZ Molecular Modelling Database - NCBI
- PDB - Protein Database of 3-D Structures of Biological Macromolecules
- PIR - Protein Information Resource Database - NBRF
- PRESAGE - Database and Search Tools for Structural Genomics - Stanford U
- SCOP - Structural Classification of Proteins Database

16.8. PROTEIN FUNCTION PREDICTION

Protein sequence determines protein structure determines protein function. We first try to predict protein structure. Then use what we learned, both on the way to structure prediction, and from the predicted structure itself to predict function. Predicting protein function from sequence adds two additional problems in comparison to the unsolved task of structure prediction:

1. Function is not entirely determined by sequence; the environment is crucially important.
2. 'Protein function' is a rather intuitive but ill defined term. Function is a complex phenomenon associated with many mutually overlapping levels: chemical, biochemical, cellular, physiological, organism mediated, and developmental.

These levels are related in complex ways, e.g., protein kinases can be related to different cellular functions (such as cell cycle), and to a chemical function (transferase) plus a complex control mechanism by interaction with other proteins.

Labeling for most protein sequences has been done in, e.g., the yeast genome. However, it is possible to label only proteins for which we find similarities in other proteins of experimentally known function. Also, even for those we label, our knowledge is mostly quite restricted to rough details. Predictions of active sites, binding sites, etc. are usually not successful. Labeling also does not imply understanding the detailed mechanism. Often we need knowledge about protein structure to manipulate functions.

Summary of different approaches in protein structure prediction

	Single residue statistics	Explicit rules	Nearest-Neighbors	Neural-Networks based prediction
First Generation (information is coming from a single residue, of a single sequence)	Chou and Fasman 1974 GOR1 1978	Lim 1974		
Second Generation (Local interactions are taken into account)	GOR3 1987		Levin et al 1986 Nishikawa and Ooi 1986	Holley and Karplus 1989 Qian and Sejnowski 1988
Third Generation (Information coming from homologous sequences is incorporated)	Zvelebil et al 1987	PREDATOR 1996	Yi and Lander 1993	
			NNSSP 1995	
	DSC 1996			PHD1993 Inet 1999 PSIPRED 1999

There are some approaches based on HMMs also.

16.9. ACCURACY OF PREDICTION

Several indices of prediction expected accuracy have been designed.

$$Q_i^{pred} = P_i \, / \, (P_i + O_i)$$

P_i is the number of residues predicted in the i state, effectively in the i state and O_i is the number of residues predicted in the i state, but not actually in the i state (*Overpredicted*). P_i+O_i therefore represents the total number of residues predicted in the i state.

$$Q_i^{obs} = P_i / (P_i+U_i)$$

U_i is the number of residues actually in the i state, but not predicted as such (*Underpredicted*). P_i+U_i therefore represents the number of residues actually in the i state. Q_i^{obs} is an index of accuracy.

$$Q_3 = (P_\alpha + P_\beta + P_{coil}) / T$$

where T is the total number of residues. Q_3 represents therefore the global accuracy. The theoretical random value for the Q_3 is theoretically 33% (although due to the bias in the actual distribution between the three states, the random is about 38%).

The *Matthew* coefficients

$$C_i = (P_iN_i-U_iO_i) / [(P_i+U_i)(P_i+O_i)(N_i+U_i)(N_i+O_i)]\pi^{1/2}$$

The value 0 represents the random prediction, 1 being the perfect prediction. The most used is the Q_3. This accuracy coefficient is not a perfect one. The following prediction is an extreme example of its pitfalls. The prediction is rather good : The two structures are correctly localised and assigned. However the Q_3 is very low.

```
Target      CHHHHHHHHHCCCCEEEECC
            |  | | | |       | | | | |     Q3 = 45%
Prediction  CCHHHHCCCCEEEEEEEEEC
```

Gene Mapping, Sequence Assembly and Gene Expression

17.1. INTRODUCTION

A genome is the completely determined DNA sequence of the genetic material (chromosomes as well as any plasmids, mitochondrial DNA etc) of an organism. A genome isn't the same as 'all genes', it is rather the 'sequence of all DNA' wherein all genes can be found. The first genome of a living organism (viruses aside) was that of *Haemophilus influenzae* published in 1995.

What is the importance of complete genomes? At the basic level, we want to know the complete set of genes that an organism has. The genome of an organism is in a certain sense the blueprint for that organism. Many observations and experiments in biology involve mutations, and knowing the complete set of genes for an organism can help with the analysis. For example, we may want to be sure that a knocked-out gene does not have a backup copy somewhere in the genome.

Also, knowing the complete genome for an organism is only the first step in the complete mapping of the constituents and processes of the organism. The complete genome is a necessary (but not sufficient) requirement for understanding an organism.

The technique of locating the genes is called "Genetic Mapping". A "genetic map" shows the positions of the genes relative to each other, and relative to the ends and centre of the chromosomes. The genetic map is amenable to "gene sequencing". Gene sequencing deals with deciphering the exact sequence of bases that compose a gene. As there can be millions of these bases in a gene and hence this process, if done without automation can take a number of years.

For example, mapping human genes involves :

1. dividing the chromosomes into smaller fragments that can be propagated and characterized
2. ordering (mapping) them to correspond to their respective locations on the chromosomes

After mapping the next step is to sequence each of the ordered DNA fragments. The ultimate goal is to find all the genes in the DNA sequence. A genome map describes the order of genes or other markers and the spacing between them on each chromosome.

Human genome maps are constructed on several different scales or levels of resolution. At the coarsest resolution are genetic linkage maps, which depict the relative chromosomal locations of DNA markers (genes and other identifiable DNA sequences) by their patterns of inheritance. Physical maps describe the chemical characteristics of the DNA molecule itself.

The availability of more and more complete genomes allows entirely new kinds of comparisons to be made between organism. New types of analysis can be applied to old questions in biology, involving problems in evolutionary history the interactions between species.

The list of currently determined genomes is growing rapidly. There are a number of web sites that try to keep track of the status of the various genome projects:

- GOLD (Genomes OnLine Database), maintained by the company Integrated Genomics, which is selling annotation services for companies that have in-house genome projects (primarily bacterial genomes).
- TIGR Microbial Database, published microbial genomes, and projects in progress. Lists maintained by TIGR, The Institute for Genomics Research.
- EBI Completed Genomes web site, links, resources. Contains sequence data for organelles (mitochondria), phages and viruses.
- Genome Monitoring Table at EBI.
- NCBI Genomic Biology web site, with links and search resources.

There are a number of web sites that focus on data for specific genomes. Usually, these sites contain more data than just the DNA sequence of the genome, such as predicted transcripts (ORFs, Open Reading Frames), verified transcripts and tentative identifications or classifications of the predicted proteins. For an illustration, please see the table given below. Please note that the number of ORFs given below for each genome is tentative. The numbers depend on the exact procedure used to identify known genes and predict previously unknown genes.

Table 17.1.

Organism	Type	Size	Comment
H. influenzae	Bacterial	1.83 Mb, 1850 ORFs	First genome of a free-living organism. <u>1995</u>
E. coli	Bacterial	4.64 Mb, 4289 ORFs	Most studied bacterium. <u>1997</u>
R. prowazekii	Bacterial	1.11 Mb, 834 ORFs	First genome sequenced in Sweden <u>1998</u>
M. jannaschii	Archaeal	1.66 Mb, 1750 ORFs	The first sequenced Archaea. <u>1996</u>
S. cerevisiae	Eukaryote	12.1 Mb (16 chromosomes), 6294 ORFs	The first sequenced eukaryote. <u>1997</u>
C. elegans	Eukaryote, nematode	97 Mb (6 chromosomes), 19,099 ORFs	The first sequenced multicellular organism.
Drosophila	Eukaryote, insect	137 Mb (excluding heterochromatin, 6 chromosomes), 14,100 ORFs	Publicly available. <u>2000</u>
Homosapiens	Eukaryote, primate	3000 Mb (24 chromosomes), ? ORFs	

17.2 GENE MAPPING

Mapping

Like geographical maps, maps of target DNA molecules give locations of 'landmarks'. Maps of DNA are composed of special features, or *markers*, along the molecule, and are useful in sequencing and in homing in on genes. There are two main classes of mapping techniques: *genetic mapping* is based on statistical analysis of inheritance patterns, and gives a relative ordering of markers used; and, *physical mapping* is based on physical and biochemical experiments on DNA sequences. In general, there are many different physical mapping techniques that have varying degrees of resolution.

We will discuss some of these techniques, then introduce the STS mapping problem, and describe the PQ-Tree Algorithm, which solves the problem in the case of perfect data.

Outline of Maps

A wide variety of mapping strategies are in use. Major ones are as follows:

- Fluorescence *in situ* Hybridization (FISH) Maps (resolution: @ 10 Mb)
- Genetic Maps
- Radiation Hybrid Maps
- STS Clone Maps (resolution: @ 100 kb)
- Optical Restriction Maps
- Multiple Complete Digest Restriction Maps (resolution: @ 1 kb)

Genetic Mapping

In a population, several alternative forms, or *alleles*, of a gene or a DNA sequence may be present at a given locus. Loci that possess two or more alleles are said to be *polymorphic*. Polymorphisms occur on average once every 300 to 500 bp of DNA. Variations within exon sequences can lead to observable changes, such as differences in eye color, blood type, and disease susceptibility. Most variations occur within introns and have little or no effect on an organisms appearance or function, yet they are detectable at the DNA level and can be used as markers.

Examples of these types of markers include:

1. Restriction fragment length polymorphisms (RFLPs), which reflect sequence variations in DNA sites that can be cleaved by DNA restriction enzymes
2. Variable number of tandem repeat sequences, which are short repeated sequences that vary in the number of repeated units and, therefore, in length (a characteristic easily measured).

The initial step in identifying the chromosomal sequence that codes for a particular gene is to genetically map the gene. Genetic mapping is based on *linkage analysis*. This is a process which takes as the input the patterns of inheritance and gives the outputs as relative positions of loci on the same chromosome. Loci that tend to be inherited together more often than would be predicted by chance are said to be *linked*. For example, we would expect different alleles at two loci on *different* chromosomes to be inherited independently. Different alleles on *one* chromosome, however, would be linked, and the degree of linkage would depend on the distance between them. This is because loci that are close together are less likely to be separated by a recombination event, or *crossover*, during meiosis.

Overview of meiotic recombination

Let A, B, C, and D be four polymorphic loci on a pair (one from each parent) of homologous chromosomes. During meiosis, the segments that contain the B locus are switched, resulting in two "nonparental" genotypes which may be inherited. Since loci C and D are tightly linked, they are essentially inherited as a pair, with either both having allele 1 or both having allele 2.

To be informative in linkage analysis, genetic markers must be polymorphic. Different alleles, and how they are inherited, are used to determine which markers a particular gene is close to. For example, if a given disease gene tends to be co-inherited with a given marker, then they are likely to be near each other on one chromosome. In this way, the region in which the gene is believed to lie can be narrowed down relative to previously mapped markers.

Human Genetic Mapping

As geneticists cannot construct testcrosses and backcrosses with humans, they must instead rely on existing family trees for analysis. Though individual phenotypes are usually easily observed (at least in living individuals), corresponding genotypes must often be inferred. An additional difficulty is that there is not necessarily a one-to-one correspondence between genotypes and phenotypes, as illustrated by blood type given the table below.

Table 17.2.

Genotype	Phenotype
A/A or A/O	A
B/B or B/O	B
A/B	AB
O/O	O

The human genetic linkage map is constructed by observing how frequently two markers are inherited together.

Two markers located near each other on the same chromosome will tend to be passed together from parent to child. During the normal production of sperm and egg cells, DNA strands occasionally break and rejoin in different places on the same chromosome or on the other copy of the same chromosome (i.e., the homologous chromosome). This process can result in the separation of two markers originally on the same chromosome. The closer the markers are to each other the more tightly linked the less likely a recombination event will fall between and separate them. Recombination frequency thus provides an estimate of the distance between two markers.

On the genetic map, distances between markers are measured in terms of centimorgans (cM), named after the American geneticist Thomas Hunt Morgan. Two markers are said to be 1 cM apart if they are separated by recombination 1% of the time. A genetic distance of 1 cM is roughly equal to a physical distance of 1 million bp (1 Mb). The current resolution of most human genetic map regions is about 10 Mb.

The value of the genetic map is that an inherited disease can be located on the map by following the inheritance of a DNA marker present in affected individuals (but absent in unaffected individuals). It is not necessary that the molecular basis of the disease is clearly understood or the responsible gene identified. Genetic maps have been used to find the exact chromosomal location of several important disease genes, including cystic fibrosis, sickle cell disease, Tay- Sachs disease, fragile X syndrome, and myotonic dystrophy.

One short- term goal of the genome project is to develop a high- resolution genetic map (2 to 5 cM); recent consensus maps of some chromosomes have averaged 7 to 10 cM between genetic markers. Genetic mapping resolution has been increased through the application of recombinant DNA technology, including in vitro radiation- induced chromosome fragmentation and cell fusions (joining human cells with those of other species to form hybrid cells) to create panels of cells with specific and varied human chromosomal components. Assessing the frequency of marker sites remaining together after radiation- induced DNA fragmentation can establish the order and distance between the markers. Because only a single copy of a chromosome is required for analysis, even nonpolymorphic markers are useful in radiation hybrid mapping. In meiotic mapping, two copies of a chromosome must be distinguished from each other by polymorphic markers.

Physical Mapping

After genetic mapping, the next step in identifying the sequence that codes for a gene is to construct a physical map of the region. Physical mapping is also an important preliminary step in many sequence assembly strategies. Physical mapping involves experimental procedures which select, separate, replicate, combine, and measure DNA molecules.

There can be different types of physical maps and they vary in their degree of resolution:

- The lowest resolution physical map is the chromosomal (sometimes called cytogenetic) map, which is based on the distinctive banding patterns observed by light microscopy of stained chromosomes.
- A cDNA map shows the locations of expressed DNA regions (exons) on the chromosomal map.
- The more detailed cosmid contig map depicts the order of overlapping DNA fragments spanning the genome.
- A macrorestriction map describes the order and distance between enzyme cutting (cleavage) sites
- The highest resolution physical map is the complete elucidation of the DNA sequence of each chromosome in the genome.

As discussed in an earlier chapter, there are five fundamental techniques that help produce "fingerprints" and physical maps of DNA segments:

1. DNA cloning
2. Hybridization
3. Polymerase Chain Reaction (PCR)
4. Restriction enzymes
5. Gel electrophoresis

There are two basic approaches : Top-down physical mapping and bottom-up physical mapping strategies. The top-down approach produces maps with few gaps, but map resolution may not allow location of specific genes. The bottom- up strategies generate extremely detailed maps of small areas but leave many gaps. A combination of both approaches is usually applied.

17.3. APPLICATIONS OF MAPPING

Using the above techniques, compound processes are created which produce different kinds of physical maps of target DNA segments. Some of the applications are :

1. DNA fingerprinting
2. Clone mapping
3. STS mapping

DNA Fingerprinting

A *fingerprint* of a DNA sequence is a pattern of size-fractionated segments. Such a pattern can be compared with fingerprints of different DNA molecules to determine sequence similarities. However, the sizes of fragments, and not their order or the sequences between restriction sites determine the fingerprint.

The steps to fingerprinting a given DNA segment include:

- Clone the segment.
- Completely digest it with chosen enzyme.
- Separate and measure the resulting fragments using gel electrophoresis.

As with any application involving the separation of restriction fragments, the original order of the fragments is lost.

Clone Mapping

Sequencing extremely large chunks of DNA is often a laborious and impractical task. To break the problem into pieces of manageable size, a divide-and-conquer strategy is employed in which a coarse map is first constructed using a *clone library*, where each portion of a DNA segment is covered by a clone.

The steps to creating a map of DNA clones include:

- Construct a clone library covering each portion of the target DNA multiple times.
- Fingerprint each clone.
- Computationally infer the arrangement of clones, based on the fact that clones that overlap significantly should have features in common.

A probabilistic analysis is used to decide the number of clones that are needed to ensure coverage of a given percentage of the target DNA. In practice, clone mapping is applied to sequencing by constructing a *tiling path* of clones, i.e. a collection of clones that completely covers the target, while minimizing the portion of it that is redundantly covered. Sequencing the target DNA is then reduced to sequencing each of the clones in the tiling path.

STS Mapping

A *sequence-tagged site*, or STS, is a sequence of about 200 nucleotides in length. It is believed that STS occurs exactly once on the entire genome. Because of this perceived uniqueness, STS's are often used as markers on physical maps; they are considered landmarks for locating other interesting sites, and are not genetically meaningful themselves.

Given a clone library and a set of STS's on a DNA segment, hybridization or PCR can be used to determine the occurrences of the STS's on the clones. Once it is discovered which STS's overlap which clones, it is possible to compute the ordering of the STS's. (This is only under the assumption that the data is perfect). Of course, many factors may contribute to an imperfect data set. For example, the STS's may not be unique, or the clones may not represent contiguous stretches of target DNA. However, in the case of perfect data, computing an ordering of the STS's is achieved by noting that STS's that overlap the same clone must occur consecutively in the ordering. In the figure below, let A-G be seven STS's on a DNA segment that is covered by six overlapping clones.

```
                              5
                    _____

                                    3
                          _____

                    2
              _____

        1              4         6
    _____    _____ _____
    _____

    E   B        F   A   C   G        D
```

We can represent the segment by a matrix M which has a row for each STS and a column for each clone. An "X" is placed in entry M[i,j] if the STS in row i occurs on clone j. The matrix for the segment above is:

	1	2	3	4	5	6
A			X	X	X	
B	X	X				
C			X	X	X	
D						X
E	X					
F		X	X		X	
G			X			X

X's in a given column represent STS's on a single clone, which are of course consecutive. Hence, if we rearrange the rows in the above matrix so that they occur in the same order as the STS's occur, then in each column all the X's are next to each other. So, any rearrangement of the rows that puts all X's in a column in consecutive positions is a possible map. For example:

	1	2	3	4	5	6
E	X					
B	X	X				
F			X		X	
A			X	X	X	
C			X	X	X	
G			X			X
D						X

The resulting ordering of STS's is EBFACGD, which is in sync with the ordering in the original figure. Note that EBFCAGD also achieves this property, and so is also consistent with the data.

The PQ-Tree Algorithm

The STS mapping problem (in the case of perfect data) can be solved by the "PQ-Tree Algorithm" using the information from the matrix M . A PQ-Tree is a data structure that represents a certain class of permutations.

A *P-node* is one whose children may be re-arranged in any order, and a *Q-node* is one whose children remain consecutive, but may be arranged in reverse order.

The PQ-Tree Algorithm computes the tree representing all orderings of rows in M such that the X's in each column are consecutive. The tree is initialized to be a root P-node with a child node for each row, A through G. At each iteration, a column is selected, which places a constraint on some subset of the leaves. The algorithm proceeds, column by column, until all constraints have been added.

In the case of the example matrix M, four orderings can be read off the final tree: EBFACGD, EBFCAGD, and their reversals DGCAFBE, and DGACFBE.

Imperfect Data

In real-life experiments, errors do creep in. In general, there are three kinds of errors that can contribute to an imperfect data set in the STS mapping problem:

1. False positives – hybridization or PCR data suggest that an STS overlaps a particular clone when it actually doesn't.
2. False negatives – hybridization or PCR data suggest that an STS does not overlap a particular clone when it actually does.
3. Chimeric clones – clones do not represent contiguous stretches of DNA.

Such imperfections usually result in a matrix M lacking the "consecutive ones property"—one whose rows cannot be rearranged to obtain the condition of consecutive X's in each column. One way of dealing with this case is to formulate the problem as an optimization problem. The objective is to find a "best" answer in the presence of noisy data, i.e. to find a small number of (presumably erroneous) data values to change so as to create a matrix having the consecutive ones property.

17.4. DNA SEQUENCING

Introduction

DNA sequencing, regardless of whether it is done on an automated sequencer or by autoradiography, relies on the Sanger method of DNA replication with dideoxy chain termination and separation of the resulting molecules by polyacrylamide gel electrophoresis. In simple terms, this means that in order to be sequenced, a DNA molecule must be copied in a test tube (in vitro) by a DNA polymerase enzyme.

The DNA fragment to be sequenced must first be cloned into a vector (such as a plasmid) to obtain a sufficient quantity of the fragment to be sequenced. Another limitation imposed by the technology is that sequences can only be determined in approximately 500 base pair (bp) chunks known as "reads". This is due to both the biochemistry of the DNA polymerase reaction and the resolution of polyacryla-mide gel electrophoresis. Yet most genes contain many thousands of bp and many modern sequencing projects are intended to produce complete sequences of large genomic regions or even entire chromosomes (many millions of bp). As a result, all sequencing projects must involve the division of the target DNA into a set of overlapping 500 bp fragments. Once the sequences of these fragments are determined, they must be pieced back together into "contigs" (lab slang for "contiguous sequenced regions") by computer "assembly" programs.

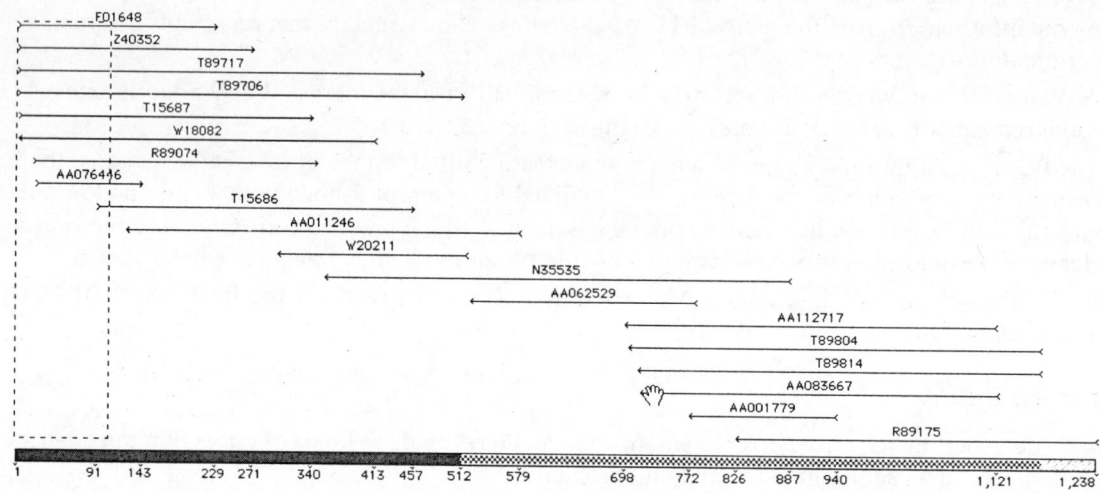

Fig. 17.1. DNA sequencing

DNA sequencing methodologies

There are three basic methods of DNA sequencing methodologies :
1. Clone-based sequencing
2. Shot-gun sequencing
3. Primer walking

Clone-based sequencing

The process is summarised as follows :
- First generate stable clones of rather large segments of DNA from the organism under study. The size of the segments depends on the technique used. The most commonly used are cosmids (max 45 kb), BACs (max 300 kb) and YACs (max 400 kb).
- The clones are selected so that they cover the genome (on a per-chromosome basis) in as complete but non-redundant fashion as possible, thus defining a so-called tiling path. So-called physical mapping does this.
- For selected clones, sequence it by fragmenting the DNA in them randomly, sequencing about 500-700 bases, and reassembling the complete clone sequence from the data.
- The complete genome is then reassembled from the known tiling path and the clone sequences.

Shotgun sequencing

The process is summarised as follows:
- Obtain a pure sample of the entire genome of the organism (all chromosomes), and split it up into

small fragments. The DNA of interest is sheared physically to make random small inserts of size 1 to 2 kb which are then cloned into M13 or plasmids. The subclones are not mapped.

- Clone these small fragments, thus creating a genomic library. Sequence as many of the clones as necessary. These subclones are then sequenced using automated DNA sequencing. This involves a number of steps. The sequencing "reads" vary from 300–900bps in length and the coverage is around 6 to 10 times (i.e., each base of the cosmid, BAC, or YAC clone is covered by 6–10 reads).

- Reassemble the genome by computational analysis of the sequence fragments. For this to work, an oversampling of the genome is required, so that the residual number of unclosed gaps is as low as possible.

- After the assembly is done, there will often be gaps in the sequence—segments where reads did not cover the clone, or where all reads were of low quality. As a result, we might get two or more contigs. In the *finishing phase* additional subclones spanning the gaps are obtained and sequenced. The goal is to allow all data to be joined into a single contig with an error rate of 10 or better.

- Annotation/Identification: Once the sequence of piece of DNA is known, comparing to other sequences in the database can identify it. Finding genes, regulatory elements and repeats, etc., using various available tools will tell about the biology of the sequence.

Primer Walking

The third strategy known as "primer walking" requires very fast and accurate analysis of sequence reads since each sequencing reaction uses information from the previous read. Again, assembly problems are minimized since both the order and the amount of overlaps of the reads are known.

It was long believed that the shotgun strategy would not work on such large DNA molecules as chromosomes. It was thought that the frequency of gaps in the final assembly (due to uncovered segments) and the problems that repetitive DNA sequences caused, would render shotgun sequencing useless for large DNA molecules. However, Craig Venter formed The Institute for Genomics Research (TIGR) in order to use shotgun sequencing in a systematic fashion for determining entire bacterial genomes.

The strategy developed by TIGR, and subsequently used by the company Celera has another important component. The DNA fragments are generated as BAC clones (100-150 kb), of which some are randomly chosen to be fully sequenced by the shotgun method. Other BAC clones are then sequenced only at their ends, so that it becomes possible to choose which of them should be sequenced next. This extra information ('mates') helps considerably in reassembling the entire genome.

Many sequencing projects use approaches that involve a mixture of these three basic strategies. Large sections of genomic DNA are first carefully sub-cloned into overlapping megabase-sized fragments (YACs), which are then carefully sub-cloned into overlapping 20-40 KB fragments (cosmids or lambda clones), and then these fragments are shotgun sequenced. Primer walking then fills gaps in the assembled sequences.

Problems in sequencing

There are two important problems inherent in any known sequencing strategy:
- The law of diminishing returns.
  There are parts of a genome that are more difficult to sequence than others. For example, the DNA sequence may cause problems in the bacterial system used to maintain the clones, so that such clones are eliminated or strongly underrepresented in the genomic libraries. This also applies to

gap-finishing: Some gaps are more difficult than others. The final 5% of sequence is more expensive to obtain than the first 50%.

- The existence of intractable regions in the genomes.

    It is not possible to sequence heterochromatin as the technology to handle it is not there. In *Drosophila melanogaster* the entire genome has a size of about 180 Mb, of which about 120 Mb is euchromatin, and was sequenced by Celera.

There are a number of computational problems faced by sequence assembly programs:

1. The 500 bp reads of sequence data produced in the lab have errors of both incorrectly determined bases and of insertions and deletions.
2. The error rate is highest at the beginning and ends of the reads - precisely the regions that must be overlapped. The quality of the data is low towards the end of the read for several reasons:
    - These are the longer fragments, and obviously there is a smaller proportionate difference in length between large fragments that differ by one base.
    - The fluorescent signal strength is weaker, since fewer long molecules are created during the reaction. (Random incorporation of ddNTPs results in a geometric distribution of concentration versus size.)
    - The longer times until these fragments pass the laser detector allow more diffusion of the molecules in the gel. Usable reads extending over 800 bases are routinely obtainable, but the above factors (among others) currently prevent dramatically longer reads.
    - There are other factors like polymerase, sequencing reaction, etc., which influence the quality of the data. For example, compression in peaks is observed because of self annealing of some part of the (single-stranded) fragment.
3. DNA fragments are frequently cloned into plasmids or other vectors, but some sequence from these vectors is often included at the ends of sequence reads.

Error probabilities

Since there is a lot of variation in quality, it is important to assign "quality values" to each base. For each base call, we estimate the probability that it is correct. This is very valuable during sequence assembly since it allows us to use the entire read length during assembly of the sequence. Also, reads can be put together more accurately if we know the probability attached with each base. Additionally, it helps to create a more accurate consensus sequence, by focusing on the high quality traces, rather than averaging over lower quality data.

Method for defining error probabilities

Error probabilities are estimated by the following procedure:

1. Determine three key parameters visible in the traces that seemed to correlate to erroneous base calls.
2. Obtain a large set of reads covering accurately known sequences, so that it was possible to classify each base call as correct or incorrect.
3. Given the trace parameters for these reads, for each choice of parameter threshold, determine empirical error rates.
4. Resulting data are summarized in a lookup table.
5. For a new read for which error probabilities are to be estimated, compute the trace parameter values and determine the estimated error rate from the lookup Table.

Parameters for defining the error probabilities

The following parameters, calculated from the fluorescence intensity traces, seem to be most critical in determining base calling error rates.

1. *Distance from the nearest unresolved peak* : It may be difficult to resolve successive peaks when they overlap significantly. Base calls tend to be more accurate if they are well-separated from unresolved peaks. The *distance parameter* for each base is the distance (number of bases) from it to the nearest unresolved peak.

2. *Spacing criterion* : Ideally, peaks will be evenly spaced, and the more even the better. We quantify this by computing the spacing between the peaks in a window of seven bases centered on the peak of interest. The *spacing parameter* is the ratio between the smallest and largest spacings observed in this window.

3. *Size criterion* : With good data, one of the four fluorescence signals will clearly dominate the other three (presumably background noise) at each peak. This is quantified in the *size parameter*: the ratio of the heights of the largest uncalled to the smallest called peak, again measured over a window of seven bases centered on the base of interest. Empirically, there is good agreement between these numerical parameters and read quality, as judged by human experts.

Computer tools for Sequencing

A wide variety of different computer tools have been created to aid DNA sequencing projects.

The GCG fragment assembly tools

The GCG Fragment Assembly System is a series of related programs (based on the Staden package) that allow data entry, and assembly of overlapping nucleotide sequence fragments into one continuous sequence. The sequence project tools include:

SEQED: a single sequence editor (based on the VMS EDT editor)

GELSTART: creates fragment assembly projects, initializes work sessions on existing projects

GELENTER: adds individual sequences (reads) to an assembly project, allows input of new sequences from keyboard, digitizer, or import of existing text files

GELMERGE: assembles individual sequences into contigs, can automatically remove vector sequences

GELASSEMBLE: multiple sequence editor for viewing and editing contigs, allows manual alignment of fragments (even those that won't align with GELMERGE), insertion/deletion of gaps and changing of individual bases

GELVIEW: displays contigs as a schematic display of overlapping fragments

GELDISASSEMBLE: breaks up contigs into individual sequences within a project

Sequencher

Sequencher is a assisting researchers with DNA sequencing. In addition to the features common to GCG, MacVector, and GeneWorks such as sequence entry and a multiple sequence alignment editor, Sequencher offers specialized tools for working with the output from automated sequencers, especially Applied Biosystems machines.

Sequencher can import the electropherograms (graphical representations of the fluorescent intensity of each band in the sequencing gel) directly from the ABI machine. So, rather than just looking at a text file of the sequence data, the quality of the sequence at each base can be assessed - much like an autoradiogram. When multiple sequences are aligned and mismatches are found, the electropherograms can also be aligned and decisions can be made based on the quality of the sequence rather than just which base occurs more often in multiple reads. Sequencher also offers impressive automated tools for removal of vector sequences and low quality sequence data from the ends of reads.

17.5 ALGORITHM FOR ALIGNMENT OF SEQUENCING FRAGMENTS

Sequence assembly process

Sequence Assembly is the process of constructing the "best guess" clone (cosmid or BAC) sequence from a set of overlapping reads of the clone. The problem is complicated by the fact that there could be errors in read sequences and the fact that there could be many repeats in the clone sequence. The broad outline of the sequence assembly process is described as below:

1. Compare reads pairwise to determine potentially overlapping reads.
2. Determine layout, *i.e.* the pattern of overlaps.
3. Determine the consensus sequence.

The essence of building contigs is identifying and aligning fragments that overlap. This is done with the same basic algorithms that we have already discussed for similarity searching and pairwise/multiple alignment. The only difference is that alignment should be found in short regions at the ends of fragments.

Because the reads are overall fairly accurate (about 99 % accurate), finding matches is much simpler than finding simple subtle sequence similarities. We can assume that two overlapping reads will have perfectly matching words of significant lengths in common.

General Method

Each fragment in the sequencing project database is part of a contig. A contig contains either a group of aligned sequences associated together or a single, unaligned fragment.

GelMerge finds the two contigs with the longest overlap and then aligns them to assemble a single contig. The program then finds the next two contigs with the longest overlap and aligns them to assemble a single contig. GelMerge repeats this process of overlap determination and contig assembly until there are no remaining overlaps among the contigs in the project database.

The result of GelMerge may either•be a single contig or several contigs (if none of the remaining contigs share significant overlap). As you add new fragments to the sequencing project database, they may connect separate contigs to form larger assemblies.

Finding Overlaps

In finding overlaps among the contigs, GelMerge represents each contig by its consensus sequence. GelMerge uses a modification of the approximate alignment procedure to determine the amount of overlap between any two consensus sequences. In GelMerge, each alignment must contain at least one long block of contiguous sequence identities. You can set the minimum length for each long block with the /MINIdentity command-line parameter (default length is 14). The requirement for at least one long block of identities allows the program to exclude trivial overlaps from consideration. This requirement also limits the extent of gapping permitted in the approximate alignment. The alignment cannot get out of phase by more than 10 registers of comparison from diagonals containing long blocks of sequence identities. (Use the /MAXGap command-line parameter to adjust this default of 10 registers of comparison.) This effectively prevents the alignment from wandering too far away from registers of comparison with significant sequence identity.

GelMerge determines all of the possible distinct alignments between the two contig consensus sequences being compared. Each alignment corresponds to a different overlap between the same two contig consensus sequences. After finding all of the distinct alignments between a pair of contigs, GelMerge counts the number of exact nucleotide matches in the best alignment. If this overlap does not meet the identity criterion (80% by default), the next best alignment is checked. If no alignment of two contig consensus sequences meets the identity criterion, then the two contigs do not overlap.

Aligning Contigs

Once GelMerge determines the pair of contigs with the longest overlap, it aligns them using the method of Needleman and Wunsch. This method, originally used to align individual sequences, has been extended for use with contigs of aligned sequences. When the program inserts gaps into a contig to produce an alignment, they are inserted at the same position in all of the sequences of the contig.

Recognizing Vector Sequences

GelMerge searches for vector sequences in single-fragment contigs using a two-step approach. First, GelMerge finds approximate alignments between vector and contig sequences using a modification of the method of Wilbur and Lipman. You can fine tune the vector searching by adjusting some parameters of the approximate alignment procedure. For vector searching, the minimum length for each short block of sequence identities is the same as the length used to find overlaps among the contigs; you can set the minimum length in response to the What word size program prompt (default length is 7). The minimum length of each long block of sequence identities in vector searching can be set with the /VECTORMINIdentity command-line parameter (default length of 12). The alignment cannot get out of phase by more than 5 registers of comparison from diagonals containing long blocks of sequence identities. (This default of 5 registers of comparison can be adjusted with the /VECTORMAXGap command-line parameter.)

Each of the approximate alignments indicates the position of possible vector sequences in the contig. In the second step of vector recognition, GelMerge refines these alignments using the method of Smith and Waterman. By default, if the aligned portions of the contig and vector sequences share greater than 80% sequence identity, the contig bases in the alignment become candidates for excision. (You can adjust this value using the /VECTORSTringency command-line parameter.) Additionally, by default, the vector sequences must begin within 12 bases of either end of the contig in order to be excised. (This value is the same as the minimum length for each long block; you can adjust it with the /VECTORMINIdentity command-line parameter).

Analysing a genome

The analysis of a genome covers many different aspects. Some of the common aspects are as follows :
- Define the location of genes (coding sequences, regulatory regions): gene prediction (identification).

- Gene prediction *ab initio* using software based on rules and patterns. Find Open Reading Frames (ORFs), with some additional criteria. Although it is simple for bacteria, it is very difficult for eukaryotes.
- Gene identification through alignment with known proteins and EST sequences.
- Gene prediction through similarity with proteins or ESTs in other organisms.
- Gene prediction through comparison with other genomes; conserved regions may be coding or regulatory regions.
- Annotation of the genes: Identify with known genes, similarity with genes in other organisms. Essentially: labelling the gene.
- Functional classification. Broad groups of functional characterization, such as 'ribosomal proteins', 'nucleotide metabolism', 'signal transduction'.
- Metabolic pathways.
  - Are any common pathways missing?
  - Are there any 'gaps' (missing enzymes) in some pathways?
  - Compare identified pathways with the life style of the organism.
- Evolutionary history
  - Internal genome duplications can sometimes be detected.
  - Gene decay can sometimes be characterized: genes that are on their 'way out' after duplication, or because the life style of the organism has changed.

Comparing genomes

One of the most interesting new fields that the availability of the complete genomes has created is the science of genome comparison. Comparing complete genomes can give deep insights about the relationship between organisms, as well as shedding light on the function of specific genes in each single genome. This is a nascent field (truly post-genomics era), and one of the most promising.

Some examples of issues that have been investigated to some degree:

- It is now possible to investigate which sets of genes are common to many different organisms, or groups of organisms. Is there a common core of genes necessary for all life? Is that core sufficient for life?
- Are all the ribosomal proteins really similar between all known species, or have there been inventions during the course of evolution in this specific, but fundamental system?
- Which genes are necessary for multicellular life forms; which set of genes are only found in multicellular organisms but not in unicellular ones?
- The rate of horizontal gene transfer (genes that have jumped the species barrier) among bacteria can now be investigated. How often, and under what circumstances do bacteria exchange genes? Has anything similar happened with higher organisms?
- Where and how have new genes emerged in evolutionary history? Can precursors of some gene families be found in distant relatives of a species?
- The problem of identifying and characterizing orthologous genes versus paralogous genes becomes easier to address (but not necessarily solve).

The recent complete genome projects, and the results in the form of analysis and comparison, have driven home the idea that the completeness of the data gives an entirely new dimension to biological science. New types of analysis can be made and new kinds of experiments can designed which simply could not be done before. The realization that the completeness of a data set can be extremely useful has made the biological scientific community look into the possibilities of obtaining other such complete data sets. It has even spawned a number of new buzzwords, some of which are less elegant than others:

	Description	Time dependence	Manipulation in the cell	Measurement in the cell
Genome	The complete DNA sequence of the organism	First approximation: none	Genetic manipulation; site-directed mutagenesis, genetic screens	Routine. High accuracy and completeness
Transcriptome	The complete set of mRNA transcripts in a cell or tissue of the organism.	Reflects the state of gene expression	Indirectly via genetic manipulation	Routine, or nearly so. cDNA microarrays, SAGE, Northern blots. Quantification in accurate. Approximate completeness.
Proteome	The complete set of proteins present in a cell or tissue, including variants due to covalent modifications. Sometimes also the the associations with other molecular component (complexes)	Responsive to all manner of influences throughout the life cycle	Indirectly through genetic manipulations. Small molecules as inhibitors of enzymes	Not routine. 2D-gels with mass spectrometry. Fusions with reporter proteins (GFP). Yeast two-hybrid system. Quantification very difficult. Completeness far away, and very difficult
Metabolism	All metabolites and their concentrations. Defined as organic small molecules, not protein, RNA or DNA	Responsive to all manner of influences throughout the life cycle	Difficult	Not routine. NMR, mass spectrometry, a few other special methods for specific molecules. Quantification and resolution difficult. Completeness far away, but may be reachable

Of these four kinds of datasets, only the genome and transcriptome can be routinely measured today. The proteome and metabolome are much more difficult.

17.6. DNA MICROARRAYS

Definitions

Sequences derived from one-pass sequencing of libraries are referred to as Expressed Sequence Tags, or ESTs. EST is an exon-specific sequence, 50-500 bp, from a cDNA. It represents a gene. There are tissue-specific libraries of ESTs, eg. DbEST. An overlap of ESTs, gets resulted in formation of "contig" of single cDNA eg. UniGene database. The existence of large sets of ESTs opens the door for studying gene expression on a large scale.

Introduction to Microarrays

The term microarray has come to refer to a series of high density DNA spots bound to some solid support. Basis is the Southern Blot technique as devised by Edwin Southern. While capillary transfer of DNA to a support membrane (nylon or nitrocellulose) does a Southern blot, microarrays bind DNA to a solid support, such as glass, using automated processes. This allows for much higher and more consistent spot densities to be realized, thus increasing the number of samples that can be probed at once. The immobilized DNA molecules can be probed with labeled complementary sequences of DNA.

Microarrays have many uses in the research lab. The key applications are :
- Gene Expression Profiling
- Identifying New Targets for functional genomics and drug development
- Single Nucleotide Polymorphism (SNP) mapping
- Mapping of Genes
- Genotyping

The ideas behind modern microarrays can be broken into two parts:
1. The manufacture of microarrays and
2. Subsequent analysis of hybridization results.

The analysis of microarrays is the more fundamental aspect and is essentially the same regardless of the way they were fabricated.

Craig Venter at the NIH realized that a rapid survey of genes in an mRNA population could be identified by doing single sequencing reactions on clones from a cDNA library as a rapid means of identifying the different classes of genes present in an mRNA population. Although sequence data from a single reaction is likely to contain errors, the error rate of automated sequencing methods is now far less than one error per hundred bases, more than good enough to identify a sequence, from several hundred bases of sequence.

1. How do gene arrays work?

Gene array experiments are sometimes referred to as "reverse Northerns". In Northern blots, RNA is blotted onto a filter and hybridized with a probe to detect a particular species of mRNA as a distinct band or spot. In gene array hybridization, cDNAs are spotted onto a filter and hybridized with a probe made from an mRNA population. Usually, probes are made by reverse-transcribing mRNA into single-stranded cDNA in the presence of labeled nucleotides. The labeled probe, therefore, is a population of cDNA molecules representing the original mRNA population. Probes are hybridized with filters containing cDNAs spotted in a 2-dimensional array. The amount of hybridization to a given clone represents the amount of mRNA present for the corresponding gene. A typical gene array experiment is illustrated below (Fig. 17.2):

Filter arrays

To minimize the risk of errors, it is essential to keep bacterial cultures in an array format, corresponding to the intended positions of the genes on the array. Cultures can be stored as glycerol cell stocks at -80°C. Since all clones usually come from a single library, or several libraries using the same cloning vector, it is usually possible to amplify any insert by PCR using primers specific for the multiple cloning site in the vector. Typically, a small number of bacterial cells are transferred to microtiter plates contiaining PCR reaction

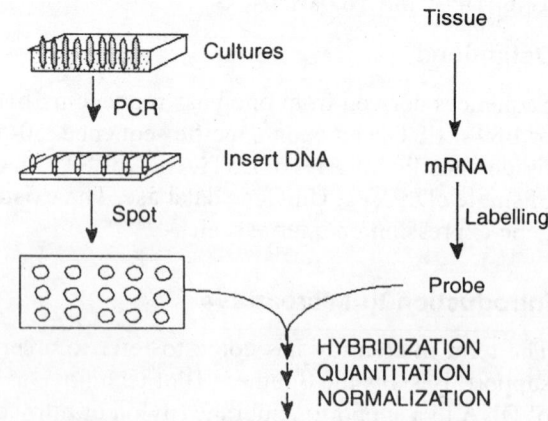

Fig. 17.2. Gene array experiment design

components, and inserts amplified by direct PCR on bacterial cells. The result is a PCR product, of only the insert and a small region of the vector. There DNAs can be directly spotted onto either nylon filters or glass microarray slides.

cDNA probes

Gene array experiments typically attempt to compare gene expression levels in different tissues of conditions, or at different times after a treatment. RNA is extracted from each tissue, condition, or traatment and RNA samples are diluted so that each sample contains the same concentration of RNA. To create a single-stranded probe, RNA is added to a reaction mix containing oligo dT primers, which can base pair with the polyA tail on mRNA, Reverse Transcriptase (RNA-dependent DNA polymerase) and labeled nucleotides. Commonly, labeled nucleotides are either tagged with fluorescent labels such as Cy3 and Cy5, or digoxygenin (DIG), which can be detected using chemiluminescent detection. In principle, for every mRNA molecule in the original RNA population, a single-stranded labeled cDNA will be produced, complementary to the mRNA. The higher the concentration of a particular mRNA, the more cDNA will be present.

Hybridization and washing

Incorporation of label into each probe is quantified, and probes are diluted so that all are at an equal concentration. Usually, a duplicate filter or microarray is prepared for each probe to be assayed. Probes are hybridized separately with each array. Filter arrays are incubated with probe and washed in much the same way as is done for Southern or Northern blotting. For glass microarrays, hybridization is done under a coverslip, and slides are washed by dipping into wash solutions.

Data acquisition

Hybridized probe is detected by either chemiluminescence for DIG label, or direct UV fluorescence for microarrays. The raw intensity of each spot is measured by a CCD camera, and the data acquired as a TIF image.

Double label

Another approach to comparing expression between two conditions is double label experiments. For example, in work from Patrick Brown's lab at Stanford, cDNA probes were made from yeast cells grown in the presence of either galactose or glucose. To distinguish between signals from the two probes, different fluorescently-tagged nucleotides, either Cy3 or Cy5 were added during reverse transcription. Cy3 has emission maxima at 565 and 615 nm, while Cy5 has an emission peak of 670nm. Replicate experiments were done in which dyes were switched. By scanning the arrays twice, once for Cy3 and once for Cy5, a composite image can be generated in which the ratio of the two dyes, and hence, the ratio of transcripts in the two growth conditions, can be measured. In pseudocolor images, spots in the array representing genes that are more strongly expressed in the presence of galactose are shown in green, and spots representing genes more strongly expressed in the presence of glucose are shown in red.

2. What are we trying to learn from gene arrays?

The primary goal of gene array experiments is to generate expression information for every gene in the array, under some set of conditions. Expression may be studied in :

- different tissues
- different developmental stages
- different genotypes
- different treatments
- different times after a treatment.

The kind of results that are sought in gene array experiments can be illustrated as follows (Fig. 17.3):

In the example, timecourse data are generated for each gene in an array. The raw data consists of a series of expression curves for timecourses, or histograms where other types of treatments are being compared. The goal is usually to find which groups of genes have the most similar expression patterns. In the example, two genes in the array (hatched background) show a gradual induction over the period of the timecourse. Two other genes (shaded background) show a biphasic response with two distinct periods of strong expression.

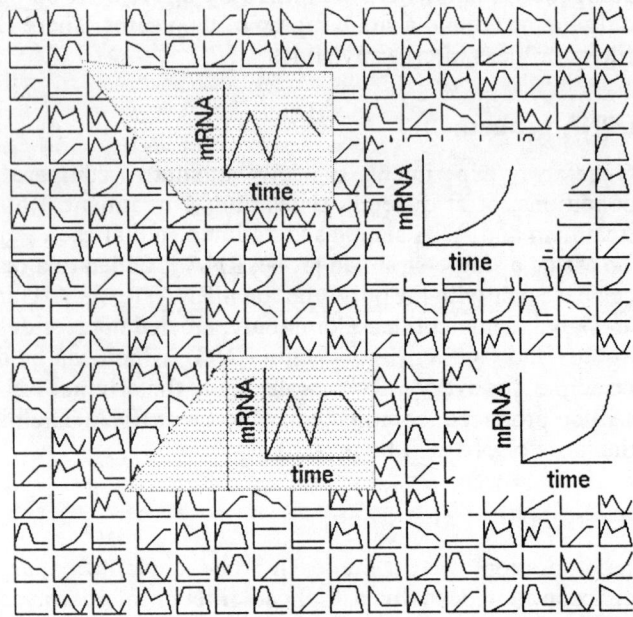

Fig. 17.3. Results of gene array experiments

17.7. MICROARRAY EXPERIMENT DESIGN AND DATA ANALYSIS

It is critical to realize that every experimental step in a procedure contributes to the final experimental error. Therefore, one should conceptualize the data as a set of observations each with a measurable amount of variation. The objective is to set up the experiment in a manner as to minimize the final standard error in the observations.

For some timepoints in which there is little true difference, a difference can only be detected when the standard error for both treatments is small. For other timepoints where the differences are large, higher standard errors will still allow the detection of the difference between two treatments.

Sources of experimental variation

Making a list of factors that contribute to experimental error follows steps in the gene array experiment. Some of these are discussed below :

- Treatments
  - Experimental conditions
  - Tissue preparation
- Probes
  - RNA isolation - use identical amounts of tissue, identical extraction methods; use minimum number of steps; measure amount of RNA and normalize concentration
  - labeling - measure incorporation of label and normalize samples to same concentration
  - amount - add same amount of label to each hybridization

- Arrays
  - PCR products - amplify directly from bacterial cells, rather than isolated plasmids; add same amount of product to each spot on filter
  - Uniformity of spotting - use arraying tool for filter arrays or robot for microarrays.
  - treatment of filters or slides
- Hybridization and washing
  - Long hybridization to ensure that hybridization goes to completion.

In any hybridization experiment, the time required for hybridization to go to completion is proportional to the concentration of the probe (Fig. 17.4). High abundance transcripts will hybridize to completion in very short times, so the signal should be roughly the same regardless of how long hybridization is done. For moderately abundant transcripts, it takes longer for hybridization to proceed to completion, so the amount of transcript for that mRNA will be underestimated unless a long hybridization time is used. Finally for rare abundance transcripts, the hybridization curve will still be in the linear phase after a long time.

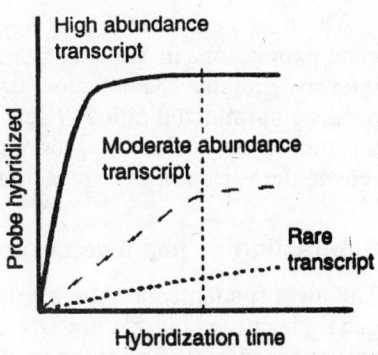

Fig. 17.4. Hybridization plot.

For genes that are members of multigene families, hybridization results could vary depending on hybridization and washing stringency. Hybridization under low stringency conditions might allow cross hybridization between members of a gene family, and all members would be expected to give roughly the same signal. Hybridization under high stringency conditions would allow for more discrimination between genes, because each transcript would only hybridize with its orthologous gene on the array.

However, it also needs to be noted that most of the errors in microarray experiments are systematic and not random. Physical parameters inherent in the production of microarrays can be used to approximately measure these systematic effects. The influence of these systematic factors can be corrected mathematically. Normalisation of the data is a process for correcting data that usually substantially reduces measurement error.

Data acquisition

- Image acquisition - The acquisition of the image data carries similar built in sources of variation, as does hybridization. Within a certain intensity range, the amount of signal detected is linearly proportional to the time of exposure. Usually, data acquisition entails accumulation of signal by a CCD camera. Data is saved as a TIFF image, where intensity of a given pixel is proportional to the amount of signal coming from part of the filter or slide. For highly abundant transcripts beyond a certain amount of signal, there may be little increase in intensity per unit time, and the spot will be saturated in the image. Moderately expressed genes may yield signal within the linear range of the camera's detection range. For rare transcripts, it may not be possible to expose long enough for signal from the transcript to shoulder out. It is important to recognize that these errors of detection are compounded on top of the errors associated with hybridization time.
- Spot and background detection. Software has to delineate each spot in the array, and to choose areas outside of spots for background estimation. Spots diameter can vary, and spot morphology may be irregular, rather than being perfectly circular.

Normalization

The term normalization has a meaning that is unique to this context. The term normalization does not necessarily refer to the assumptions of normality here. The raw intensities of signal from each spot on the array are not directly comparable. Normalisation is the re-scaling and correction of two data sets prior to comparison. Depending on the types of experiments done, a number of different approaches to normalization may be needed. Not all types of normalization are appropriate in all experiments. Some experiments may use more than one type of normalization.

There are many methods of normalization and each method makes assumptions about the biology of gene expression. In general, normalization methods calculate a scaling factor or function to correct intensity effects. These factors or functions are then applied to the measure of relative abundance to produce normalized ratios or scaled intensities. There are various mathematical approaches including mean correction, linear regression etc. for doing normalisation. The effect in most of the cases is to reduce the variation of expression measures.

Subtraction of negative controls from gene signals (Fig. 17.5)

The most fundamental type of normalization is to subtract negative controls from the signal for each gene. Negative controls are DNAs which are not present in the mRNA population. For example, an array of plant genes might contain several vector spots.

Ratio of signal to positive control (Fig. 17.6)

To allow comparison of genes from one filter to the next, it is often useful to spike the labeling reaction with some foreign RNA or DNA that is not normally in the RNA population. While in principle some presumably "constitutive" genes like actin, tubulin, or ubiquitin might serve, careful experiments often show that these genes are not really constitutive. Therefore, foreign gene sequences, known not to be present in the species being studied, are better controls. For example, a human RNA population might be spiked with plant RNA, and plant genes used as positive controls on the array. The signal s_i for gene i would therefore be raw counts g_i divided by the median of the counts for the vector spots. Normalization of signal for each gene to a ratio makes it possible to compare ratios between experiments, provided that the spiked controls are the same in all experiments. Normalization to a positive control is typically used in single-label experiments. Comparison of one experiment to another can either be

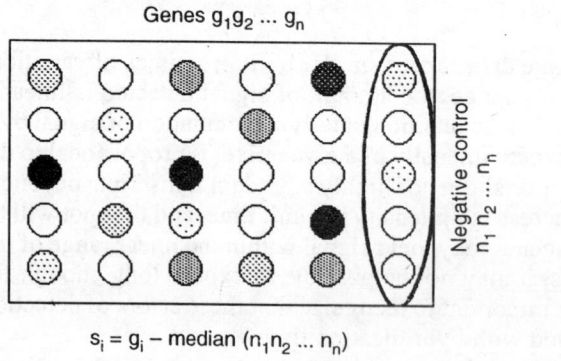

$$s_i = g_i - \text{median}(n_1 n_2 \dots n_n)$$

Fig. 17.5. Results of negative control experiment.

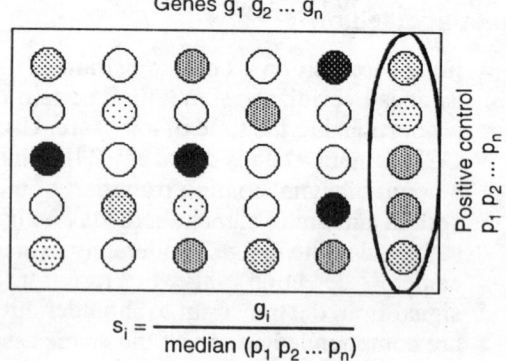

$$s_i = \frac{g_i}{\text{median}(p_1\, p_2 \dots p_n)}$$

Fig. 17.6. Results of positive control experiments

done by plotting signal s_I directly on a graph, or signals from two experiments can be converted into a ratio, usually by choosing one treatment as a control. For example, in a timecourse, a 0 hour timepoint might be chosen, and signal from all other timepoints divided by the signal for the 0 hour timepoint, to give a ratio.

Ratio of each gene to its control level

Because of the many sources of variation from experiment to experiment, one of the best possible controls is to choose some experimental condition as a baseline, to use as a control against all other experimental conditions or treatments. For example, the level of expression in a wild type organism might be the baseline, for comparison with expression levels in mutants. An excellent control can then be implemented by labeling the control RNA population with one dye (eg. Cy3) and all other RNA populations with a different dye (eg. Cy5). Each labeled experimental population is then mixed with an equal quantity of the labeled control RNA, and the mixed probe is hybridized with a gene array. The array is scanned at the wavelengths for each dye, and the ratio of the experiment to the control is the ratio of the intensities for each dye (corrected for background) for the two dyes. This approach is illustrated below (Fig. 17.7):

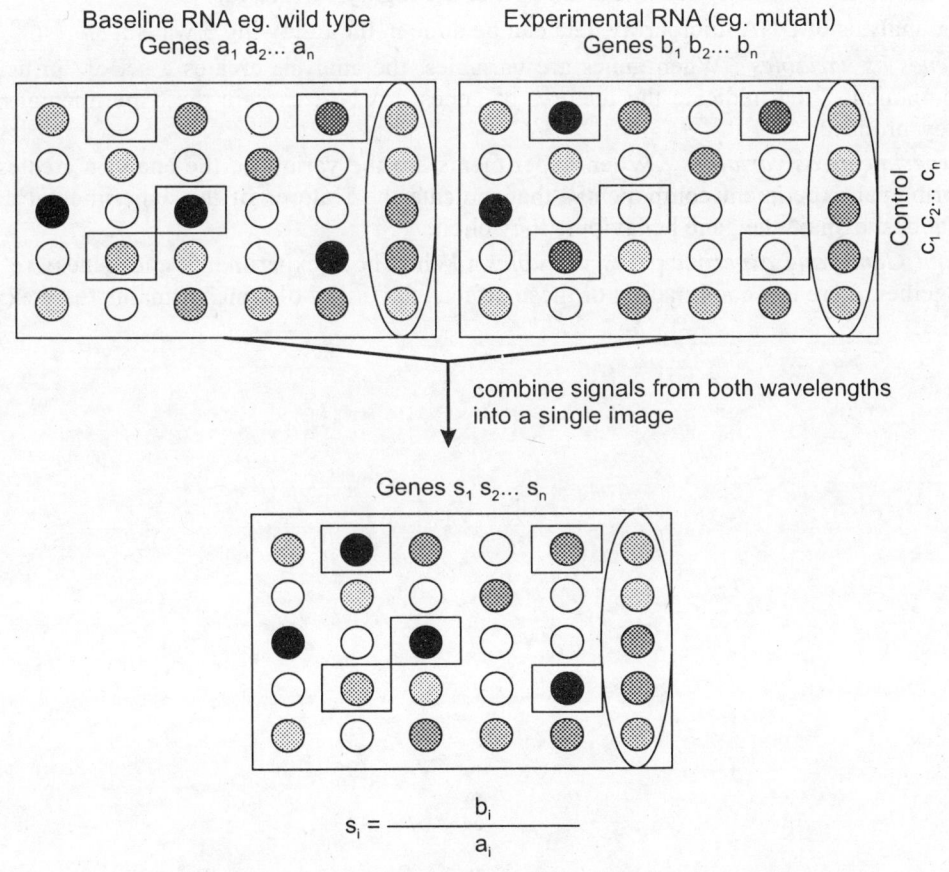

Fig. 17.7. Combining signals from both wavelengths

Normalized ratios are usually expressed as logs

To facilitate easier mathematical handling of the data, as well as comparisons over a wide range of expression levels, ratios are usually expressed as logs. For example, if a gene is expressed at 100-fold greater level in the control than in the mutant, $\log_{10}(1/100) = -2$. A log ratio of 0 is therefore indicative of a gene whose expression is the same in either conditions or treatments.

Exploratory techniques

PCA (discussed in an earlier chapter) is an exploratory multivariate statistical technique for simplifying complex data sets. Given m observations on n variables, the goal of PCA is to reduce the dimensionality of the data matrix by finding r new variables, where r is less than n. There r set of variables are termed as principal components, these r new variables together account for as much of the variance in the original n variables as possible while remaining mutually uncorrelated and orthogonal.

PCA has been extensively used for the analysis of microarray data in search of outlier genes as well as the analysis of other types of expression data. DNA microarray data sets are analysed by characterizing the waveform of gene expression over time, and in clustering genes based on this waveform or other features. When genes are clustered based on expression information, it is important to determine if the experiments have independent information or are highly correlated.

A PCA analysis of DNA microarray data can be done in the following 3 ways :

1. *Genes as variables* : When genes are variables, the analysis creates a set of "principal gene components" that indicate the features of genes that best explain the experimental responses they produce.
2. *Experiments as variables* : When experiments are the variables, the analysis creates a set of "principal experiment components" that indicate the features of the experimental conditions that best explain the gene behaviours they elicit.
3. *Both Genes and experiments as variables* : When both experiments and genes are analyzed together, there is a combination of these affects, the utility of which remains to be explored.

Proteomics Technology

18.1 INTRODUCTION

The term 'proteomics' stands for the systematic analysis of the *entire* protein complement produced by a genome, or by a cell or tissue type. *Proteome* refers to all proteins produced by a species, much as the genome is the entire set of genes. Unlike the genome, the proteome varies with time and is defined as "the proteins present in one sample (tissue, organism, cell culture) at a certain point in time".

Proteomics is a much bigger field than genomics. Genomics deals with one genome per organism. However, there are a large number of proteomes in an organism. Also, while the genome is a constant feature of an organism, the proteome varies with nature of tissue, the state of development, health or disease and effect of drug treatment. Genomics starts with the gene and makes inferences about its products (proteins), while proteomics begins with the functionally modified protein and works back to the gene responsible for its production.

There is an increasing interest in proteomics technologies now because DNA sequence information provides only a static snapshot of the various ways in which the cell might use its proteins, whereas the various processes in a cell are dynamic processes. Hence, DNA or RNA sequences are not enough for the clear identification of a therapeutic target because proteins, and not DNA or RNA are the basis of mode of action of drugs.

Types of proteomics

Proteomics can be broadly divided into three categories:

1. Expression proteomics
2. Functional proteomics
3. Structural proteomics

Expression proteomics

Expression proteomics is the approach that involves the creation of quantitative maps of expressed proteins from cell or tissue extracts, similar to cDNA arrays for transcription profiling. This comparative profiling of proteins regarding cataloguing their presence or absence under different cellular or physiological states, is often carried out by separating the proteins via two-dimensional (2-D) gel electrophoresis and identifying them by mass spectrometry. New approaches to address the limitations of 2-D gels by detecting less abundant proteins through the use of protein chips arrayed with specific capture molecules like antibodies or aptamers are being pursued actively. However, these approaches do not provide direct functional information on a particular protein that is expressed differentially. To infer functional information from differences in expression is difficult, because it is not possible to conclude which differences have true causal relationships to biological function.

Functional proteomics

Functional proteomics is the systematic perturbation or functional inactivation of proteins within a given physiological environment to address the potential role of the target protein in a cellular process, akin to gene disruption to elucidate the function of a gene. It is becoming clear that proteins can perform a multitude of functions depending on their cellular location; cell types where they are to be expressed, multimeric state and the bound substrate. Approaches in functional proteomics include the use of specific blocking molecules such as neutralizing antibodies and aptamers, pharmacological inhibitors, transdominant mutations and chromophore-assisted laser inactivation. Arraying functional proteins on a chip is another strategy for defining protein function. This has been demonstrated successfully with soluble yeast proteins on a proteomic scale. Preliminary results have been published that set the stage for arraying recombinant human proteins for functional studies with miniaturized assays.

Furthermore, significant progress has been made by using functional membrane proteins, an important class of protein targets for drug development. Finally, chemical genetics can be classified under this category since small synthetic organic molecules or natural products are used to modulate the function of proteins.

Structural Proteomics

Structural Proteomics is the large-scale determination of the three-dimensional (3-D) structure of proteins. The appropriate term is structural proteomics because it is the structure of proteins that are being determined and not the nucleic acids corresponding to the gene sequence. Identification of all potential protein folds should provide the structural framework for understanding how a protein executes its function. However, identification of all protein folds only represents the first step. Since proteins can have multiple structural domains, each specifying functional properties, it will be necessary to link these two types of information. Due to the lack of understanding of protein structure-function relationships, it is still not possible to deduce all possible functions from a protein's 3-D structure with high confidence. This becomes more complicated in humans, wherein most genes are fusions of different structural domains, providing further functional diversity. The use of computational techniques to infer protein structure, as well as to design protein ligands, falls under this category.

Unlike genomics, which deals with one genome per organism on which to focus, there is a very large number of proteomes in an organism. Therefore, proteomics is a much bigger field than genomics. In bacteria, a single gene codes for one or two protein spots on 2-D PAGE; in yeast one gene codes for three protein spots, and in humans one gene codes for three to more than 6 protein spots. The human body may contain more than two million different proteins (3-D structures), each having different functions. Genomics starts with the gene and makes inferences about its products (proteins), while proteomics begins with the functionally modified protein and works back to the gene responsible for its production. Proteomics thus runs parallel to functional genomics in a manner.

18.2 METHODS OF PROTEOME ANALYSIS

Proteins in an organism change during growth, disease, and the death of cells and tissues. Modifications of proteins that occur during and after their synthesis, such as the attachment of sugar residues or lipids, change the proteome complement. The minimum proteome size can be calculated from the size and 2-D polyacrylamide gel electrophoresis (2-D PAGE) separated proteins. Proteomics is based on leading edge technological capability for undertaking the mass screening of proteins and their post-translational modifications in whole organisms as well as in their tissues in normal and diseased states.

Proteomics enables correlations to be drawn between the range of proteins produced by a cell or tissue, and the initiation or progression of a disease state. Proteome research helps the discovery of new protein markers for diagnostic purposes and of novel molecular targets for drug discovery. The abundance of information provided by proteome research is complementary to the genetic information generated by genomic research. However, proteomics is not the study of individual proteins; it is a study of proteins on a large-scale using automation and new technologies. Proteomics at a broad level attempts to catalogue and characterize these proteins, compare variations in their expression levels in health and disease, study their interactions, and identify their functional roles. Fig. 18.1 provides an overall view of steps in proteome analysis.

There are five main steps in proteome analysis:

1. Sample collection, handling and storage
2. Separation of individual proteins by 2-D electrophoresis
3. Protein characterization
4. Identification by mass spectrometry or other methods
5. Storage, manipulation, and comparison of the data using bioinformatics

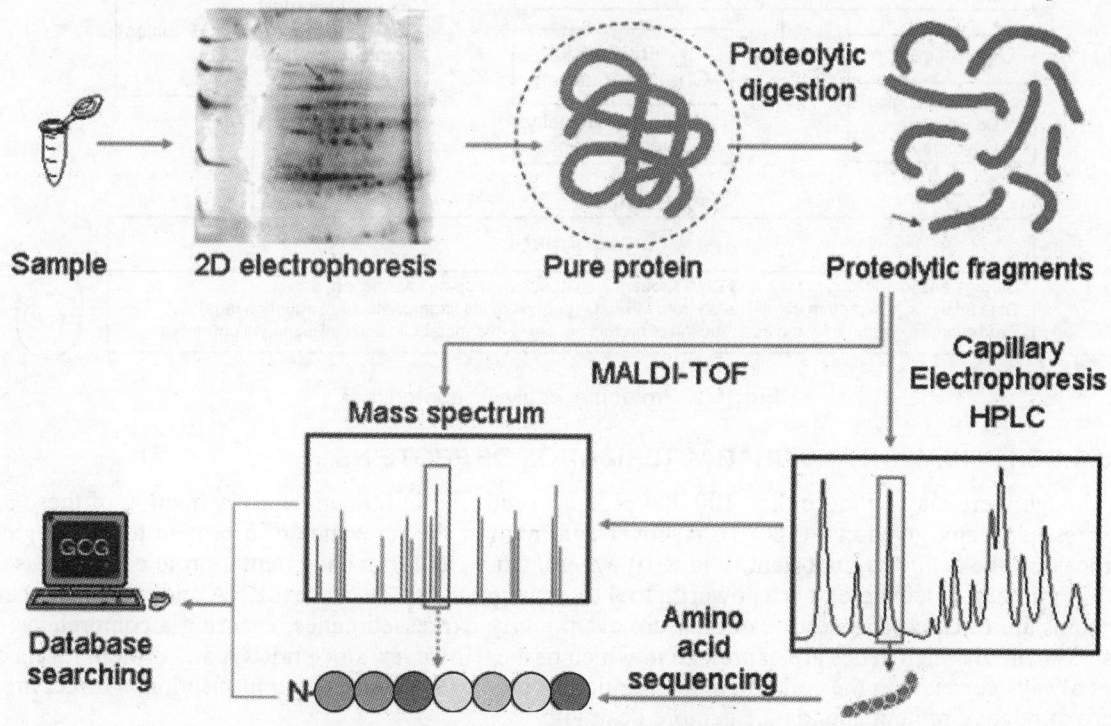

Fig. 18.1. Steps in proteome analysis.

The proteome can be analyzed using the two approaches in the Fig. 18.2. While one approach focuses on the analysis of proteome sample and the other approach does the analysis for understanding the interaction of various proteins. The first approach leads to quantitation and characterization of the protein and the second approach leads to the understanding of the protein-protein interactions.

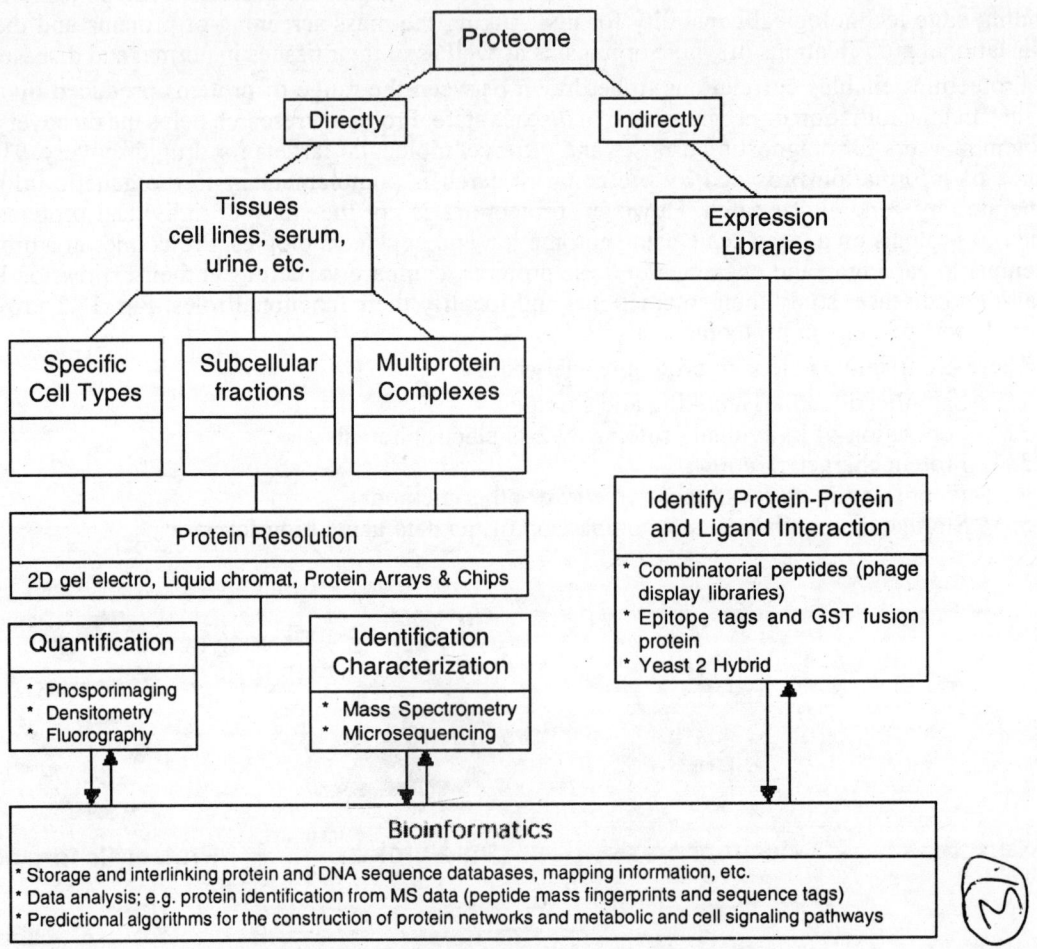

Fig.18.2 Proteome analysis approaches.

18.3 IDENTIFICATION AND CHARACTERIZATION OF PROTEINS

Although there may be more than 100,000 proteins produced in humans, only a fraction of these are expressed in any given cell type. To discover and monitor the relevance of a protein to a biological process in the cell, it is important to identify where, when, and to what extent a protein is expressed. DNA microarray technology is a powerful tool to accomplish this, because mRNA and protein concentrations are often correlated. It can measure even poorly expressed genes, ensuring a comprehensive assessment of which genes are expressed in which tissue. However, since mRNA and protein levels do not always correlate in the cell and many regulatory processes occur after transcription, a direct measure of relative protein abundance is more desirable.

A variety of proteomics technologies are now being used to measure differences in various proteins expressed by a cell. Currently, the primary method is electrophoresis or chromatography coupled with mass spectrometry (MS). In this method, mixtures of proteins in cellular extracts are resolved and then individual proteins are identified using MS peptide fingerprinting. Although in theory MS approaches have the potential to characterize the entire protein complement of a cell, in practice it has proved difficult to identify proteins of low abundance, because cell extracts, and a few hundred abundant proteins dominate the resulting mass spectra.

Defining the protein composition of a cell must also take into account the fact that mRNA splicing and covalent modifications generate protein isoforms that might contribute to important regulatory processes in the cell. Several approaches are being used to study post-translational modifications on a proteome-wide scale. Again, the most popular approach couples MS, which can detect even subtle covalent modifications, with methods to specifically enrich for modified proteins. Other strategies include the use of modification-specific antibodies.

The techniques that catalog changes in gene expression, protein levels, or modification due to disease or other cellular perturbations are powerful methods of identifying potential targets for drug discovery. However, they do not reveal the biochemical mechanism of *how* a gene product is related to disease or whether the protein is likely to be amenable to drug development. To address these issues, proteomics approaches that link protein function are required.

Quite often, proteins having identical functions share structural homology in the absence of obvious sequence homology. As a result, many of the newly sequenced proteins share unrecognized structural and functional homology with known proteins. On the basis of current estimates, structural information is predicted to provide functional clues for a large proportion of unannotated proteins. The principle that structure underlies function is known as *structural proteomics*. The aim of structural proteomics is to provide three-dimensional information for all proteins.

Protein characterization and quantitation can be done using the following methods :

1. Mass spectrometry
2. Protein fingerprinting
3. 2-D gel electrophoresis

Mass Spectrometry (MS)

Mass spectrometry is used for protein identification. It is useful to obtain structural information like peptide mass sequences. It is also useful in identifying type and location of protein modifications. MS can be used to characterize as little as picomoles of proteins at high resolution.

A mass spectrometer separates proteins according to their mass-to-charge (m/z) ratio. The molecule is first ionized. Ion flights must be observed *in vacuo* in order to avoid collisional scattering. The process of ionization of proteins forces them to move towards the analyzer because of the charges on ions. Mass spectrometery can provide molecular weight and structural information. Samples (M) with molecular weights greater than 1200 D give rise to multiple charged ions like $(M+nH)^{n+}$. Proteins or peptides have many suitable sites for protonation as all the backbone amide nitrogen atoms could be protonated theoretically, as well as certain amino acid side chains such as lysine and arginine that contain primary amine functionality.

We may now study the sequence of activities in mass spectrometry.

Ionization

The atom is ionized by knocking one or more electrons off to give a positive ion. This is true even for things that you would normally expect to form negative ions (chlorine, for example) or never form ions at all (argon, for example). Mass spectrometers always work with positive ions.

Acceleration

The ions are accelerated so that they all have the same kinetic energy.

Deflection

The ions are then deflected by a magnetic field according to their masses. The lighter they are, the more they are deflected. The amount of deflection also depends on the number of positive charges on the ion - in other words, on how many electrons were knocked off in the first stage. The more the ion is charged, the more it gets deflected.

Detection

The beam of ions passing through the machine is detected electrically.

This sequence is shown in the Fig. 18.3.

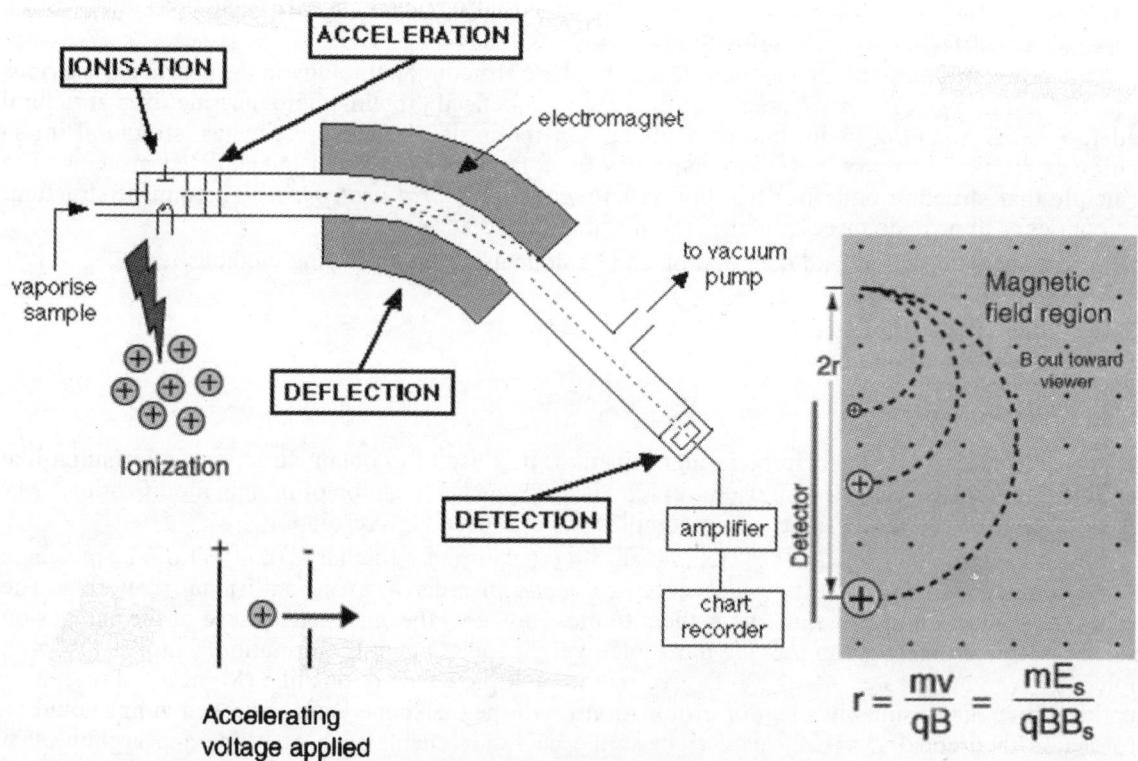

Fig. 18.3. Sequence of activities in MS.

The process of ionization can be done by techniques like *MALDI* and *ESI*. (*MALDI is matrix-assisted laser desorption/ ionization and ESI stands for electrospray ionization*). The ion is then propelled across the analyzer by an electric field that resolves each ion according to its m/z ratio. These are discussed below.

MALDI

Ionization by MALDI is done by having a protein suspended or dissolved in a crystalline structure (the matrix) of small, organic, UV-absorbing molecules. The crystal absorbs energy at the same wavelength of the laser that is used to ionize the protein. The laser energy strikes the matrix to cause rapid excitation of the matrix and subsequent passage of matrix and analyte ions into the gas phase. The ionized protein is accelerated by an electrostatic field and expelled into a flight tube. As it exits the flight tube the mass analyzer is encountered. The analyzer is often a time-of-flight analyzer (TOF). This is based on the principle that when accelerated by application of a constant voltage, the velocity with which an ion reaches the detector is determined by its mass. MALDI is able to analyze proteins down to femtomole quantities. MALDI is able to tolerate small amounts of contaminants; therefore, sample preparation is not as tedious as with ESI mass spectrometry. The information obtained from MALDI analysis can be automatically submitted to a data base search for further examination.

The sample that you want to analyze is spotted onto a target plate and allowed to dry. The plate is then put inside the machine. With MALDI-TOF the sample needs to be ionized and vaporized in some way and in this case a laser is used to provide the energy requirement.

Once the sample has been ionized it is accelerated through an electric field. The inside of the spectrometer is a vacuum and the ions are able to pass along a straight length of analyzer where their time of flight is measured. This measures the mass/charge ratio (m/z) of the fragment and smaller fragments move faster than larger ones, therefore allowing them to be measured. In MALDI the peptide fragments generally only have a single charge so that the m/z normally represents the mass of the fragment. Schematic diagram of MALDI-TOF is shown in Fig. 18.4.

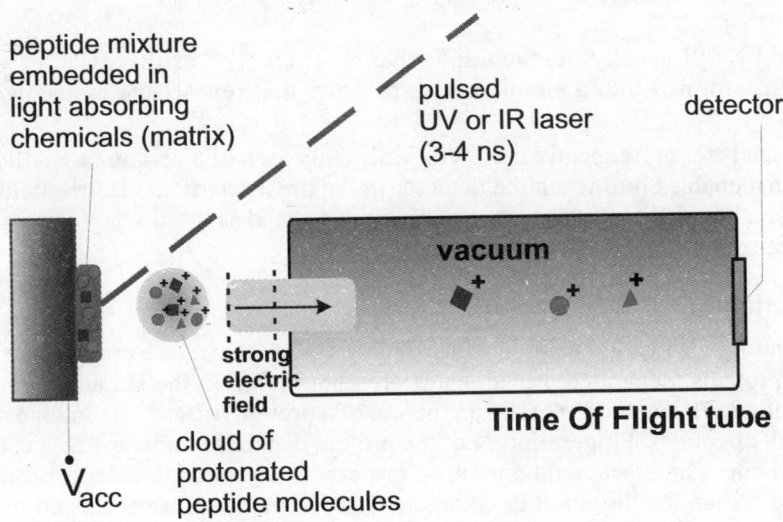

Fig 18.4. Schematic of MALDI-TOF.

Electrospray ionization (ESI)

Electrospray ionization (ESI) involves the production of gaseous ions by application of a potential to a flowing liquid resulting in the formation of a spray of small droplets with solvent-containing analyte. Solvent is removed from the droplet by heat or any other form of energy such as collision with a gas, and multiple charged ions are formed. As the droplet size further decreases, they reach a point at which they become unstable and explode into even finer droplets (Fig. 18.5). Finally electrostatic repulsion is sufficiently high to cause desorption of the analyte ions which are then passed to the mass spectrometer.

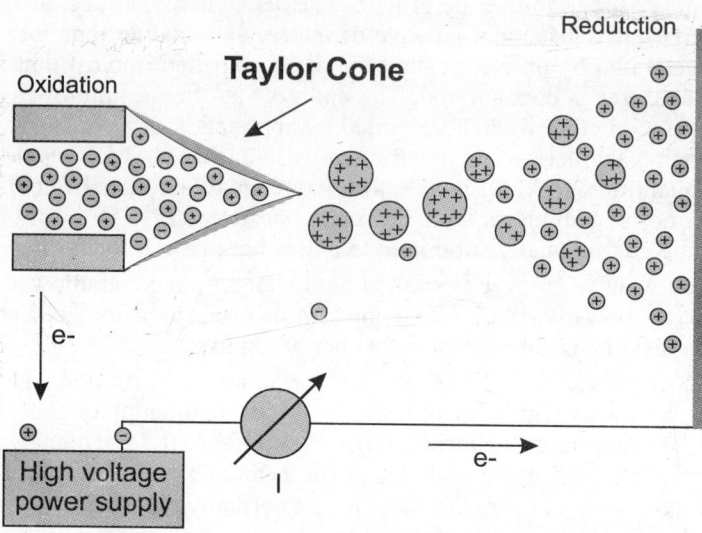

Fig.18.5. Schematic of Electrospray ionization.

Ions generated by ESI usually bear multiple charges $(M+nH)^{n+}$ as discussed earlier. This can be mathematically transformed into a simple mass spectrum that reveals the molecular weights of the fragments

A quadropole analyzer is frequently used with ESI. Only ions of a certain m/z will have the correct oscillation path that enables it to reach the detector in the presence of an electric field. One benefit of this method is that a liquid chromatography column may be used as the source for the proteins entering the ESI mass spectrometer, facilitating automation.

Protein Fingerprinting

Protein fingerprinting, also called peptide mass fingerprinting or peptide mapping, is a technique for identification of proteins. Separated protein spots are obtained from the gel and then identified using protein fingerprinting. The method is based on the use of a proteolytic enzyme to digest the protein into a number of smaller peptides. Fingerprinting of the protein depends on the protease used, but is always the same for each one. The most commonly used protease is trypsin, which cuts protein at lysine and arginine positions. When the digestion in complete, a set of peptides are produced of varying masses that are unique to that protein. The mass of each peptide will be the sum of the amino acids present including any modifications that those amino acids might have undergone.

Following are the steps in protein fingerprinting used for analyzing haemoglobin :

1. Take out haemoglobin from normal RBC and a sickle cell RBC.
2. Use trypsin to digest each sample.
3. Spot the two trypsin digested proteins on strips of filter paper.
4. Perform electrophoresis at pH 2.1.
5. Remove and dry the paper.
6. Perform paper chromatography using butanol : water : acetic acid in 4 : 5 : 1 ratio. The peptides

separate depending on their *partition coefficient*, which is dependent on their hydrophilicity and hydrophobicity. (Partition coefficient is a measure of the relative hydrophobicity/hydrophilicity of a compound. A partition coefficient of 0.1 means that the compound is distributed with 10% in the solvent and 90% in the aqueous solution). The most hydrophobic peptide will move the maximum and most hydrophilic peptide would move the least. Peptides would have hence partially separated.

7. Remove, dry and stain with ninhydrin reagent. Ninhydrin reacts with amino acids to form a blue stain.
8. This reveals that all the peptides except one are identical in normal and sickle cell haemoglobin.
9. The non-overlapping peptide are eluted and sequenced.

Protein fingerprinting is a better technique compared to pI (isoelectric pH) or molecular weight determination. One can also use the amino acid sequence to identify the protein, however, obtaining sequences is a time and effort intensive job. Protein fingerprinting is quicker than using sequences and better than using pI and molecular weights in terms of accuracy as fingerprinting is unique to a molecule.

Protein fingerprinting technique has been modified to compare the whole protein patterns in normal and abnormal cells by two-dimensional gel electrophoresis technique developed by O'Farrel.

Two-dimensional Gel Electrophoresis (Fig. 18.6)

2 D gel electrophoresis a method for the separation and identification of proteins in a sample by displacement in 2 dimensions. It is used for the isolation of proteins that are further characterised by mass spectroscopy techniques.

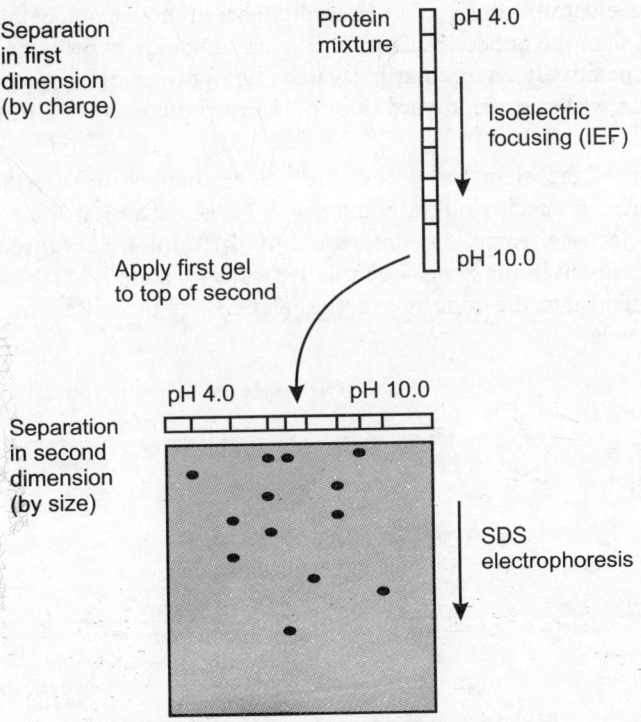

Fig. 18.6 (a). Separation in two dimensions.

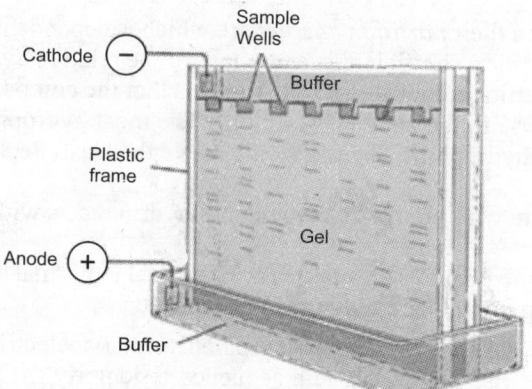

Fig 18.6 (b). Equipment for SDS-PAGE. The sample is put in the small "wells" at the top.

The first dimension of 2 D gel electrophoresis is the *isoelectric point (pI)*. The protein is first separated out according to the pI characteristics in a thin gel. After incubation in a detergent solution for some time, the proteins are then separated in a second dimension according to their size.

In simple electrophoresis, the movement of proteins is due to their charge, which is pH dependent. At pI, a protein has no charge and hence shows no movement on application of an electric field.

Isoelectric focusing (IEF)

IEF can be described as electrophoresis in a pH gradient set up between a cathode and anode with the cathode at a higher pH than the anode. Because of the amino acids in proteins, they have *amphoteric properties* and will be positively charged at pH values below their pI and negatively charged above. This means that proteins will migrate toward their pI. Most proteins have a pI in the range of 5 to 8.5 (Fig. 18.7).

Under the influence of the electrical force, the pH gradient will be established by the carrier ampholytes, and the protein species migrate and focus (concentrate) at their isoelectric points. The focusing effect of the electrical force is counteracted by diffusion that is directly proportional to the protein concentration gradient in the zone. Eventually, a steady state is established where the electro-kinetic transport of protein into the zone is exactly balanced by the diffusion out of the zone. IEF is performed in thin tube gels.

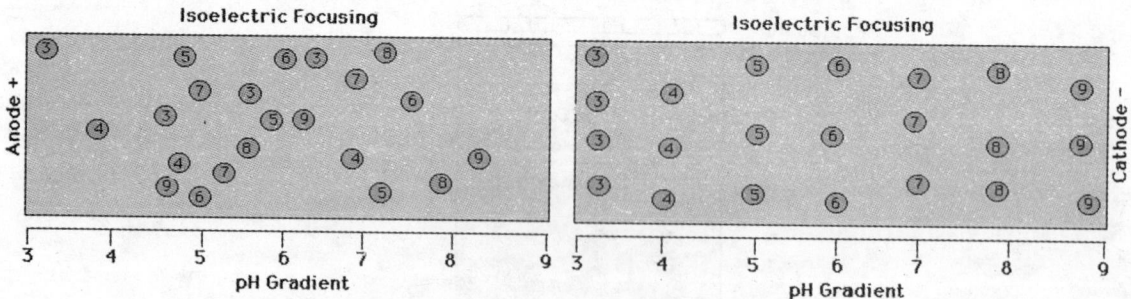

Fig. 18.7. IEF process – before and after.

Sodium Dodecyl Sulphate Polyacrylamide Gel Electrophoresis (SDS-PAGE) is a protein separation method used for separating peptide and protein mixtures. It is used with IEF. In the first step, an IEF tube gel is run, and the resulting gel is placed horizontally across the top of the stacking gel of a SDS-PAGE gel. The proteins in SDS-PAGE are separated by their molecular mass. Both the techniques are high-resolution techniques and hence the cumulative effect is a very high resolution separation of proteins.

The gels are then stained with dyes that bind to proteins (Fig 18.8). Examples of such dyes are Coomassie blue, silver stain and fluorescent dyes. Specially designed scanners that provide high-resolution images of these then scan the stained gels.

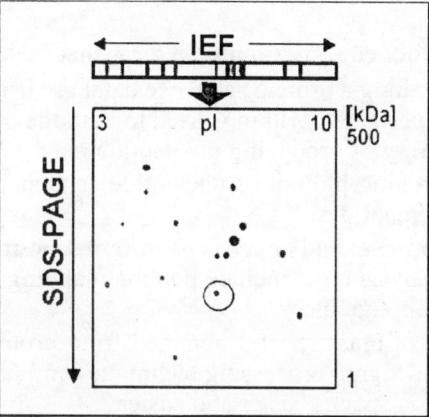

Fig. 18.8. Output of 2-D gel electrophoresis, showing excision of spots of interest. Subsequently proteins corresponding to the selected spots are identified.

Advantages and disadvantages of these techniques are summarized in the Table 18.1.

Table 18.1 Advantages and disadvantages of various techniques

Method	Advantages	Disadvantages
2-D PAGE	Can resolve up to 10,000 proteins. Widely used technique	Labour and time intensive with high variability between runs. It is biased toward display of cystolic and hydrophilic proteins
MALDI-TOF MS (for PMF)	Spectra are simple to interpret. The mass range is large and it is a sensitive technique	Success of PMF depends on access to complete, non-redundant and annotated DNA sequence databases. PMF can fail because of unanticipated peptide pos-translational modifications
MS/MS (for peptide fragmentation)	Derived peptide sequence tags facilitate accurate and large-scale protein identification	Sequence-specific peptide fragmentation spectra may be difficult to interpret. The success depends on access to complete, non-redundant DNA sequence databases.
Liquid Chromatography MS/MS	Complex peptide mixture can be analysed. The technique can be used for high-throughput analysis	Same as MS/MS

Bioinformatics tools for protein characterization

SWISS-2DPAGE (http://us.expasy.org/ch2d/) contains data on proteins identified on various 2-D PAGE and SDS-PAGE reference maps. You can locate these proteins on the 2-D PAGE maps or display the region of a 2-D PAGE map where one might expect to find a protein from SWISS-PROT

Proteome 2D-PAGE database (http://www.mpiib-berlin.mpg.de/2D-PAGE/) provides the facility to retrieve information on a protein spot within a 2DE gel image or to retrieve the position of a protein when its protein name or search expression is given.

PepMAPPER (http://wolf.bms.umist.ac.uk/mapper/) is a PMF tool from UMIST, UK. PeptideSearch (http://www.mann.embl-heidelberg.de/GroupPages/PageLink/peptidesearchpage.html) is a similar tool. PeptideSearch uses a non-redundant protein database (nrdb) that currently contains more than 750,000 entries.

PROWL (http://prowl.rockefeller.edu/) has multiple tools that include the following :

ProFound - a tool for searching a protein sequence database using information from mass spectra of peptide maps. A Bayesian algorithm is used to rank the protein sequences in the database according to their probability of producing the peptide map.

PepFrag - a tool for searching protein or nucleotide sequences using information from fragmentation mass spectra of peptides.

ProteinInfo - a tool for retrieval and analysis of information from protein sequence databases. The capabilities of the analysis tools include peptide mapping, mass spectrometric fragmentation analysis, disulfide mapping, etc.

M/Z - a tool for analysis of mass spectra obtained from protein chemistry experiments. M/Z employs an array of digital signal processing techniques and novel interface designs that make the analysis of protein mass spectra faster and easier.

PAWS - a tool for analysis of protein sequences and post-translational modifications.

ProteinProspector (http://prospector.ucsf.edu/) is an even more extensive server, with the following tools :

Sequence Database Search Programs

MS-Fit (search with peptide-mass fingerprinting data from MS)

MS-Tag (search with fragment-ion tag data from MS/MS)

MS-Seq (search with sequence tag data from MS/MS)

MS-Pattern (search with Edman microsequence/peptide MS data)

MS-Homology (homology based searches)

MS-Bridge (linked peptide search of MS data)

MS-NonSpecific (find peptides with non-specific cleavages)

Peptide/Protein MS Utility Programs

MS-Digest (peptide masses from enzymatic digestion of protein)

MS-Product (fragment ion masses for peptide)

MS-Comp (AA compositions fitting parent or fragment mass and ammonium ions)

MS-Isotope (isotope patterns of peptides and organic molecules)

Mascot (http://www.matrixscience.com/cgi/index.pl?page=/search_form_select.html) is a very popular tool used to analyse the MS data. You can perform the following tasks with Mascot :

Peptide Mass Fingerprint - The experimental data are a list of peptide mass values from an enzymatic digest of a protein.

Sequence Query - One or more peptide mass values associated with information such as partial or ambiguous sequence strings, amino acid composition information, MS/MS fragment ion masses, etc. A super-set of a sequence tag query.

MS/MS Ion Search - Identification based on raw MS/MS data from one or more peptides.

18.4 PREDICTION OF POST-TRANSLATIONAL MODIFICATIONS (PTMs)

As mRNA and protein expression levels do not always correlate, analysis of mRNA does not provide a direct correlation with the protein content in a cell. mRNA production is the first step in synthesis of proteins (Fig. 18.9).

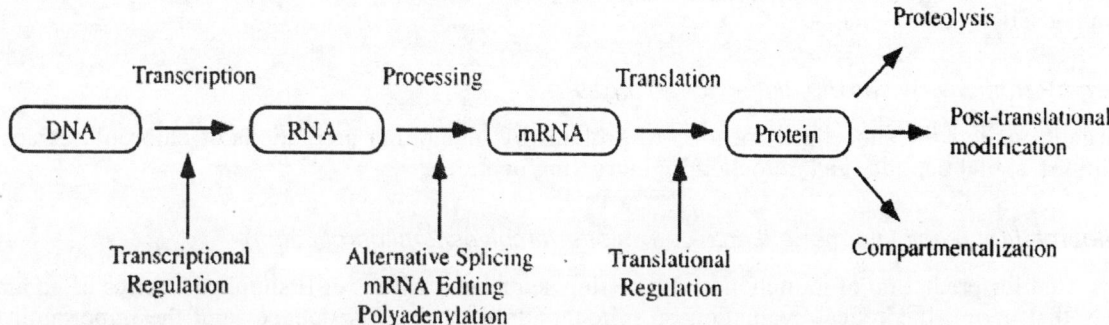

Fig. 18.9 Mechanism by which a single gene can give rise to multiple gene products (proteins).

A *protein* can undergo post-translational modification (like polyadenylation) and hence various proteins can be formed from a single gene. After transcription from DNA to RNA, the gene mRNA can be spliced in different ways prior to translation into protein. Following translation, most proteins are chemically modified through post-translational modification, mainly through the addition of carbohydrate and phosphate groups. Such modifications play a vital role in modulating the function of many proteins but is not directly coded by genes. As a consequence, the information from a single gene can encode as many as 50 different protein species.

PTM events can affect nearly all properties of 3D structure of a protein: size, charge, hydrophobicity. A phosphorylation event, or glycosylation event, or adenylation event, would change the local environment substantially, making likely changes in the 3D structure and/or secondary structure. Even a methylation or acetylation event could have a substantial change in 3D structure of the proteins

As proteomics is the elucidation of the totality of protein-related events in the cell, it also includes PTM protein variants. Such variants can be considered to be new proteins and often have very different function than the original gene product. Some of the bioinformatics tools for prediction of PTMs are discussed here.

PSORT (http://psort.nibb.ac.jp/)

It is used for prediction of protein sorting signals and localization sites. It receives the information of an amino acid sequence and its origin, e.g., Gram-negative bacteria, as inputs. Then, it analyzes the input sequence by applying the stored rules for various sequence features of known protein sorting signals. Finally, it reports the possibility for the input protein to be localized at each candidate site with additional information.

SignalP (http://www.cbs.dtu.dk/services/SignalP/)

SignalP stands for Prediction of signal peptide cleavage sites. It can predict the presence and location of signal peptide cleavage sites in amino acid sequences from different organisms. The method incorporates a prediction of cleavage sites and a signal peptide/non-signal peptide prediction based on a combination of several artificial neural networks.

ChloroP (http://www.cbs.dtu.dk/services/ChloroP/)

ChloroP is used for prediction of chloroplast transit peptides. The ChloroP WWW server predicts the presence of chloroplast transit peptides (cTP) in protein sequences and the location of potential cTP cleavage sites.

TargetP (http://www.cbs.dtu.dk/services/TargetP/)

TargetP predicts the subcellular location of proteins by integrating predictions of chloroplast transit peptides, signal peptides and mitochondrial targeting peptides.

Mitoprot II (http://bioinformer.ebi.ac.uk/newsletter/archives/2/mitoprotii.html)

It is used for prediction of mitochondrial targeting sequences. MitoProt II supplies a series of parameters that permit theoretical evaluation on mitochondrial targeting sequences and the importability. MitoProt II provides the possibility to predict mitochondrial proteins harbouring targeting sequences. Chloroplast proteins also can be studied.

Predotar (http://www.inra.fr/predotar/)

It is a tool for prediction of mitochondrial and plastid targeting sequences.

NetOGlyc (http://www.cbs.dtu.dk/services/NetOGlyc/)

This tool is used for prediction of type O-glycosylation sites in mammalian proteins The NetOglyc WWW server produces neural network predictions of mucin type GalNAc O-glycosylation sites in mammalian proteins.

NetPhos (http://www.cbs.dtu.dk/services/NetPhos/)

NetPhos is used for prediction of Ser, Thr and Tyr phosphorylation sites in eukaryotic protein produces neural network predictions for serine, threonine and tyrosine phosphorylation sites in eukaryotic proteins.

FindMod (http://us.expasy.org/tools/findmod/)

FindMod is a program for *de novo* discovery of protein post-translational modifications. It examines peptide mass fingerprinting results of known proteins for the presence of 22 types of PTMs of discrete mass: acetylation, amidation, biotin, C-mannosylation, deamidation, N-acyl diglyceride cysteine (tripalmitate), FAD, farnesylation, formylation, geranyl-geranyl, gamma-carboxyglutamic acid, O-

GlcNAc, hydroxylation, lipoyl, methylation, myristoylation, palmitoylation, phosphorylation, pyridoxal phosphate, pyrrolidone carboxylic acid, sulfatation. This is done by looking at mass differences between experimentally determined peptide masses and theoretical peptide masses calculated from a specified protein sequence.

GlycoMod (http://us.expasy.org/tools/glycomod/)

GlycoMod is a tool that can predict the possible oligosaccharide structures that occur on proteins from their experimentally determined masses. The program can be used with free or derivatised glycans and for glycopeptides where the peptide mass or protein is known. Compositional constraints can be applied to the output.

Delta Mass (http://www.abrf.org/index.cfm/dm.home)

Delta Mass is a listing of mass differences caused by modifications to amino acids or amino acid substitutions.

Scansite (http://scansite.mit.edu/)

Scansite is a tool to search a protein and predict phosphorylation sites. Scansite searches for motifs within proteins that are likely to be phosphorylated by specific protein kinases or bind to domains such as SH2 domains, 14-3-3 domains or PDZ domains.

18.5 PROTEIN-PROTEIN INTERACTIONS

Establishing protein interaction networks is crucial for understanding cellular operations. Detailed knowledge of the *interactome* (*interactome* is the whole set of molecular interaction in cells) in model cellular systems can provide new insights into the structure and properties of these systems.

Protein–protein interactions lie at the heart of most cellular processes, including carbohydrate and lipid metabolism, cell-cycle regulation, protein and nucleic acid metabolism, signal transduction, and cellular architecture. A complete understanding of cellular function depends on a full characterization of the complex network of cellular protein–protein associations.

Here we shall delve into some methods to study protein-protein interactions.

Y2H system for protein-protein interaction

The yeast protein interactome analysis was achieved first by using yeast two-hybrid (Y2H) system in a proteome-wide scale, and subsequently by large-scale mass spectrometric analysis of affinity-purified protein complexes. Most of the yeast two-hybrid systems utilize the reconstitution of an active transcription factor to assay for protein-protein interactions.

The Y2H system uses the transcription process to make predictions about protein interaction. This method is based on the ability of an interacting protein pair to bring together the DNA binding domain and activation domain of a transcription factor *in vivo* to produce a functional activator of transcription. The interaction can be detected by expression of the linked reporter genes.

The system requires that two yeast hybrids be prepared – called "bait-prey" system. The "bait" protein is fused to a transcripton factor DNA binding domain. The other "prey" protein is fused to a transcription factor activation domain. When expressed in a yeast cell containing the appropriate reporter gene, interaction of the "bait" with the "prey" brings the DNA binding domain and the activation domain into close proximity, creating a functional transcription factor. This triggers transcription of the intended reporter gene (e.g., ß-galactosidase). The "bait-prey" nomenclature has applied to *in vitro* methods used to study protein interactions. *In vitro* methods for protein interaction analysis are often employed to confirm interactions indicated by the Y2H method.

The natural affinity of binding partners for each other is the principle for *in vitro* methods and is used for both interaction discovery and confirmation. *In vitro* methods span a broad range of techniques. Some of the popular methods are summarised in Table 18.2.

Table 18.2. *In vitro* methods for protein interaction analysis

In vitro Methods	*Description*
Co-Immunoprecipitation (Co-IP)	This method uses total cell extracts to analyze putative protein-protein interactions in eukaryotic cells. One can also use nuclear extracts as a source. An immunoprecipitation (IP) experiment is designed to purify a bait protein antigen together with its binding partner using a specific antibody against the bait.
Cross-linking reagents	Bifunctional chemical cross-linking reagents and the intramolecular and intermolecular cross-linking of proteins and protein complexes have been used in the structural and functional characterization of proteins. The cross-linking reagents are a proxy of molecular rulers that provide information on distances between the cross-linked amino acid residues that are pertinent to both the tertiary and quaternary arrangements of proteins. Such distance determinations are useful in membrane proteins and other proteins that cannot be crystallized and frequently lead to important advances in mapping the protein topography.
Far-Western analysis	Similar to Western blotting method with a difference. The antibody probe used in standard Western blot detection is substituted with an appropriately labeled bait protein as the probe. Detection can be radio-isotopic, chemiluminescent or colorimetric, depending on the probe label.
Label transfer	This method involves a specialized cross-linking agent with several important features. These include heterobifunctionality for step-wise cross-linking, a detectable label and reversibility of the cross-link between binding partners. Upon reduction of the cross-linked complex a binding partner (prey) acquires the label from a bait protein that was first modified with the reagent. The label is typically used in the detection process to isolate or identify the unknown prey protein.
Protein arrays/ Protein chips	Antibody-based or bait-based arrays that allow for screening and detection of specific interactions of proteins from complex mixtures. Primary applications include high-throughput assays of protein expression profiling, protein-protein interaction and enzyme activity.
Protein Interaction mapping	Utilizes an "artificial protease" on a bait protein to initiate contact-dependent cleavages in the prey protein in the presence of specific reactants. The nonspecific cleavage fragments produced by the artificial protease can be analyzed to map the contact sites or interface of a known protein-protein interaction.
Pull-down assays	This is an affinity chromatography method that involves using a tagged bait to create a specific affinity matrix that will enable binding and purification of a prey protein from a lysate sample or other protein-containing mixture.

Surface Plasmon Resonance (SPR)	SPR occurs when light is reflected under certain conditions from a conducting film at the interface between two media of different refractive index. SPR can relate binding information to small changes in refractive indices of laser light reflected from gold surfaces to which a bait protein has been attached. Changes are proportional to the extent of binding. Special labels and sample purification are not necessary, and analysis occurs in real time.
NMR (Nuclear Magnetic Resonance)	Method that can provide insights into the dynamic interaction of proteins in solution.
Mass Spectroscopy	Used in concert with affinity-based methods, such as co-IPs, to isolate binding partners and complexes and identify the component proteins using standard mass spectral methods, e.g., MALDI-TOF and searching bioinformatics databases.
X-ray Crystallography	Crystallization of the interacting complex allows definition of the interaction structure.

Non-homology methods

Domain fusion (Rosetta Stone)

Domain fusion analysis is a useful method to predict functionally related proteins that may be involved in direct protein-protein interactions or in the same metabolic or signaling pathway. Domain fusion analysis exploits the fact that certain proteins in a given genome consist of fused domains that correspond to single, full-length proteins in other genomes. The proteins with fused domains in a given genome are likely to directly interact or be involved in the same metabolic and signaling pathways.

A comparison of sequence homologs from multiple organisms can reveal these fused sequences, called *Rosetta Stone sequences* because they decipher the interactions between the protein pairs. For example, consider the Fig. 18.10.

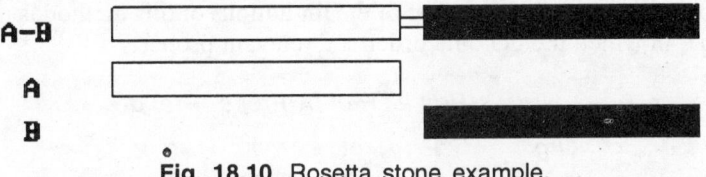

Fig. 18.10. Rosetta stone example.

Here, A-B is the Rosetta Stone protein that suggests that proteins A and B are functionally related and have a better-than-random chance of interacting.

Examples of predicted functional linkages are shown in Fig. 18.11. The sequences and domains are identified by their SWISS-PROT+TrEMBL and Pfam id, respectively, and the gene name is enclosed in brackets if applicable. The first three examples are known functional linkages in *S. cerevisiae* and *H. sapiens*, while the last one is unknown.

Conservation of gene position (Fig.18.12)

Genes of related function are often adjacent in the genome - especially in prokaryotic operons. This neighbourhood relationship becomes even more relevant when it is conserved in different species. The adjacent positions of genes in various bacterial genomes have been used to predict functional relation-

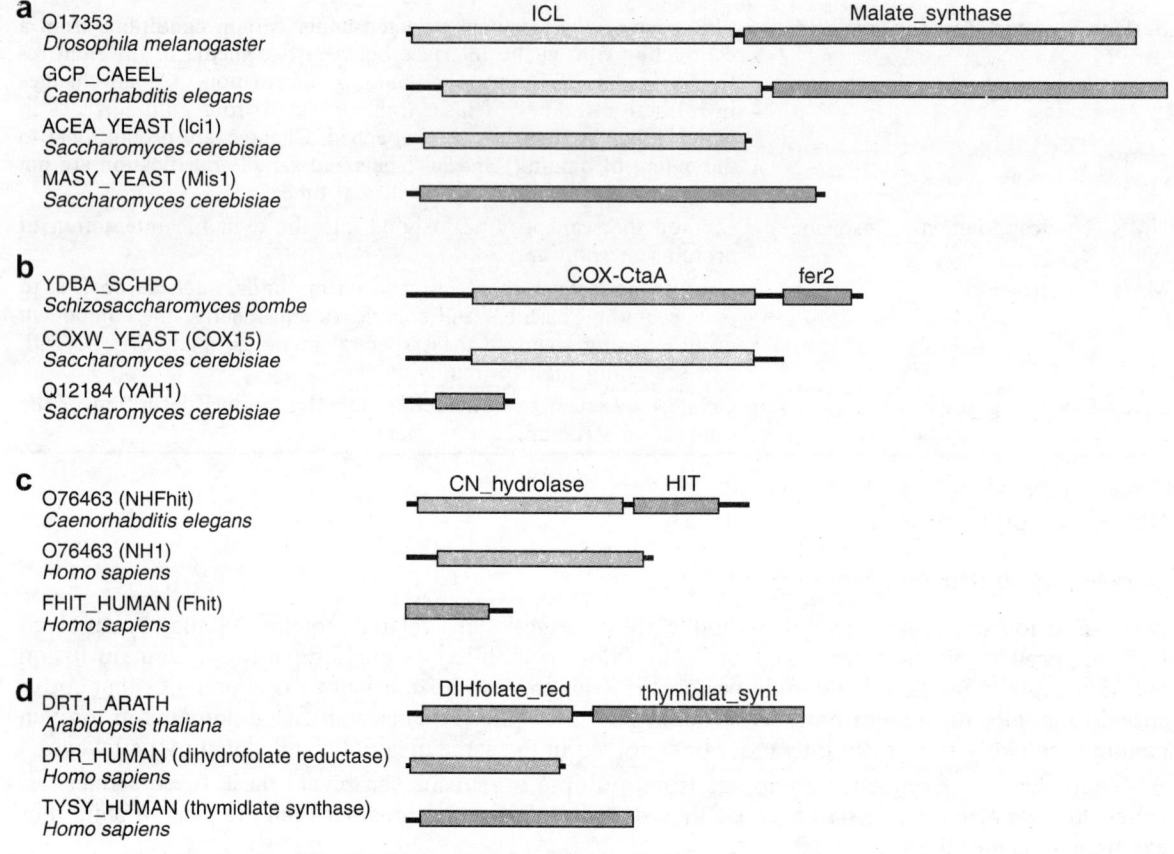

Fig. 18.11. Examples of predicted functional linkages.

ships between the corresponding proteins. One of the limitations of this method is that it is only directly applicable to bacteria, in which the genome order is a relevant property.

	Prot a	Prot b	Prot c	Prot d
Org 1	1	1	1	1
Org 2	0	1	0	1
Org 3	1	0	1	0
Org 4	1	0	1	1

Prot a ◄─► Prot c

Fig. 18.12 Conservation of gene position

Phylogenetic profiles (Fig. 18.13)

This method is based on the pattern of the presence or absence of a given gene in a set of genomes, so as to determine in which organisms the gene is present and in which it is not. Many genes are not universally conserved and are found in some genomes and absent in others, because of gene loss and horizontal transfer. Genes will tend to only occur in an organism that is using them productively, so for a set of genes that function in a particular pathway, there will be an all or none effect: either all the genes are functioning in a given organism, or none of them at all.

Similarity of phylogenetic profiles might then be interpreted as indicative of the functional need for corresponding proteins to be simultaneously present in order to perform a given function together. However, although this similarity may suggest a related functional role, a direct physical interaction between the proteins is not necessarily implied. The limitation of this approach is that it can only be applied to complete genomes (as only then is it possible to rule out the absence of a given gene). Similarly, it cannot be used with the essential proteins that are common to most organisms.

	Prot a	Prot b	Prot c	Prot d
Org 1	1	1	1	1
Org 2	0	1	0	1
Org 3	1	0	1	0
Org 4	1	0	1	1

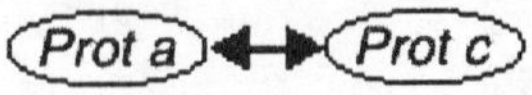

$$\boxed{Prot\ a} \longleftrightarrow \boxed{Prot\ c}$$

Fig. 18.13. Phylogenetic profiles.

All-against-all self-comparison methods

In this method, each protein in the proteome is compared against all other proteins in the same proteome. This method can identify unique proteins that have arisen from gene duplication, and can also reveal the number of protein families. The domain content of these proteins may also be analyzed.

Following sequence of steps is used :

1. Make a database of the proteome.
2. Use each protein as a query in a similarity search against the database (using BLAST, WU-BLAST or FASTA).
3. Generate a matrix of alignment scores (P or E value).

In this analysis, each protein is used as a query in a similarity search against the remaining proteome. (Fig. 18.14).

Cluster analysis

Cluster analysis sorts out the relationships among all the proteins. Clustering organises the proteins into groups by some objective criterion. One such criterion can be the statistical significance of their alignment score (P or E value). Another criterion can be the distance between each pair of sequences in a MSA. The distance is the number of amino acid changes between the aligned sequences.

Clustering by single linkage

This method is based on the distance criterion for sequence relationships. First, a group of related sequences found in the all-against-all proteome comparison is subjected to a MSA (ClustalW). A distance matrix that shows the number of amino acid changes between each pair of sequences is then made. This matrix is then used to cluster the sequences by a neighbour-joining algorithm. This forms a phylogenetic tree called a minimum spanning tree that minimizes the number of amino acid changes that would generate the group of sequences (Fig. 18.15). GeneRage (http://www.ebi.ac.uk/research/

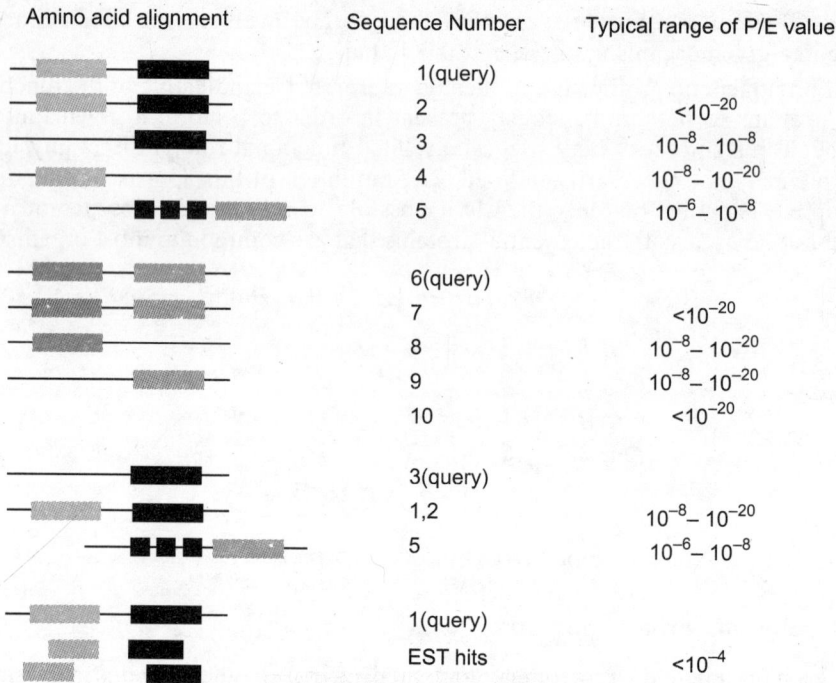

Fig. 18.14. All-against-self comparison.

cgg/services/rage/) program provides a system for classifying protein data sets by means of an iterative refinement approach using local alignments, matrix methods and single-linkage clustering.

Core Proteome

The all-against-all analysis provides an indication as to the number of protein/gene families in an organism. This number represents the core proteome of the organism from which all biological functions have diversified. For example, in *H. influenzae*, the total number of genes is 1709 and the number of gene families is 1425 (Table 18.3).

Table 18.3 Core proteome for some organisms

Between-proteome comparison methods

Organism	No. of genes	No. of gene families	No. of duplicated genes
H. influenzae (bacteria)	1709	1425	284
S. cerevisiae (yeast)	6241	4383	1858
C. elegans (worm)	18,424	9453	8971
D. melanogaster (fly)	13,600	8065	5536

This analysis is used to identify orthologs, gene families and domains. In this analysis, each protein in the proteome is used as a query in a database similarity search against another proteome or combined set of proteomes (Fig. 18.16).

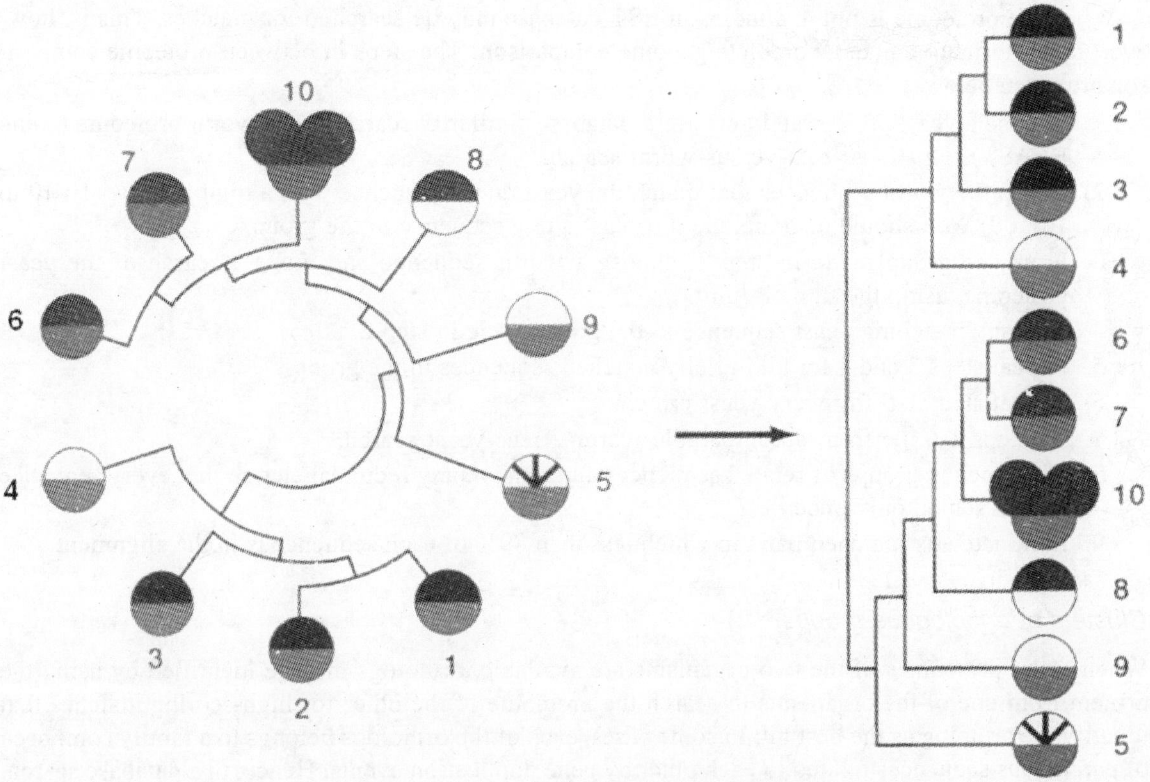

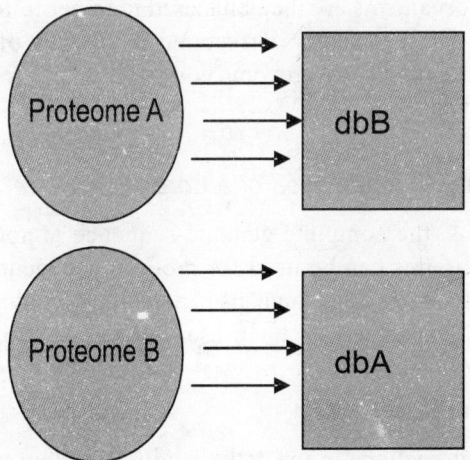

Fig. 18.15. Clustering by single linkage.

Fig. 18.16. Between proteome comparison.

When the proteome is not available, an EST database may be searched for matches. This is, however, less informative than a complete genome comparison. The steps in between-proteome comparison are given below :

1. Choose a yeast protein and perform a database similarity search of the worm proteome (using BLAST). This is a yeast-versus-worm search.
2. Group the worm sequences that match the yeast query sequence with a high P value (10-10 to 10-100). You should also include the yeast query sequence in the group.
3. From the group made in step 2, choose a worm sequence and make a search of the yeast proteome, using the same P limit.
4. Add any matching yeast sequence to the group made in step 2.
5. Repeat steps 3 and 4 for all initially matched sequences in the group.
6. Repeat steps 1-5 for every yeast protein.
7. As steps 1-6, perform a comparable worm-versus-yeast search.
8. Coalesce the groups of related sequences and remove any redundancies so that every sequence is represented only once.
9. Eliminate any matched pairs in which less than 80% of each sequence is in the alignment.

Clusters of orthologous groups

When entire proteomes of the two organisms are available, orthologs may be identified by using the protein from one of the organisms to search the proteome of the other for high-scoring matches that identify the ortholog as the best hit. In some cases, each of the orthologs belongs to a family composed of paralogous sequences related to each other by gene duplication events. Hence, in a database search, the ortholog would not only match the orthologous sequence in the second proteome but also these other paralogous sequences.

COG (Cluster of orthologous groups) is used to identify all matching proteins in the organisms, defined as an orthologous group related by both speciation and gene duplication events. Related orthologus groups in different organisms are then clustered together to form a COG that would include both orthologs and paralogs. These clusters correspond to classes of metabolic function. A COG analysis provides an initial assessment of the genome composition of prokaryotic organisms and should be followed by a more detailed analysis.

Comparison of proteomes to EST databases of an organism

For many eukaryotic organisms, the complete genome sequence is not available. In such cases EST databases can be used. EST libraries can be used for preliminary identification of genes by database similarity searches and then a more detailed analysis can be done by cloning and sequencing the intact cDNA. An EST database can be analysed for the presence of gene families, orthologs and paralogs.

Bioinformatics tools for Interactomics

Interactomics is the study of interactions in the cell – study of protein-protein interactions is also part of interactomics.

PSIbase (http://psibase.kaist.ac.kr/) is a molecular interaction database. It focuses on structural interaction of proteins and their domains. It is based on PSIMAP that is a map of protein interactome. It covers the interaction of all known 3D protein structures, based on PDB and SCOP databases.

DIP (http://dip.doe-mbi.ucla.edu/) database catalogs experimentally determined interactions between proteins. It combines information from a variety of sources to create a single, consistent set of protein-protein interactions. The data stored within the DIP database are curated.

InterPreTS (Interaction Prediction through Tertiary Structure) (http://www.russell.embl.de/inter-prets/) is a web-based tool for predicting protein-protein interactions. Given a pair of query sequences, it first searches for homologues in a database of interacting domains (DBID) of known three-dimensional complex structures.

InterDom (http://interdom.lit.org.sg/) is a database of putative interacting protein domains derived from multiple sources, ranging from domain fusions (Rosetta Stone), protein interactions (DIP and BIND), protein complexes (PDB), to scientific literature (MEDLINE).

Analyzing Metabolic Pathways

19.1 INTRODUCTION

Cellular metabolism is often described in terms of the biochemical reactions that make up the metabolic network. Study of genomics has provided us a lot of information regarding the genes and proteins participating in cellular metabolism for a number of organisms. As the fundamental functional units of metabolic systems are its pathways, we can define and analyse complete metabolic pathways. Biochemical pathways such as genetic, metabolic, regulatory or signal transduction pathways can be viewed as interconnected processes forming an intricate network of functional and physical interactions between different molecular species in the cell (Fig. 19.1).

The amount of information available on such pathways for different organisms is increasing very rapidly. Analyzing these networks is complex owing to the nature of the databases, which are often heterogeneous, incomplete or inconsistent. Pathway analysis is hence a challenging problem in bioinformatics.

19.2 GENE TRANSCRIPTION NETWORKS

Since the development of the microarray technology in 1995, there has been an enormous increase in gene expression data from several organisms. Based on the view of gene systems as a logical network of nodes that influence each other's expression levels, scientists dream of reconstruct the precise gene interaction network from the expression data obtained with this large scale arraying technique.

The transcription factors are themselves are part of a network, the *transcription network* or *gene regulatory network*, in which transcription factors regulate the expression of other transcription factors in addition to structural genes, and determine the transcriptional *state* of the cell. A gene regulatory network (GRN) is a collection of DNA segments in a cell which interact with each other and with other substances in the cell, thereby governing the rates at which genes are transcribed into mRNA. Genes can be viewed as nodes in

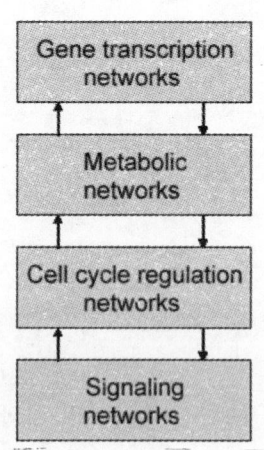

Fig. 19.1. Cellular pathways.

such a network, with input being proteins such as transcription factors, and outputs being the level of gene expression. The node itself can also be viewed as a function which can be obtained by combining basic functions upon the inputs.

The basic drivers within cells are levels of proteins, which determine *spatial* (tissue related) and *temporal* (developmental stage) parts of the cell. Mathematical models of GRNs have been developed to allow predictions of the models to be tested. Various modeling techniques have been used, including boolean networks, Petri nets, Bayesian networks, and sets of differential equations.

One gene can affect the expression of another gene by binding of the gene product of one gene to the promoter region of another gene. If we have a large number of measurements of the expression level of a number of genes, we can model the regulatory network that controls their expression level. The problem can be resolved in two different ways: using time-series data and using steady-state data of gene knockout.,

GRNs act as analog biochemical computers to specify the identity and level of expression of groups of target genes. When active transcription factors associate with the promontory region of target genes, they can function to specifically repress (down-regulate) or induce (up-regulate) synthesis of the corresponding RNA. The immediate molecular output of a gene regulatory network is the constellation of RNAs and proteins encoded by network target genes. The resulting cellular outputs are changes in the structure, metabolic capacity, or behavior of the cell mediated by new expression of up-regulated proteins and elimination of down-regulated proteins.

GRNs function as the on-off switches of a cell operating at the gene level. A simple GRN would consist of one or more input signaling pathways, regulatory proteins that integrate the input signals, several target genes, and the RNA and proteins produced from those target genes. The networks may also include dynamic feedback loops that provide for further regulation of network architecture and output.

GeneNet (http://wwwmgs.bionet.nsc.ru/mgs/gnw/genenet/) is a system designed for formalized description and automated visualization of gene networks.

A collection of artificial gene networks can be found at http://mendes.vbi.vt.edu/AGN/.

19.3 METABOLIC PATHWAYS

The rapid development in genome sequencing has provided a large amount of genome data. The analysis of this information for understanding the organization principle of genetic and metabolic networks is one of the important research areas in the post-genome era.

From gene annotation information, the genes are classified into different functional groups. A great number of gene products are enzymes that catalyze cellular reactions forming a complex metabolic network. The study of metabolic networks has gained increasing attention in recent years. Several methods and metabolic databases are available to reconstruct an organism's specific metabolic network from genome information, such as KEGG (http://www.genome.ad.jp/kegg), and EcoCyc (biocyc.org/ecocyc/). These databases can be used for further analysis of the global metabolic network.

Methods of analysis of metabolic networks

There are several methods developed for conducting analysis of metabolic networks.

Flux Balance analysis

Flux balance analysis has been used for predicting the flux distribution in a whole metabolic network under certain physiological conditions. However, this method gives little information about the overall network structure.

Elementary Flux Mode Analysis

Elementary Flux mode analysis (EFM) is a method to analyze small networks. Elementary flux modes can be computed to fragment or breakup the biochemical network into minimal parts which fulfill the steady state condition and represent essential structural features of the biochemical network. No kinematic parameters of enzymes are involved in EFM and the focus is on structural rather than kinetic properties of biochemical reactions

Extreme Pathway analysis

Extreme pathway analysis is another method to analyse small networks. In network-based pathway analysis, a biological network of interacting components is represented by a stoichiometric matrix which relates reactions and metabolites. An algorithm that computes a set of routes satisfying specified conditions can be used to analyze this matrix.

For a route to be a valid elementary mode, three conditions are required:

1. *A pseudo steady-state condition* i.e. none of the metabolites must be consumed or accumulated.
2. *A feasibility condition* i.e. no negative flux is allowed for irreversible reactions.
3. *A non-decomposability condition* i.e. no subset of the route can hold the network in a steady-state with non-zero fluxes.

Extreme pathways require an additional condition :

4. *Systemic independence condition,* i.e. no extreme pathway can be represented by a non-negative linear combination of other extreme pathways.

For this reason the set of extreme pathways is minimal and always a subset of the set of elementary modes. In a mathematical multidimensional representation where each axis corresponds to a reaction flux, all possible steady-state flux distributions lie within a *multidimensional flux cone*, and extreme pathways form the edges of this cone. The additional elementary modes may lie on the surface or the interior of the cone. These structure-oriented approaches have lead to a significant number of applications, and they can help predicting key aspects of functionality, robustness and gene regulation. For example, the number of elementary modes can serve as a measure of network robustness and fragility towards disturbances such as mutations or drug inhibition, and allow the prediction of gene expression patterns.

Decomposition Methods

Metabolic networks are organized in a modular, hierarchical manner. Methods for a rational decomposition of the metabolic network into relatively independent functional subsets are essential to better understand the modularity and organization principle of a large-scale, genome-wide network. For large-scale networks reconstructed from genome information, *decomposition methods* should be first used to divide the whole network into small subsystems. The pathway structure of these subsystems may then be properly analyzed by the methods for small networks.

Graph Theory

Another set of methods is based on *graph theory*. In these methods the metabolites correspond to nodes in the graph, and reactions correspond to connections between these nodes. Using such a graphic representation, the structure of metabolic networks using methods adopted from studies of the world wide web. It has been found that metabolic networks exhibit characteristics of *small world networks*. This implies that most of the nodes have a low connection degree, while few nodes have a very high connection degree. The connection degree distribution follows a *power law*. The high degree nodes dominate the network structure and are called *hubs* of the network. A relatively short path connects most of the nodes. For metabolic network this has been calculated as the average path length (AĽ). AL is defined as the shortest path length averaged for every pair of metabolites in the whole network. It has been found that AL is almost the same (about 3.2) for 43 organisms that have been studied. This means that most of the metabolites can be converted to each other in about only 3 steps.

In this study, ATP, ADP and other metabolites are regarded as nodes in the network. This results in an unrealistic definition of the path length in many cases as illustrated with a part of the glycolytic pathway in Fig 19.2 (a) and (b). It is obvious that the path length (number of reaction steps in the pathway) from glucose to pyruvate should be nine in terms of biochemistry. Hence, this calculation of path length is obviously biochemically not meaningful.

Another characteristic of metabolic pathways is the irreversibility of many reactions. Information about reaction reversibility is important in network analysis. However, until now there is no metabolic reaction database available that gives clear and enough information about it.

Bioinformatics tools to study metabolic pathways

KEGG (Kyoto Encyclopedia of Genes and Genomes) (www.genome.jp/kegg/)

The objectives of KEGG are as follows:

1. Organizing knowledge of molecular and genetic pathways from experimental observations.
2. Maintenance of the catalogue of all organisms that has been sequenced and mapping each gene product onto a component in the pathway.
3. Development of techniques for comparing and computing pathways.

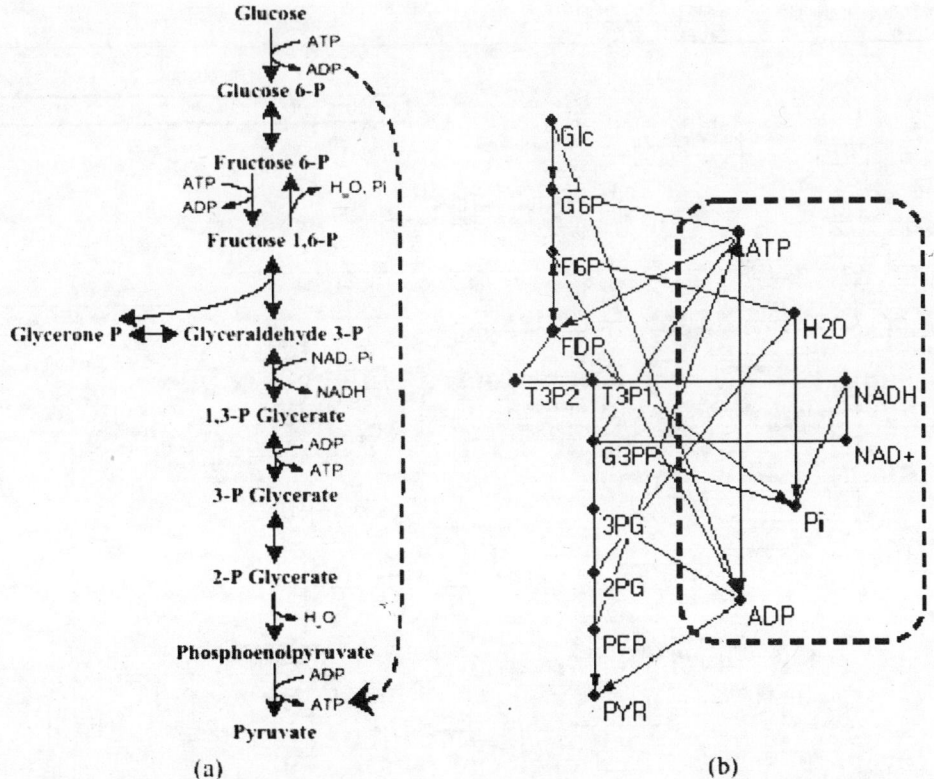

(a)   (b)

Fig. 19.2. (a) Biochemical pathway of glycolysis (b) Graph view of glycolysis.

The KEGG pathway database consists of three databases:
1. Pathway database
2. Gene database
3. Ligand database

An enzyme is denoted by a rectangle in KEGG. For each pathway diagram there is one reference diagram that is manually drawn and updated, and matching the enzyme objects and the corresponding genes in the gene catalogue computationally derives all organism-specific diagrams. In this way KEGG is able to immediately reconstruct organism-specific pathways for an increasing number of complete genomes. The enzyme object is hyperlinked to the ENZYME section of the LIGAND database containing, among others, the enzyme nomenclature, the reaction scheme, the chemical compounds involved, and additional links to molecular and biological information.

For example, Fig. 19.3 shows the Pentose and Glucoronate interconversions pathway. The enzyme 3.1.1.11 is represented in a rectangle in the Fig. The enzyme object is hyperlinked to the information shown in Fig. 19.4.

Matching the reference pathway diagram and the gene catalogue according to the EC number automatically generates an organism-specific pathway. When the gene for an enzyme exists in the gene

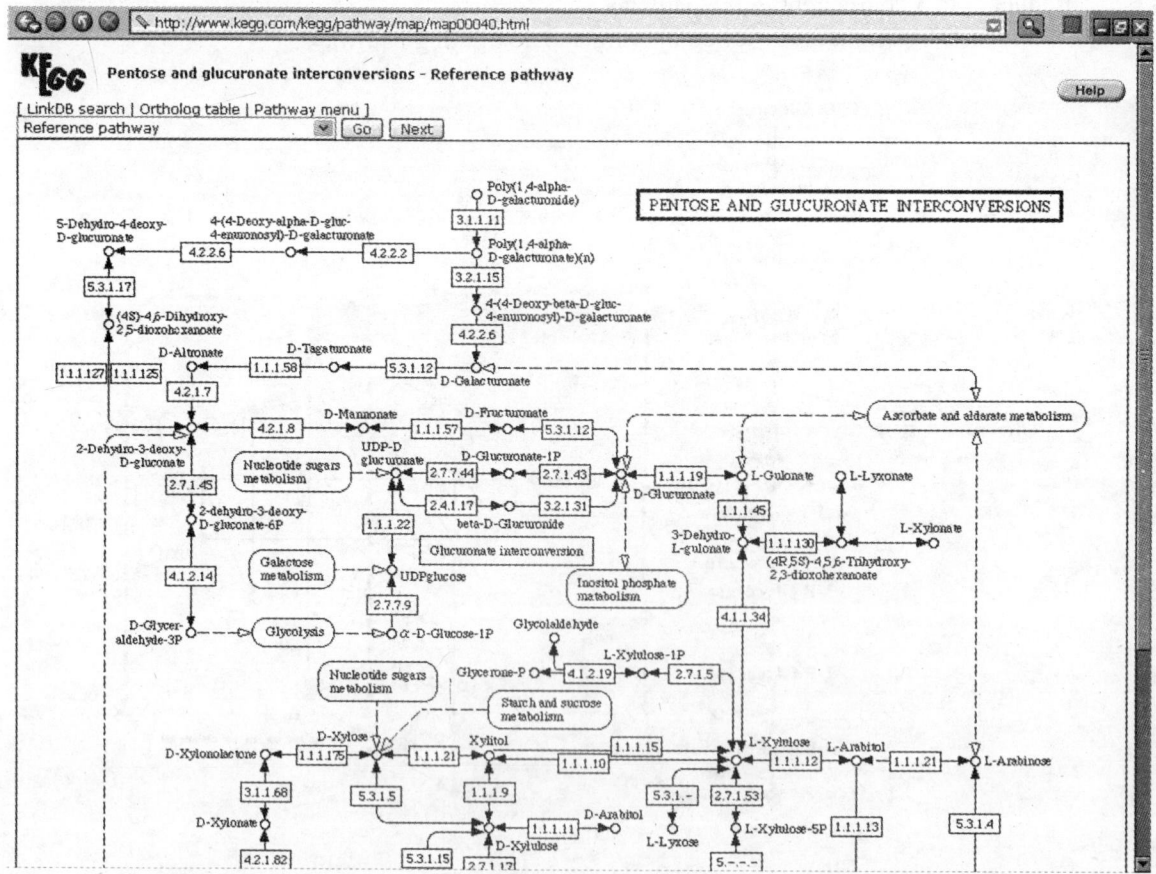

Fig. 19.3. Pentose and Glucoronate interconversions pathway from KEGG.

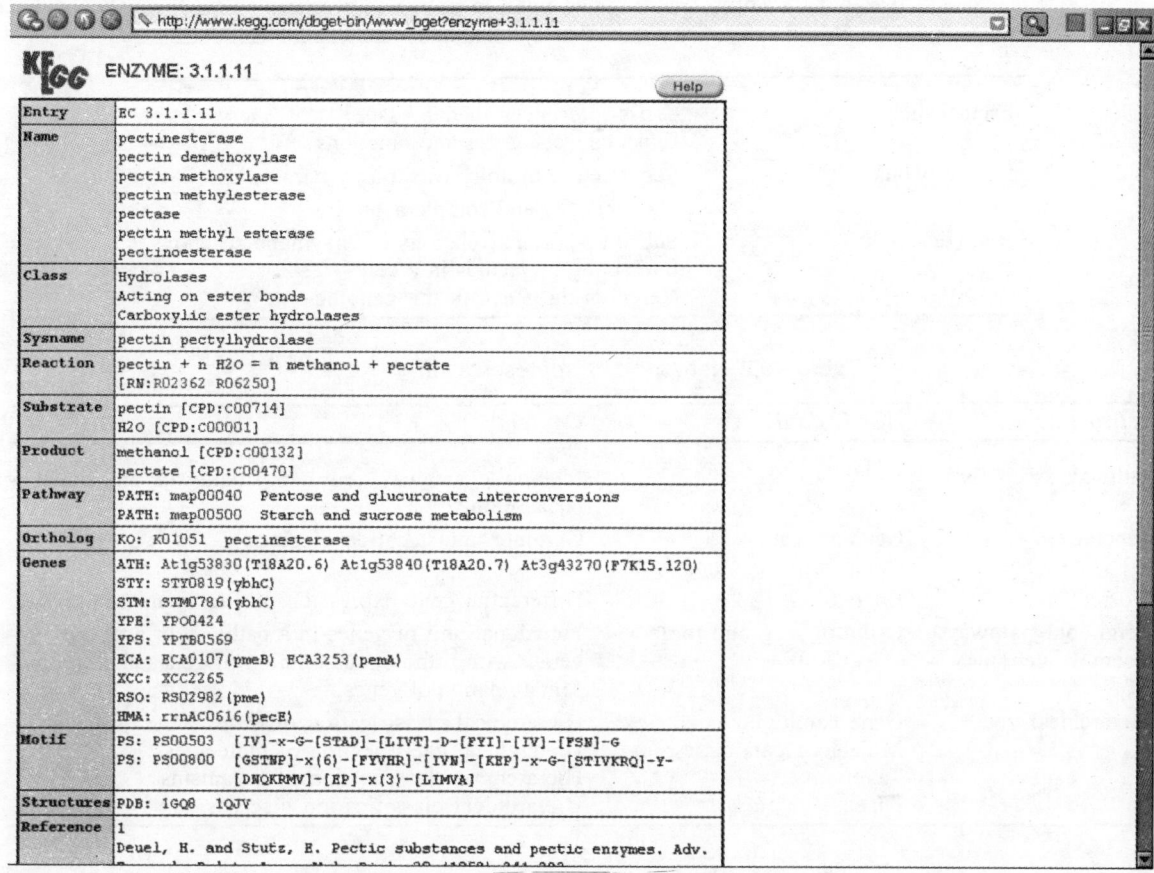

Fig. 19.4. Information linked to enzyme 3.1.1.11.

catalogue, the box representing the corresponding enzyme is marked by colour on the pathway. The consecutive appearance of the coloured boxes would then be considered an organism-specific pathway. For this procedure to be successful, the reference diagram should contain all known alternatives of reaction paths and not just the consensus alone. Different organisms have different sets of metabolic pathways that reflect the living environment and the strategy of adaptation.

In general, an enzymatic reaction involves multiple substrates and multiple products. In KEGG a reaction is represented by a collection of binary relations between all possible substrate-product pairs. Various kinds of reasoning steps during *in silico* analysis taken by biologists often involve sophisticated navigation across many links among biological entities. The nature of these links would be classified into three categories shown in the Table 19.1: factual, similarity, and biological links. Automation of the reasoning steps by path computation of these links is one of the major objectives of the KEGG project.

Network data representation in KEGG is given in Table 19.2.

Enzymes and Metabolic Pathways (The EMP Project at http://www.empproject.com/ /) database is another comprehensive source of biochemical data. The format allows different types of tables and stoichiometric matrices to encode metabolic pathways, reaction mechanisms, rate laws and a very wide spectrum of numeric data. Search for the enzyme 3.1.1.11 gives the information shown in Fig. 19.5.

Table 19.1 Three type of links used in path computation.

Type	Example
Factual link	Cross-references in databases Links between genes and functions
Similarity link	Sequence homology (orthology/paralogy) 3D similarity and complementarity
Biological link	Substrate-product relations in enzymatic reactions Interacting molecules in a cell Neighboring genes in the genome

Table 19.2 Network data representation in KEGG

Network type	KEGG data	Content
Pathway assembly	Pathway map	Metabolic pathway, regulatory pathway, and molecular assembly
Genome	Genome map Comparative genome map	Chromosomal location of genes
Cluster	Expression map	Differential gene expression profile by microarrays
Neighbour pathway assembly genome	Orthologue group table	Functional unit of genes in a pathway or assembly, together with orthologous relation of genes and chromosomal relation of genes
Hierarchical tree	Gene catalogue Molecular catalogue Taxonomy Disease catalogue	Hierarchical classification of genes Hierarchical classification of molecules Hierarchical classification of organisms Hierarchical classification diseases

BioCyc (http://biocyc.org/intro.shtml) is a collection of databases that provides electronic reference sources on the pathways and genomes of different organisms. As on end-December 2004, detailed organism-specific databases are available for 14 species. In addition, the MetaCyc metabolic pathway database contains literature-derived metabolic pathway data for 160 species.

PathDB (http://www.ncgr.org/pathdb/) is a data repository and a system for building and visualizing cellular networks targeted for the gene expression, proteomics, and metabolic profiling communities.

19.4 SIGNALING NETWORKS

Signaling networks are another kind of pathways that are of central importance in understanding cellular metabolism. Metabolic and signaling networks are viewed as different entities. In metabolic networks the flow of mass and energy is the essential purpose of the machinery. In signaling networks the purpose is the regulation of other processes, and the use of energy and mass flow is a requirement.

Living cells can be viewed as signal processors. The cells receive signals from the environment in the form of specific molecules (e.g. hormones, transmitter substances), nutrient levels (e.g. glucose, lipids) or stress (e.g. osmotic pressure, poisons, heat, cold). The cells also produce signals internally, e.g. in the cell cycle, where such events as DNA damage or failures in chromosome duplication generate signals that stop cell division from occurring, and may also start repair processes or to begin apoptosis.

An essential mechanism in regulation is feedback. The result of a process feeds back signals to

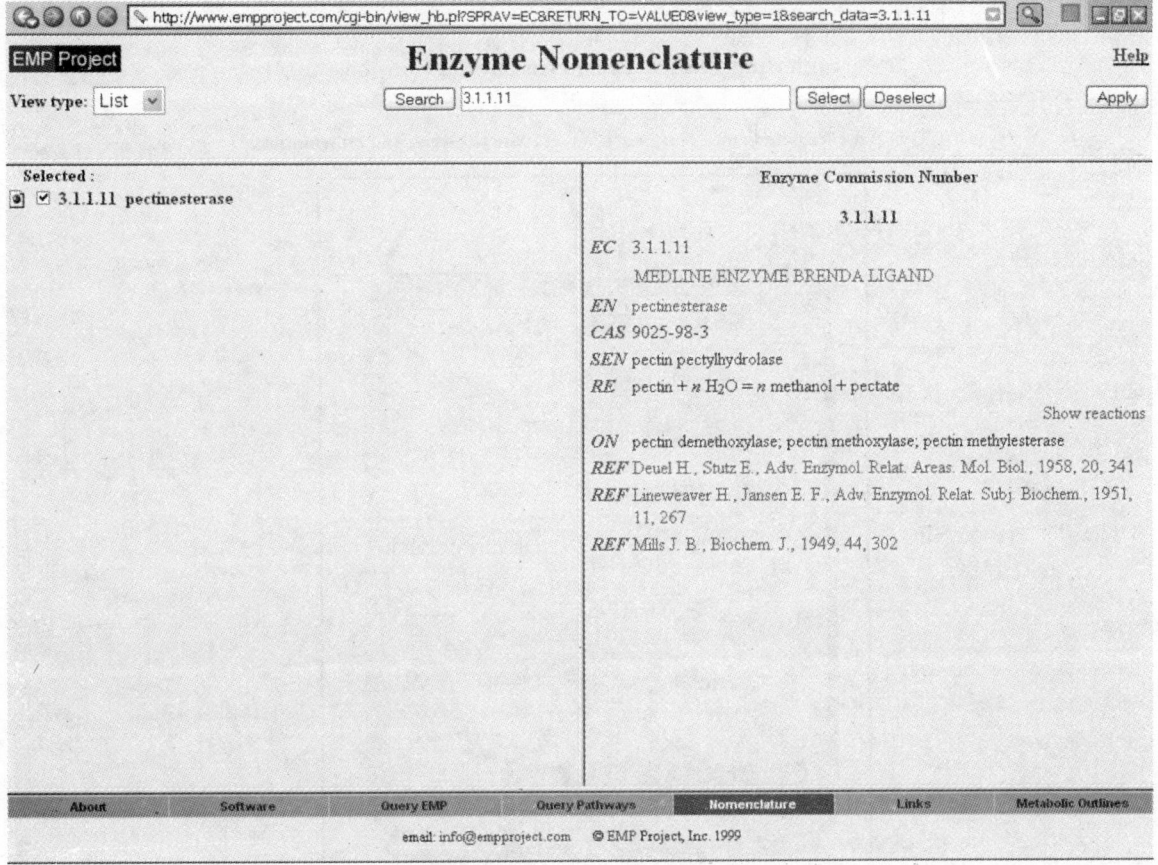

Fig. 19.5. Information on 3.1.1.11.

control the process itself. This makes the process self-monitoring to some degree. Feed-back can be positive or negative. Negative feed-back is a system where the product or resulting signal down-regulates the process. This may be useful to keep the level of a substance at a steady state. This is very common in the metabolism, since the organism only wants to produce as much as is needed of some particular compound, and no more. For example, many pathways for compounds such as amino acids are regulated by negative feedback, where the final product of the pathway influences some early step in the pathway negatively by inhibiting an enzyme. This is called retro-inhibition.

Positive feedback is a signaling loop where the product reinforces the process. This is found in systems that have to maintain one chosen state among several alternatives, e.g. the specific state of a differentiated cell, or to commit a cell towards a chosen development path. The starting point is an undecided state, which by some process (influence from the outside, or purely stochastic events) starts to tilt over in one particular direction. This small, initial bias is then reinforced by the regulatory system, so that a final, fixed, stable state is reached.

A special class of regulatory networks generates cyclic processes. These are processes that never reach a steady state, but move between stages or states in an ordered fashion. There are many important examples of cyclic processes. Examples are the cell cycle and the circadian clock (the changes following the time of day) in many plants and animals. These systems require complex networks.

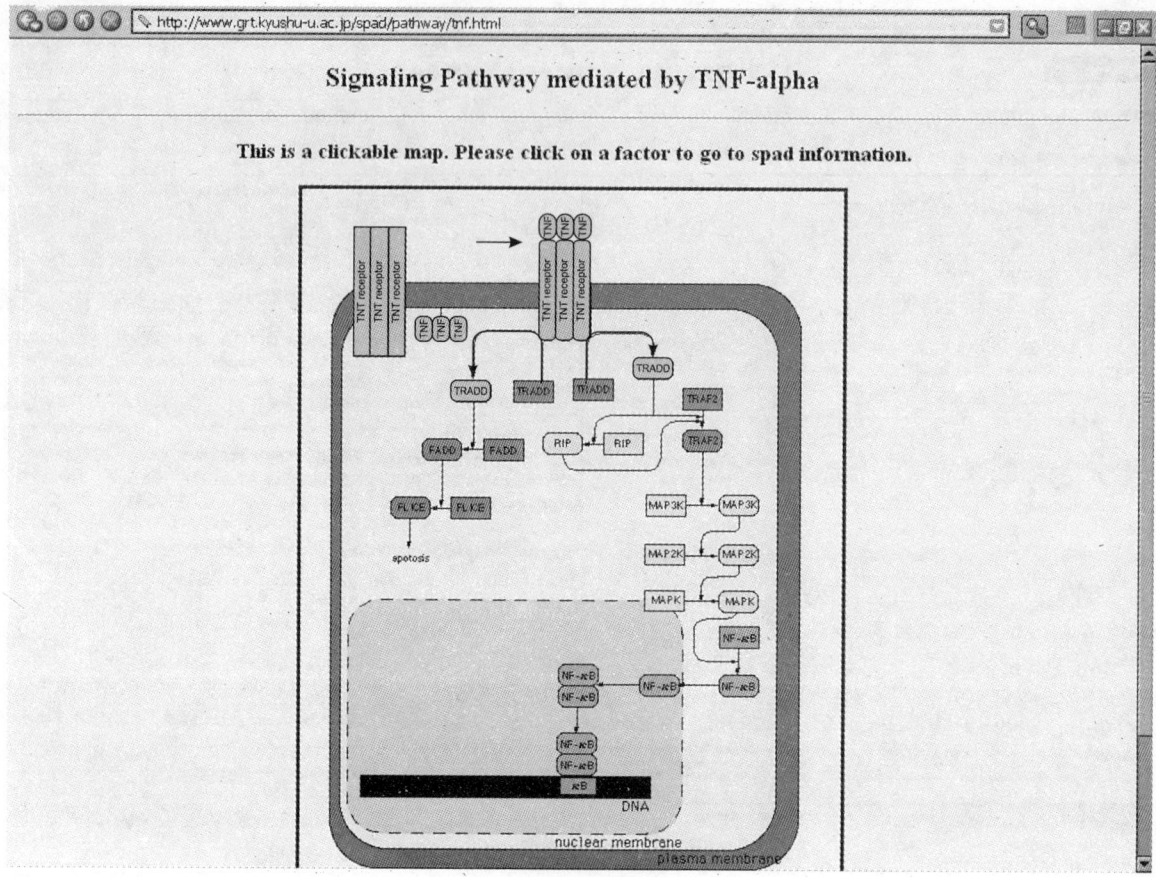

Fig. 19.6. Output from SPAD.

SPAD, the Signaling PAthway Database (http://www.grt.kyushu-u.ac.jp/spad/) is a database of signaling networks. An output for TNF-alpha is shown in Fig. 19.6.

Biocarta (http://www.biocarta.com/genes/CellSignaling.asp) also lists signaling pathways. A sample pathway is shown in Fig. 19.7.

19.5 SIMULATION OF CELLULAR METABOLISM

Simulation models are used to analyze the dynamic nature of cellular regulatory networks.

Simulations can be used for following purposes :

1. To identify design principles for the biochemically based logic;
2. To understand the dynamic response of both normal and mutant cells to environmental and internal signals;
3. To predict quantitative effects of mutations on regulatory outcomes;
4. To verify consistency and completeness of hypothesized reaction systems.

A realistic simulation requires modeling approximations that have a rationale traceable to physical and chemical mechanisms. For example, genetic networks have many attributes commonly associated with computing (Table 19.3).

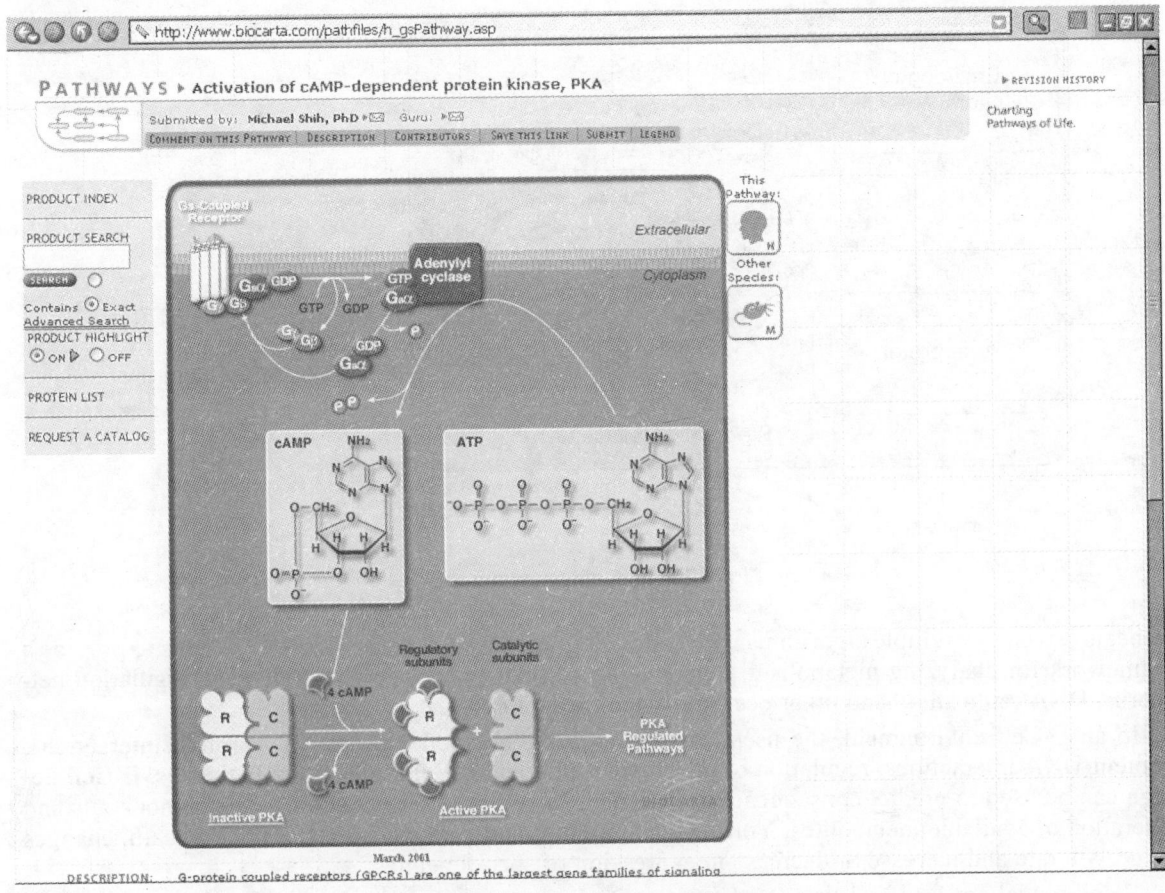

Fig. 19.7. Pathway from BioCarta

Table 19.3 Genetic networks and electronic networks have common features

	Electronic logic	*Genetic logic*
Signals	Electron concentrations	Protein concentrations
Distribution	Point → point (by wires or by electrically encoded addresses	Point → point (movement by diffusion or active transport by encoded reaction specificity)
Organization	Hierarchial	Hierarchical
Logic type	Digital, clocked sequential logic	Analog unlocked (can approximate asynchronous sequential logic)
Noise	Inherent noise due to discrete electron events and environmental effects	Inherent noise due to discrete chemical reaction events and environmental effects
Signal/noise ratio	Signal/noise ratio high in most circuits	Signal/noise ratio low in most circuits
Switching speed	Fast ($> 10^6$ sec^{-1})	Slow ($< 10^{-2}$ sec^{-1})

E-Cell Simulation Environment (E-CELL SE) (http://ecell.sourceforge.net/) is an object-oriented software suite for modeling, simulation, and analysis of biological cells. E-Cell is a deterministic simulator based on differential equations (Fig. 19.8). E-Cell Simulation environment allows for many com-

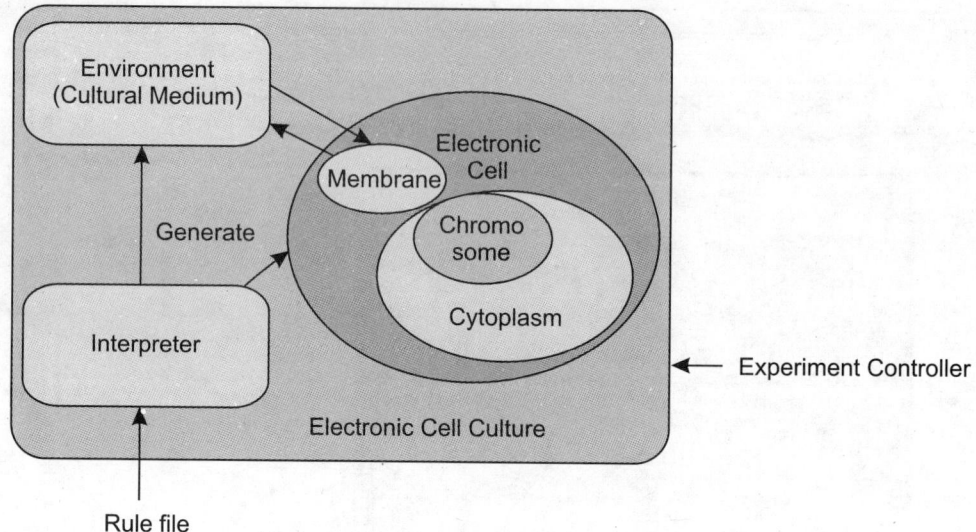

Fig. 19.8. E-Cell environment.

ponents driven by multiple algorithms with different time-cales to coexist. E-Cell attempts to provide a framework for analyzing metabolism, higher-order cellular phenomena such as gene regulation networks, DNA replication, and other occurrences in the cell cycle.

In an E-Cell environment, the users can define protein functions, protein - protein interactions, protein-DNA interactions, regulation of gene expression and cellular metabolix pathways. E-Cell design can be used to predict consequences of changes in cell or environment, e.g. gene knockouts and alteration of available metabolites. You can design interventions that can result in cell death, changes in growth rate and increase or decrease in expression of specific genes.

E-cell model consists of 3 lists for the design by the user:

1. Substance list, which defines all objects making the cell and culture medium (substrates, products, catalysts).
2. Rule list, which defines all the reactions that can take place within the cell.
3. System list, which defines spatial and/or functional structure of the cell and its environment.

State of cell at each time frame can be expressed in form of :

1. Concentrations of all substances in cell
2. Cell volume, pH & temperature

In a single time interval, each rule in the rule list is called upon to compute the change in concentration of each substance (proteins, DNA, RNA & small molecules) to generate next state of the cell.

E-Cell can be used for the following applications :

Assessment of the metabolic requirements of the cell

E-Cell can be used for many purposes such as assessment of the metabolic requirement of the cell. For example, *M. Genitalium* is grown on complex material containing fetal bovine serum, yeast extracts etc. and E-Cell can help formulate chemically-defined synthetic medium. Also, comparison of experimental and computed results could result in identification of new enzymes or transporters

Understanding gene regulatory networks

E-Cell can be used as an important model to understand gene regulatory networks. Specific mechanisms for control of transcript levels can be identified by comparison of parallel *in vitro* and *in silico* experiment. It is also used to modify non-essential genes by gene transcription.

Definition of the minimum set of genes required under specific set of conditions

Non-essential genes can be modified by gene disruption.

20

Methods of Statistical Analysis

20.1 INTRODUCTION

Statistics is the collection and interpretation of quantitative data and the use of probability theory to estimate population parameters. Statistics has two main branches : descriptive statistics and inductive statistics. Descriptive statistics deals with the reduction of large data sets to few parameters. Inductive statistics, also known as inferential statistics, inductive statistics draws conclusions from suitable data sets (samples) to general laws, which are valid for the whole population and not just the sample. Inductive statistics is based on probability theory (Fig. 20.1).

Some definitions

The subset of population used for a survey is called a sample. The characteristic that is studied and found to be varying from one object to another is termed as a variable. Types of variable are as follows:

Nominal (qualitative). Nominal variables are classifiable by some quality like colours of flower, forms of peas etc. For nominal variables, order and distance are not interpretable.

Ordinal (comparative). Ordinal variables are graduated by intensity- the order is important. Distance is not interpretable for ordinal variables.

Metric (quantitative). Metric variables are numerical and recordable. Order and distance are important. Ratio can be calculated for metric variables. Metric variables can be of continuous and discrete types. Continuous variables can have any value in a given range, while discrete variables can only take integer values.

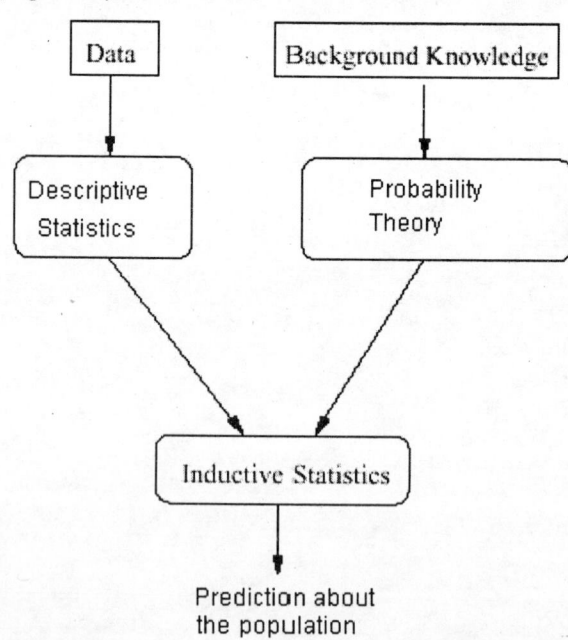

Fig. 20.1. Various branches of statistics study.

344

20.2 FUNDAMENTALS OF PROBABILITY AND STATISTICS

Probability theory

The *probability* of an event is the true relative frequency of that event. A *Venn diagram* can be used to describe the probabilities of different events graphically. The area of the figure marked A is equal to the probability that A will occur; the area of the figure marked B is the probability that B will occur (Fig. 20.2(a)).

$A \cap B$: The *intersection* of A and B means A *and* B (Fig. 20.2(b)).

$A \cup B$: The *union* of A and B means A *or* B (Fig. 20.2(c)).

If there is no possibility of A and B both being true, then they are said to be *mutually exclusive*. Here $A \cap B = 0$ (Fig. 20.2(d)).

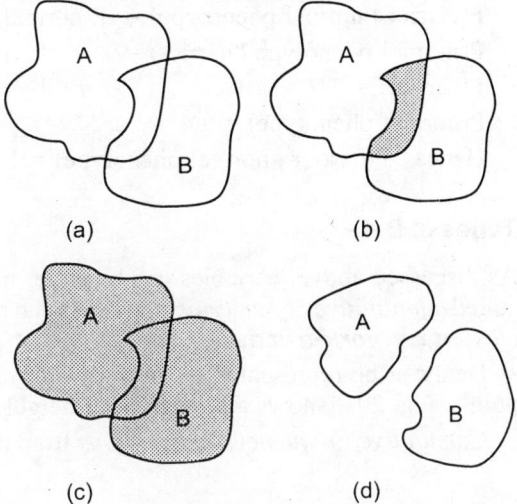

(a)   (b)

(c)   (d)

Fig. 20.2. Venn diagrams.

A *probability tree* is a useful device for calculating the probabilities of combinations of events. Two events are said to be *independent* if $P(A \cap B) = P(A) P(B)$.

Some of the relations in probability are as follows :

1. The probability of A or B involves addition.
2. $P(A \text{ or } B) = P(A) + P(B)$ if the two are mutually exclusive.
3. The probability of A and B involves multiplication
4. $P(A \text{ and } B) = P(A) P(B)$ if the two are independent
5. $P(\text{Not } A) = 1 - P(A)$
6. $P(\text{At least one}) = 1 - P(\text{none})$
7. $P(\text{none}) = P(\text{each event not happening})^{\# \text{ of events}}$

The *frequency* is the count of the number of times that a particular combination occurred in a data set. The *relative frequency* is the proportion of the total that the combination occurred.

Conditional probability is the probability of an event, given that another fact is true. $P(X \mid Y)$ means the probability of X if Y is true. It is read as "the probability of X given Y."

The probability of an event is its conditional probability, times the probability of the condition, summed over all conditions.

$$P[A] = \sum_{\text{all } Y} P[A \mid Y] P[Y]$$

Bayes' Theorem

According the Bayes' theorem :

$$P(X \mid Y) P(Y) = P(Y \mid X) P(X)$$

Both of these are equal to $P(X \text{ and } Y)$. Hence $P(X \mid Y) = P(Y \mid X) P(X) / P(Y)$

Example : An individual is known to have parents that are both heterozygous for alleles at a locus that causes phenylketonuria. This individual has a normal phenotype. What is the chance that she is a carrier (i.e. a heterozygote) for the disease?

P(carrier | normal phenotype) = P(normal phenotype | carrier) P(carrier) / P(normal phenotype)

P(normal phenotype | carrier) = 1

P(carrier) = 1/2

P(normal phenotype) = 3/4

Hence : P(carrier | normal phenotype) = 1 (1/2) / (3/4) = 2/3.

Types of Data

As discussed above, variables can be either metric type or non-metric type. Metric variables are also called *quantitative* or *numerical* variables and non-metric variables (ordinal and nominal) are also called *class* or *categorical* variables.

Data can be represented in the form of graphs, e.g. a histogram shows frequency of various data points. Fig. 20.3 shows a histogram of height in a specific population.

Cumulative Frequency Distributions from this histogram can be plotted in the graph as in Fig. 20.4.

Methods to describe the data

Central tendency is a description attribute that describes where the center of the distribution is located. There are several descriptions of the central tendency of a distribution. Mean, mode and median are used to describe central tendency.

The mean is the center of gravity of a distribution. The median is the value which has half the data above and half the data below. The mode is the highest peak in frequency of the distribution. Arithmetic mean (A.M) is the simplest calculation of the mean. A.M is the sum of all the data points, divided by the total number of data points. Mean is represented by a bar over the letter for that variable like *x*.

The sum of a series of variables can be written in the following notation :

$$\overline{X} = \frac{\sum\limits_{i=1}^{N} X_i}{N}$$

The $\sum\limits_{i=1}^{N} X_i$ in this equation means "the sum of all x_i from i = 1 to i = N."

The arithmetic mean is also said to be the *expected value* of a variable, and can be written as E[x].

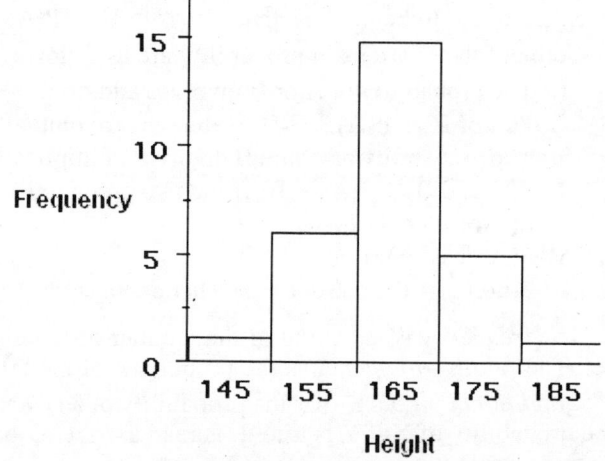

Fig. 20.3. Histogram.

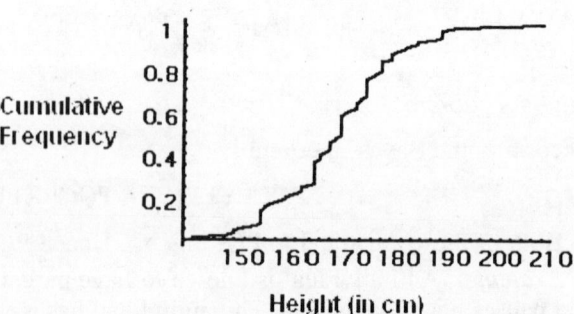

Fig. 20.4. Cumulative distribution frequency histogram.

The *median* is the middle measurement in a set of ordered data. For example, if there are an even number of data points, the median is usually given as the average of the two middle data points. The *mode* is the most frequently occurring measurement in a data set or distribution.

The simplest measure of the dispersion of a data set is its *range*. The range is the difference between the maximum and minimum measurement. The range is very sensitive to sample size - larger samples tend to have a larger range even if they are drawn from the same distribution. This makes the range an unsatisfactory measure of the dispersion of a distribution.

The most commonly used measure of spread is the *variance*. Variance is defined as the average squared deviation from the mean, or

$$Var[x] = E[(x - \mu)^2]$$

where μ is the true mean of the distribution of x. This can also be written as

$$Var[x] = \frac{\sum_i \{x - \mu\}^2}{N}$$

In practice, to estimate the variance of a distribution from a sample of data points, we have to calculate the *sample variance*:

$$s^2 = \frac{\sum_{i=1}^{n} (x - x)^2}{n - 1}$$

where s^2 is the sample variance, and *n* is the number of individuals in the sample.

Because $\dfrac{\sum_{i=1}^{n} (x - x)^2}{n} = \dfrac{\sum_i (x^2)}{n} - x^2$, an easy method to calculate a sample variance is :

$$s^2 = \left(\frac{n}{n - 1} \right) \left(\frac{\sum_{i=1}^{n} X^2}{n} - x^2 \right)$$

The *standard deviation, S.D.,* is the positive square root of the variance. It expresses exactly the same information as the variance, but re-scaled to be in the same units as the mean. The sample standard deviation, represented by *s*, is the square root of the sample variance.

The *Coefficient of Variation*, CV is another way of expressing the information in the variance, but standardized to the mean value of the variable. The CV is usually expressed as a percent.

Some of the results on mean and variance are as follows :

1. The mean of the sum of two variables: $E[X + Y] = E[X] + E[Y]$
2. The mean of the sum of a variable and a constant: $E[X + c] = E[X] + c$
3. The mean of a product of a variable and a constant: $E[c X] = c E[X]$
4. The mean of a product of two variables: $E[X Y] = E[X] E[Y]$ if and only if X and Y are independent.
5. The variance of the sum of two variables: $Var[X + Y] = Var[X] + Var[Y]$ if and only if X and Y are independent.

6. The variance of the sum of a variable and a constant: $Var[X + c] = Var[X]$
7. The variance of a product of a variable and a constant: $Var[c \, X] = c^2 \, Var[X]$

Basic Probability Distributions

There are many probability distributions which can be described mathematically.

Binomial Distribution

The binomial distribution describes the distribution of "success" in a series of trials, i.e., out of N tries, what is the probability that X of them succeed? This type of a distribution can be seen in coin tosses, number of fatalities per number of drug applications etc. The binomial distribution is a discrete distribution (i.e.) the number of successes can only take integer values.

The probability of x successes of N trials, P(x)), is

$$P(x) = \binom{N}{X} P^x (1 - P)^{N-x}$$

$$\binom{N}{x} = \frac{N}{(N-x)! \, x!}$$

where

P is the probability of "success"

N is the number of trials

X is the number of successes out of N trials.

The mean number of successes of a binomial distribution is $\mu = N \, p$ and the variance of the number of successes is $\sigma^2 = N \, p \, (1 - p)$.

Poisson Distribution

The Poisson distribution describes the random occurrence of events, when the number of times that an event does not occur is infinitely large. The Poisson describes the probability of getting X successes per unit time (or per unit space). The Poisson distribution is also a discrete distribution and is applicable only for non-negative integers.

$$P[x] = \frac{e^{-\lambda} \lambda^x}{x!} \, ,$$

where e is the base of the natural log, and λ is the expected number of successes per unit time.

The mean of x over all possible samples is λ, and for the Poisson the variance is also λ.

Normal Distribution

The normal distribution is the most important probability distribution and most traditional statistical tests were designed to work with data which follows a normal distribution (bell-shaped curve) (Fig. 20.5). This graph is an example of the standard normal curve, which has been standardized to have a mean of zero and a variance of 1.

The normal distribution is a continuous distribution. The variable can take any real value.

The equation for the normal distribution is given by:

$$f(x) = \frac{1}{\sqrt{2\pi\sigma^2}} \, e^{-\frac{(x-\mu)^2}{2\sigma^2}}$$

where μ is the mean of the distribution and σ^2 is the variance.

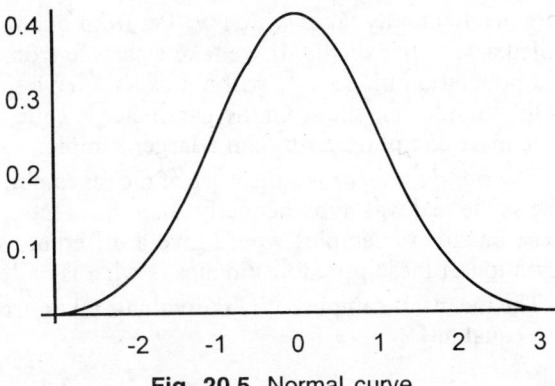

Fig. 20.5. Normal curve.

The normal curve is symmetric around the mean, with only one mode. This implies that the mean, mode, and median are all the same for the normal distribution. Approximately 2/3 of the probability density is within 1 standard deviation of the mean ($\mu \pm \sigma$) and approximately 95% of the probability density is within 2 standard deviations of the mean ($\mu \pm 2\sigma$).

A normal distribution where $\mu = 0$ and $\sigma^2 = 1$ is called a *standard normal distribution*.

The standard normal distribution is used widely as all normal distributions are shaped alike, and can be standardized to determine their properties. This standardization is called the Z-transformation.

$$Z = \frac{x - \mu}{\sigma}$$

We need to use *statistical tables* to find different probabilities for the normal distribution. We use the standard normal distribution and convert to the actual normal distribution we have.

As the standard normal distribution is symmetric around 0,

$$P[x > a] = P[x < -a].$$

If N is large, and p is not too close to 0 or 1, then the binomial distribution can be *approximated* by the normal distribution. This is useful, because with a large N calculating the exact probability of an outcome can be very time-consuming. A normal distribution with mean N p and variance N p (1 − p) is approximately equal to the binomial distribution, for large N.

The Central Limit Theorem

If we take large enough samples, the means of the samples will be approximately normally distributed even if the underlying variable being averaged is not normally distributed. This is the *Central Limit Theorem*. The phrase "large enough" in the previous sentence will vary from distribution to distribution; the further the underlying distribution is from normal, the larger the sample which is required to give a mean which is normally distributed.

The Central Limit Theorem is very important. Many statistical tests assume that means are normally distributed, and the CLT allows us to sometimes use these tests even when the underlying distributions are not normal.

Populations and Samples

We refer to the whole group of individuals about which inferences are to be made as the *population*. A *sample* is the subset of the population which are actually observed. For every value which we want to estimate has a true value in the population, which we call a *parameter*. Our best guess of the value that parameter actually takes which we get from our sample is called an *estimate*. An estimate can also be called a *sample statistic*. If we take a sample from a population, unless we measure every member of that population the sample will not exactly have the same properties as the population. This deviation of the sample statistic from the parameter is called *sampling error*. A smaller sample will on average have more sampling error than a larger sample.

The *standard error* is a measure of the repeatability of an estimate. Assume that a sample of the same size as the real was hypothetically taken from the same population an infinite number of times. Each of these imaginary samples would give a different estimate of the parameter in question. The standard deviation of these pseudo-estimates is what is called the *standard error* of the estimate.

The means of samples of N individuals taken from a normal distribution will have a standard deviation equal to

$$SE_x = \frac{\sigma}{\sqrt{N}}$$

so we say that this is the standard error of the mean. We can estimate this standard error by using our estimate of σ:

$$SE_x = \frac{s}{\sqrt{N}}$$

A sample which is *expected* to give an answer which is off in one direction is called *biased*. The average over samples of x is μ, so it is an unbiased of μ. The average over samples of s^2 is σ^2, so it is an unbiased of σ^2.

The average value over samples of $\dfrac{\sum\limits_{i} (X_i - X)^2}{n} < \sigma^2$, so it would be a *biased* estiator of σ^2. This is

why we use $\dfrac{\sum\limits_{i} (X_1 - X)^2}{n - 1} = s^2$ instead.

The size of samples used to generate an estimate is often described in terms of the numbers of *degrees of freedom* in that sample. There as many degrees of freedom in a sample for a particular estimate as there are independent terms used to calculate that estimate. For example, for a mean there are N degrees of freedom in a sample of size N; for an estimate of variance there are N-1 degrees of freedom in that same sample.

Hypotheses Testing

With hypothesis testing, we divide all possible interpretations of an experiment into two alternatives: a null hypothesis and an alternative hypothesis. A null hypothesis is the statement that there is "no effect" or the "status quo." The alternative hypothesis in turn is that there is an effect of an experimental manipulation, or that the status quo is not in fact true.

You can use the null hypothesis to generate the distribution of what sample statistics *would* look like, if the null hypothesis were true and we took many, many samples like the one we actually took. You can then compare the actual statistics we measured to this distribution of possible sample statistics to see how unusual it would be, *if this null hypothesis were true.*

What is the probability of getting a result as extreme or more in the possible range of test statistics as the one we actually got? This probability is called the *p-value* of the test (Fig. 20.6).

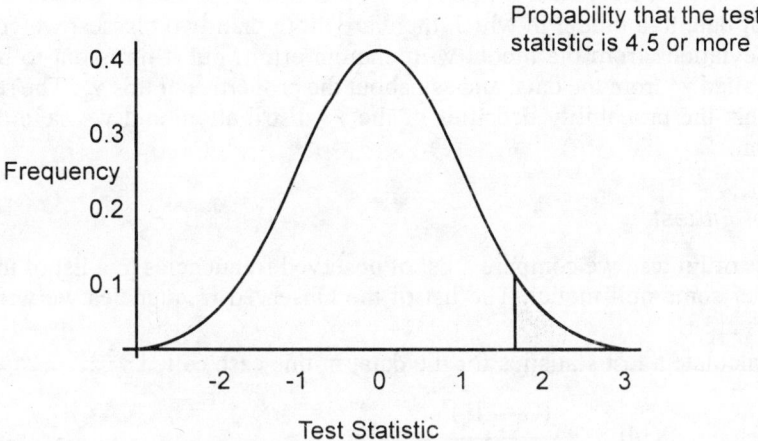

Fig. 20.6. p-value of the test.

Samples from the null distribution usually can take many of the possible values regardless of whether the null hypothesis is true. Some of these values are extremely unlikely, but still possible. Thus there is a chance that we can falsely reject a true null hypothesis. If we reject a null hypothesis which is in fact true, then we have made a Type I error. The probability of having a Type I error is α. Similarly, if we do not reject a *false* null hypothesis, we have made a *Type II error*. The probability of having a Type II error is β.

We must choose a level of að which corresponds to a Type I error rate we are satisfied with. This is called the *significance level*. A times, we are confronted with a situation in which it would be difficult to calculate directly the p-value of a particular result, but there is a similar result which is easy to calculate or look up in a table which we can use by mapping our question on to another scale. We therefore often calculate a *test statistic*. The value of this test statistic which corresponds to the point at which $p = \alpha$, we call the *critical value* of that test statistic. If we get a statistical result in which $p < \alpha$ (that is, we can reject the null hypothesis), then we can say that the result is *statistically significant*.

Parametric and non-parametric tests

With *parametric tests*, we assume that a test statistics follows a particular distribution, then use that distribution to generate a null distribution. Most of the statistical tests in use are parametric tests (often assuming the data follow a normal distribution).

Non-parametric tests do not make assumptions about the distribution that a data set is drawn from. Non-parametric tests tend to use information about the rank-order of the data to make statistical inference. They are useful because they can be calculated with general formulae and most statistical packages, and are therefore easily applied to most data sets, even when the assumptions of the parametric tests are violated.

Using test statistics

It is not always easy to calculate the probability of a given event directly. Sometimes it much easier to translate a problem into an analogous problem, for which the mathematics are easier. In these cases instead of calculating the p-value directly given the null hypothesis and the data, we calculate a *test statistic*, and then find the probability of our result using the test statistic.

To test the fit of data to a model in which there are more than two classes, we could calculate the exact chance of deviations from the model with enough effort, but it turns out to be much easier to calculate a value called χ^2 from the data, and ask about the properties of this χ^2. The reason is that there are tables which list the probability densities of the χ^2 distribution, and we save ourselves a lot of difficult calculation.

The Goodness of Fit test

With the Goodness of Fit test, we compare a list of observed frequencies to a list of the frequencies we would expect under some null model. The list of the Observed frequencies we write as O_i; the Expected frequencies are E_i.

Then we can calculate a test statistics for the data, in this case called χ^2 :

$$X^2df = \sum_i \frac{(O_i - E_i)^2}{E_i}$$

Notice that if the observed closely matches the expected, then the χ^2 value will be small, but if there is a great difference between the observed and expected, χ^2 will be large.

The "df" in the subscript of the χ^2 means "degrees of freedom," and the value of the χ^2 distribution that we expect under the null model will depend on the number of degrees of freedom a particular test has.

The χ^2 distribution

The χ^2 distribution is a continuous distribution, ranging from 0 to infinity (Fig.20.7)

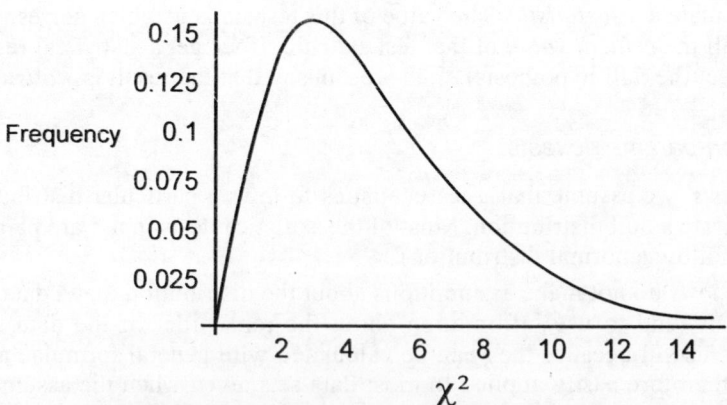

Fig. 20.7. χ^2 distribution with 5 degrees of freedom.

If there are c classes and r parameters estimated from the data to generate a null hypothesis, a c/χ^2 test has a number of degrees of freedom equal to $df = c - 1 - r$.

Sample from normal distributions

To begin with, focus on samples which are drawn from a population which has a *normal distribution*. The distribution of the population is given in Fig. 20.8.

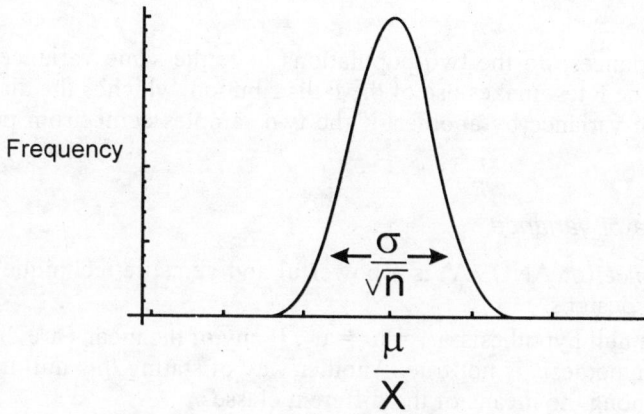

Fig. 20.8. Normal distribution curve.

The means of samples with *n* data points that come from this distribution will also be normally distributed. They will have a mean which is also equal to μ, but the standard deviation of the sample means is equal to $\sigma/\sqrt{n}$. Note that the larger the sample size (*n*), the *smaller* the variance of the distribution of sample means will be.

Note that this implies:

$$Z = \frac{x - \mu}{\sigma/\sqrt{n}} \text{ has a normal distribution with mean} = 0 \text{ and SD} = 1.$$

The problem with using this is that it implies that we know what the standard deviation of the population is. We usually only have information about the standard deviation from our sample itself, and this gives us an idea of the variance (s^2), but with sampling error. We must estimate $\sigma/\sqrt{n}$ as $s/\sqrt{n}$.

This is the statistic, t, which is defined as:

$$t = \frac{x - \mu}{s/\sqrt{n}}$$

This *t* is distributed by a *Student's t distribution* with *n*-1 degrees of freedom.

The distribution of the mean is estimated by the t-distribution:

$$t = \frac{x - \mu}{s/\sqrt{n}}, \text{ with } v = n - 1.$$

The χ^2 distribution

The χ^2 *distribution* describes the sampling properties of sample variances for normal distributions. If a variable is normally distributed, then $(n - 1)\, s^2/\sigma^2$ has a χ^2 distribution with n-1 degrees of freedom.

The χ^2 distribution starts at zero and continues to infinity. Similarly, a sample variance estimate cannot be less than zero, but can be up to indefinitely large. This relationship between the sample variance and the χ^2 distribution allows us to make inferences about the confidence we can have about our estimates of the population's variance.

The F test

Given two sample variances, do the two populations have the same variance? This question is answered by the F test. The F test makes use of the F distribution, which is the distribution you get when you divide one sample variance by another, if the two samples come from populations which have equal variances.

Single factor Analysis of variance

The *Analysis of Variance* (or ANOVA) is a powerful and versatile technique for dealing with more complex experimental designs.

Suppose we test the null hypothesis: $\mu_1 = \mu_2 = \mu_3$. If any of the means are different from any of the others, then this null hypothesis is not true. Another way of stating this null hypothesis is to say that there is no variance among the means of the different classes.

Doing an ANOVA comes down to testing whether there is more variance among the samples' means than we would expect by chance sampling error alone. This results in a comparison of two variances: the variance we *observed* among the means of the samples vs. the variance we *expected* to see due to sampling error. If we have these two, we can do an F test to compare these two variances statistically.

The variance among sample means from the same distribution is

$$\sigma_{\bar{x}}^2 = \frac{\sigma_x^2}{n}$$

where n is the sample size of each sample.

Therefore, under the null hypothesis that there is no real variance among the means of the different sets, we expect the variance among the means of the samples to be approximately equal to the variance among individuals divided by the sample size, or equivalently:

$$n\sigma_{\bar{x}}^2 = \sigma_x^2$$

σ_x^2 can be estimated by the pooled sample variance, and $\sigma_{\bar{x}}^2$ can be estimated by the variance among the samples. An F test could then resolve whether the variance we see among groups is in fact equal to the variance we expect to see by sampling alone.

The assumptions of ANOVA's are:

1. Random samples
2. Normal distributions for each population
3. Equal variances for all populations. (*Homoscedasticity*)

Kruskal-Wallis test

If the data do not come from a normal distribution, or if the variances of the different populations are very unequal, then you can use a non-parametric version of the analysis of variance, called a *Kruskal-*

Wallis test. This test is 95% as powerful as a single-factor ANOVA, and much better when the assumptions of the ANOVA are not true.

The test statistic for the Kruskal-Wallis test is

$$H = \frac{12}{N(N+1)} \left[\sum_{i=1}^{k} \frac{R_i^2}{n_i} \right] - 3(N+1)$$

where N is the total sample size and R_i is the rank sum for group *i*.

20.3 APPLICATIONS OF STATISTICAL TOOLS

Biostatistics encompasses such diverse applications as :
1. Modeling animal populations in an ecosystem
2. Designing a sample scheme to evaluate health services
3. Designing and analyzing epidemiological studies and clinical trials
4. Designing and analyzing pharmacological experiments and microorganism assays
5. Analysis of health care utilization patterns

In bioinformatics, almost all the fields that we have studied have applications of statistics. Some of these applications are discussed here.

Scoring a pair-wise alignment

The score of an alignment is the sum of the scores for pairs of aligned characters plus the scores for gaps. For example, consider the following alignment :

VAHV –––D––DMPNALSALSDLHAHKL
AIQLQVTGVVVTDATLKNLGSVHVSKG

The score for this alignment would be given by :

$$s(V,A) + s(A,I) + s(H,Q) + s(V,L) + 3r + s(D,G) + 2r...$$

where s(a,b) indicates score of aligning character a with character b, r is a constant in the linear gap function $w_x = rx$

There are

$$\binom{2n}{n} = \frac{(2n)!}{(n!)^2} \approx \frac{2^{2n}}{\sqrt{\pi n}}$$

possible global alignments for 2 sequences of length *n*.

We can thus see that using pair-wise alignment is not practical for large n.

Probabilistic model of alignments

Consider protein alignments without gaps. Given an alignment, we can consider two possibilities :

R : when the sequences are related by evolution
U : when the sequences are unrelated

Case 1 : For unrelated sequences

If we assume that each position in the alignment is sampled randomly from some distribution of amino acids and let q_a be the probability of amino acid a. The probability of an n-character alignment of x and y is given by (using Baye's theorem):

$$\Pr(x, y) \mid U) = \prod_{i=1}^{n} q_{x_i} \prod_{i=1}^{n} q_{y_i}$$

Case 2 : For related sequences

If we assume that each pair of aligned amino acids evolved from a common ancestor and let q_{ab} be the probability that evolution gave rise to amino acid a in one sequence and b in another sequence. The probability of an alignment of x and y is given by :

$$\Pr(x, y) \mid R) = \prod_{i=1}^{n} p_{x_i} p_{y_i}$$

To decide which possibility (U or R) is more likely, we can calculate the relative likelihood of the two possibilities (called the odds ratio) as follows :

$$\frac{\Pr(x, y \mid R)}{\Pr(x, y \mid U)} = \frac{\prod_i p_{x_i y_i}}{\prod_i p_{x_i} \prod_i q_{y_i}} = \frac{\prod_i p_{x_i y_i}}{\prod_i q_{x_i} q_{y_i}}$$

Taking the log, we get:

$$\log \frac{\Pr(x, y \mid R)}{\Pr(x, y \mid U)} = \sum_i \log \left(\frac{p_{x_i y_i}}{q_{x_i} q_{y_i}} \right)$$

The score for an alignment is given by:

$$S = \sum_i s(x_i, y_i) = \log \frac{\Pr(x, y \mid R)}{\Pr(x, y \mid U)}$$

The substitution matrix score for the pair a, b is given by :

$$s(a, b) = \log \left(\frac{p_{ab}}{q_a q_b} \right)$$

The probability that a and b arose from a common ancestor is given as follows :

Case 1 : diverged recently, $p_{ab} \approx 0$, for $a \neq b$

Case 2 : diverged long ago, $p_{ab} = q_a q_b$

For BLOSUM matrices,

$$p_{ab} = \frac{A_{ab}}{\sum_{c,d} A_{cd}} \qquad q_a = \frac{\sum_b A_{ab}}{\sum_{c,d} A_{cd}}$$

Significance of BLAST results

Please refer to Chapter Tools for sequence alignment for the discussion on E values and P values.

HMM approaches

There are many problems where we would like to represent the statistical regularities of some class of sequences like genes, various regulatory sites in DNA and proteins in a given family. Hidden Markov Models are well suited for these kinds of problems. Consider the Fig. 20.9.

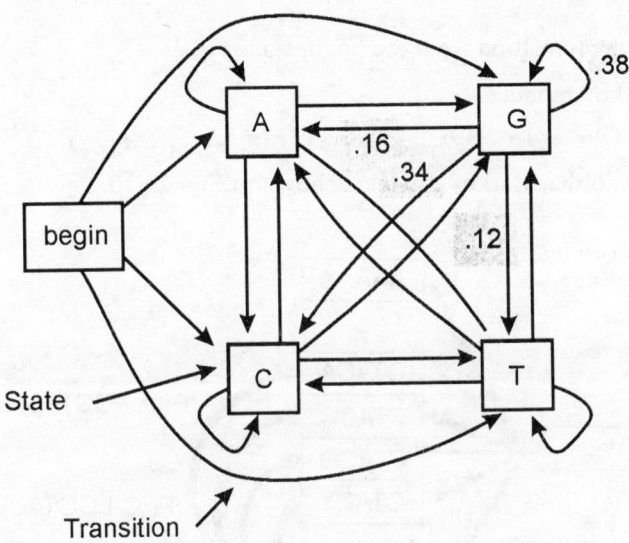

Fig, 20.9. Sample Markov chain.

The transition probabilities (using Baye's theorem) are as follows :

$$\text{Pr } (x_i = a \mid x_{i-1} = g) = 0.16$$
$$\text{Pr } (x_i = c \mid x_{i-1} = g) = 0.34$$
$$\text{Pr } (x_i = g \mid x_{i-1} = g) = 0.38$$
$$\text{Pr } (x_i = t \mid x_{i-1} = g) = 0.12$$

A Markov chain model is defined by a set of states and transitions. Some states emit symbols and some other states like the begin state are silent. There is a set of transitions with associated probabilities. The transitions emanating from a given state define a distribution over the possible next states.

Given some sequence x of length L, the probability of any sequence in the Markov model is given as follows :

$$\text{Pr } (x) = \text{Pr } (x_L, x_{L-1}, \ldots x_2, x_1) = \text{Pr } (x_L / x_{L-1}, \ldots, x_1) \text{Pr } (x_{L-1} / x_{L-2}, \ldots, x_1) \ldots \text{Pr}(x_1)$$

For the first order Markov model, value of x_i depends on the value of x_{i-1} only.

$\text{Pr } (x) = \text{Pr } (x_L / x_{L-1}) \text{Pr } (x_{L-1} / x_{L-2}) \ldots \text{Pr}(x_1)$. This is written as :

$$\text{Pr}(x_1 \prod_{i=2}^{L} \text{Pr}(x_i \mid x_{i-1})$$

For the above Markov model, the probability of a sequence cggt is given by :

$$Pr\ (cggt) = Pr\ (c)\ Pr\ (g|c)\ Pr\ (g|g)\ Pr\ (t|g)$$

For a general Markov chain, the transition parameters can be represented by $a_{x_{i-1}x_i}$

where $\qquad\qquad a_{x_{i-1}x_i} = Pr\ (x_i\ |\ x_{i-1})$

The probability of a sequence x is given by :

$$a_{Bx_1}\ \prod_{i=2}^{L}\ a_{x_{i-1}x_i} = Pr(x_1)\ \prod_{i=2}^{L}\ Pr(x_i\ |\ x_{i-1})$$

where a B_{x_i} represents the transition from the begin state.

For an nth order Markov model,

$$Pr\ (x_i\ |\ x_{i-1}, x_{i-2}, \ldots x_1) = Pr\ (x_i\ |\ x_{i-1}, \ldots x_{i-n})$$

An example of a fifth order Markov model is shown in Fig. 20.10.

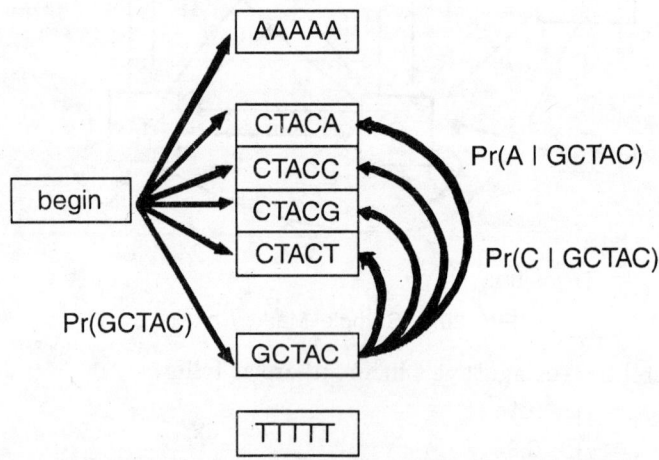

Fig. 20.10. Fifth order Markov model.

Here Pr (gctaca) = P (gctac) Pr (a|gctac)

In simple Markov model, the probabilities do not depend on where we are in a given sequence. This is a simplistic assumption. In an *inhomogeneous* Markov model, we can have different distributions at different positions in the sequence (Fig. 20.11).

GenMark (http://opal.biology.gatech.edu/GeneMark/) uses 5th order inhomogeneous Markov chain models.

Markov models are widely used in bioinformatics and several algorithms dealing with problems in gene recognition, protein family modeling and motif modeling have been developed. Also refer to Chapter gene prediction methods.

Multiple sequence and phylogenetic trees analysis

Multiple sequence and phylogenetic trees are the subjects of discussion in Chapters Alignment of multiple sequences and Phylogenetic trees.

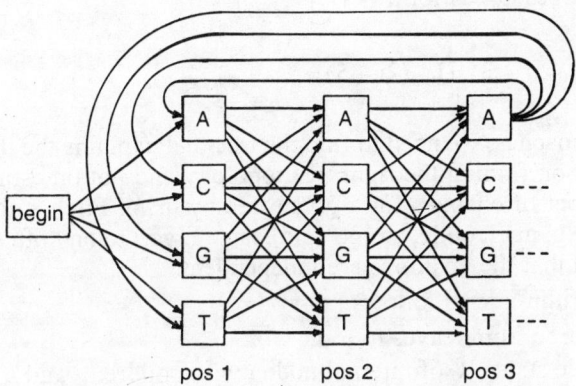

Fig. 20.11. Inhomogenous Markov chain.

UPGMA method in alignment of multiple sequences is based on arithmetic averages calculation. The generalized algorithm is discussed here. The basic idea of the UPGMA method is to iteratively pick two sequences/clusters and merge them. This creates a new node in tree for merged cluster.

Average distance d_{ij} is defined as

$$d_{ij} = \frac{1}{|C_i||C_j|}\Big|_{p\varepsilon C_i,\ q\varepsilon C_j} \Sigma\ d_{pq}$$

where C_i and C_j are the two clusters of sequences. The steps followed in the method are as follows:

1. Assign each sequence to its own cluster
2. Define one leaf for each sequence; place it at height 0
3. While more than two clusters
   a. Determine two clusters i,j with smallest d_{ij}.
   b. Define a new cluster $C_k = Ci \cup Cj$
   c. Define a node k with children i and j and place it at a height of $d_{ij}/2$.
   d. Replace clusters i and j with k.
   e. Compute distance between k and other clusters
4. Join last two clusters, i and j, by root at height $d_{ij}/2$.
5. Given a new cluster Ck formed by merging C_i and C_j, you can calculate the distance between C_k and any other cluster C_j as follows :

$$d_{kl} = \frac{d_{il}|C_{jl}|\ |C_j|}{C_i|+C_j|}$$

We have discussed the concept of rooted and unrooted trees. Given n sequences, the possible unrooted trees are as follows :

$$\prod_{i=3}^{n}\ (2i-5)$$

and the possible rooted trees are as follows :

$$(2n - 3) \prod_{i=3}^{n} (2i - 5)$$

In the parsimony approaches, we need to find the tree that explains the data with a minimal number of changes. The focus is on finding the right tree topology and not on estimating branch lengths. We can find minimum number of changes for a given tree by using Fitch's algorithm. Fitch's algorithm assumes that any state (e.g. nucleotide, amino acid) can convert to any other state, the "costs" of these changes are uniform and that the positions are independent.

The steps in this algorithm are as follows :

1. Do a traversal of tree from leaves to root.
2. Determine possible states R_i of internal node i with children j and k as follows :

$$R_i = \left\{ \begin{array}{l} R_j \cup R_k, \text{ if } R_j \cap R_k = \varnothing \\ R_j \cap R_k, \text{ otherwise} \end{array} \right\}$$

This step calculates the number of changes required. Number of changes is equal to the number of union operations.

3. Now do a traversal from root to leaves.
4. Select r_j of internal node j with parent i as follows :

$$r_j = \left\{ \begin{array}{l} r_j, \text{ if } r_i \in R_j \\ \text{arbitrary state} \in R_j, \text{ otherwise} \end{array} \right\}$$

This algorithm can be modified to include weights. Here, instead of assuming all state changes are equally likely, we use different costs for different changes.

Analysis of microarray data

Refer to the Chapter Gene mapping, sequence assembly and gene expression. Microarray analysis applies almost the entire discussion we have had on statistics and probability. Microarray analysis is a data-intensive activity and there are several computational tasks associated with the output data from microarrays like :

1. Clustering genes: which genes seem to be regulated together
2. Clustering samples: which treatments/individuals have similar profiles
3. Classifying genes: to which functional class does a given gene belong
4. Classifying samples: to which class does a given sample belong
5. Inferring regulatory networks in the cell

Microarray output data can be represented in a matrix form, represented by M_{ij} of relative expression values of gene i in condition j. It is often presented as $\log_2$ values, since this means that down-regulation of gene (e.g. ratio ½) is not construed as an interval $(0,1)$, but takes values e.g. (-1) in $(-\infty, 0)$.

The steps in analysis of microarray data are as follows :

Pre-processing

There are several sources of variation in intensity in microarray experiments other than differences in gene expression between samples. These are thought of as "noise" and we would ideally want to remove them. This is done by pre-processing. Some of the sources of noise and methods to eliminate them are outlined here.

Missing values

One of the sources of noise can be *missing values* in microarray data. Missing values are usually observations (intensities of spots) where the quantification results are missing. In microarrays, the missing values can occur because the spot is empty (intensity = 0) or because background intensity is higher than the spot intensity (background corrected intensity < 0).

Missing values can lead to problems in the data analysis, because they easily interfere with computation of statistical tests and clustering. Missing values can be replaced with estimated values in a process called *imputation*, or they can be deleted from the further analyses.

Background intensities

Sometimes background intensities can result in noise. The background intensities should not correlate highly with the spot intensities, if the spot intensities are truly independent of the background intensities. A scatter plot of background intensities against spot intensities can do this assessment. If the spot intensities are dependent on the background intensities, it is possible either not to apply any background correction to the data or discard the deviating observations from further analyses.

Expression change

After background correction, expression change is calculated. The preliminary method applied is to divide the intensity of a gene in the sample by the intensity level of the same gene in the control. Intensity ratio can be calculated from background corrected or uncorrected data.

To make the distribution look closer to a normal distribution, log-transformation can be applied. After the log-transformation, unchanged expression is zero, and both up-regulated and down-regulated genes can take values from zero to infinity. Some of the mathematical operations also become easier after log transformation.

Another method to make the distribution of intensity ratios more symmetrical is to calculate the fold change. The fold change is equal to the intensity ratio, when the expression is higher then one. Below one, the fold change is equal to the inversed intensity ratio.

Replicates

Replicates can be technical or biological in nature. If we treat a certain cell line with a cancer drug, we can set up several culture flasks, and then harvest them as biological replicates. For every culture flask, the isolated and labeled mRNA population can be hybridized to several chips making a number of technical replicates . In addition, every hybridized chip can be quantified several times or using different image analysis software – these are called software replicates.

Outliers

Outliers can occur at several levels. There can be entire chips, which deviate from all the other replicates. On the other hand, there can be an individual gene, which deviates from the other replicates of the same gene. Outliers can be removed by using a statistical model. A simple model is equality between replicates. If one replicate deviates several standard deviations from the mean of the other replicates, it can be considered an outlier and removed. The t-test measures standard deviation and gives genes, where outliers are present among replicates, a low significance. Removal of outliers can be combined with filtering also.

Normalization

There are many sources of systematic variation in microarray experiments that affect the measured gene expression levels. *Normalization* is used to describe the process of removing such variation. Normalization can also be thought of as an attempt to remove the non-biological influences on biological data.

There are several sources of systematic bias like :

1. Differences in dye (labeling) efficiencies
2. Malfunction of the scanner
3. Uneven hybridization
4. Printing tip defects
5. Slides from the same print run (or batch) often cluster together and also slides from an identical print design but different print run. This is called batch defect

The principle behind normalization is that the expected mean intensity ratio between the two channels (two-colour data) or two chips (one-colour data) is one, because only about 10–20% of all the genes in a cell are expressed at any one time. If the observed mean intensity ratio deviates from one, the data is mathematically processed in such a way that the final observed mean intensity ratio becomes one. When the mean intensity ratio is adjusted to one, the distribution of the gene expression is centered so that different arrays can be compared.

Log-transformation method is widely used for normalization. *Standardization,* the process of expanding or contracting the distribution of a statistic so that the experimental values can be compared with those from another experiment is also used. Standardization involves converting the intensity ratios to Z-scores, which are distributed as a standard normal distribution.

Centralization, the process of moving a distribution so that it is centered over the expected mean (balancing the two channels) is also used in normalisation. For the log-transformed intensity ratios, an intensity dependent centralization might help to correct the dye bias.

Some of the methods used for normalization are :

1. Mean centering
2. Median centering
3. Trimmed mean centering
4. Lowess smoothing
5. Ratio statistics
6. Analysis of variance
7. Spiked controls

Filtering

Filtering is a process where observations which do not fulfill a pre-formulated presumption are excluded from the data. For example, there is a certain limit of the scanner below which the intensity values cannot be trusted anymore. The first step of filtering is flagging. Flagging is performed at the image analysis step. The "bad" spots are flagged off for removal.

Some statistical measures can be used for filtering. Some image analysis programs give signal-to-noise or signal-to-background measurements for every spot on the array. These quality measurements can be used for filtering out bad data. Often a cut-off point of 90–95% for signal-to-noise ratio is used, at least on control channel.

Clustering

Microarray output is a large amount of data. This data needs to be meaningfully analysed - clustering provides the framework for this analysis. Clustering is used to organize the data into a small number of homogeneous groups. Cluster analysis aims to group or segment a collection of objects into subsets or "clusters", such that those within each cluster are more closely related to one another than objects assigned to different clusters.

Clustering methods can be grouped as *supervised* and *unsupervised*. Supervised methods assign some predefined classes to a data set, whereas in unsupervised methods no prior assumptions are applied.

Clustering methods include hierarchical clustering, K-means, self-organizing maps (SOMs), and principal component analysis (PCA) have been commonly used. There are also other methods, such as multidimensional scaling (MDS), minimum description length (MDS), gene shaving (GS), decision trees, and support vector machines (SVMs) that are used for clustering (Fig. 20.12).

Hierarchical clustering is a statistical method for finding relatively homogeneous clusters. The hierarchical clustering algorithm either iteratively joins the two closest clusters starting from single clusters (agglomerative, bottom-up approach) or iteratively partitions clusters starting from the complete set (divisive, top-down approach). After each step, a new distance matrix between the newly formed clusters and the other clusters is recalculated. If there are N cases, N-1 clustering steps are needed. There are several methods of hierarchical cluster analysis including average linkage (UPGMA), single linkage (minimum method, nearest neighbor) and complete linkage (maximum method, furthest neighbor). Hierarchical clustering is often applied in the analysis of patient samples to organize the data based on the cases.

Self-organizing map (SOM) is a neural net that uses unsupervised learning for which no prior knowledge of classes is required. SOMs are usually used to visualize and interpret large high-dimensional data sets. In SOM, every input is connected to every output via connections with variable weights. Also, the output nodes are highly interconnected. SOM tries to learn to map gene expression profiles to similar regions of the output array of nodes In SOMs, the number of clusters has to be predetermined. The dimensions of the two-dimensional grid or array give the value.

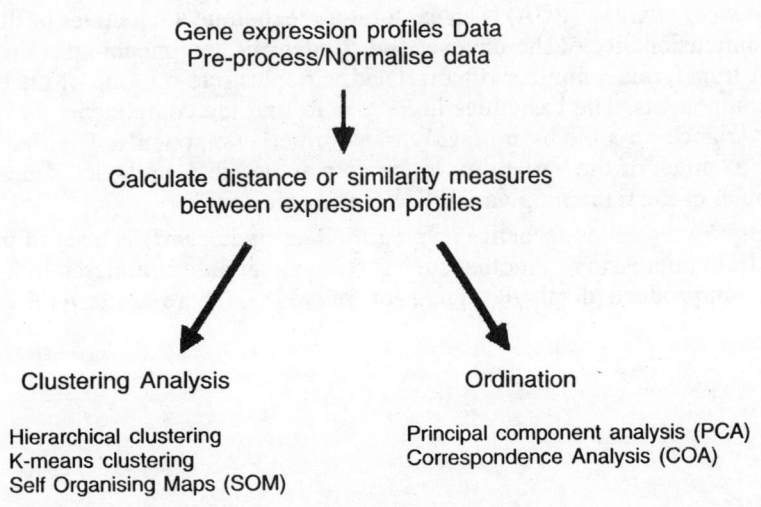

Fig. 20.12. Clustering methods.

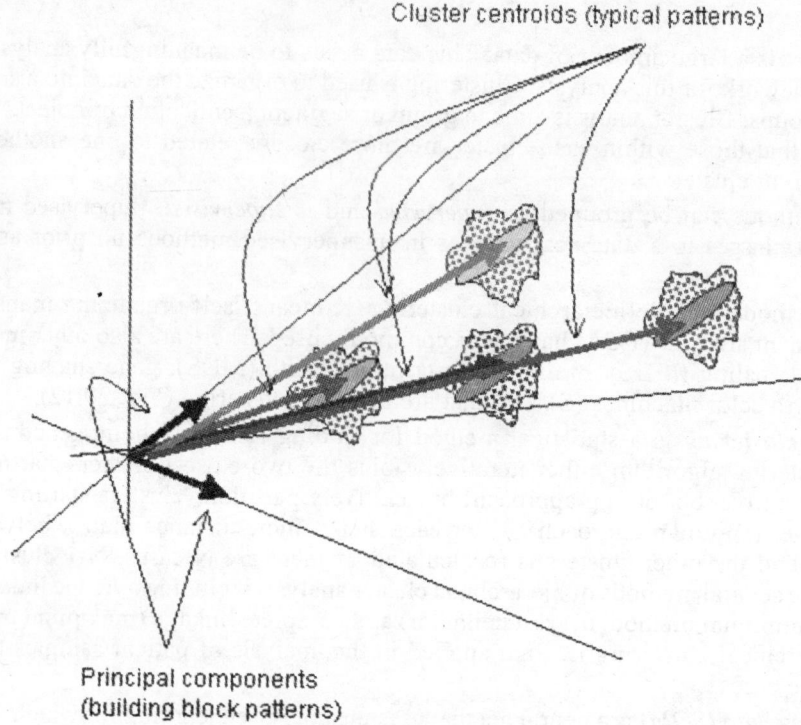

Cluster centroids (typical patterns)

Principal components
(building block patterns)

Fig. 20.13. PCA technique.

K-means clustering is a least-squares partitioning method for which the number of groups, K, has to be provided. The algorithm computes cluster centroids and uses them as new cluster seeds, and assigns each object to the nearest seed. However, it is also possible to estimate K from the data, taking the approach of a mixture density estimation problem.

Principal component analysis (PCA) is an exploratory technique. Objectives of PCA are to discover or to reduce the dimensionality of the data set and to identify new meaningful underlying variables (Fig. 20.13). PCA transforms a number of correlated variables into a group of uncorrelated variables called principal components. The basic idea in PCA is to find the components that explain the maximum amount of variance possible by n linearly transformed components. The first principal component accounts for as much of the variability in the data as possible, and each succeeding component accounts for as much of the remaining variability as possible.

GeneSpring (http://www.silicongenetics.com/cgi/SiG.cgi/index.smf) is a set of tools that can used to analyse output from microarrays. Another such software available commercially is StratGene (http://www.stratagene.com/products/displayProduct.aspx?pid=538). There are several other similar utilities available.

Problem Solving in Bioinformatics

21.1. INTRODUCTION

This chapter discusses some of the more common bioinformatics problems and the generalised approach to solve them. The approach outlined may not be the only correct approach and hence should be taken at best as one of the better ways of solving the problems. The discussion is supported with some illustrations.

21.2. GENOMIC ANALYSIS FOR DNA SEQUENCES

Genomic DNA

- Find protein encoding regions which include introns in some organisms
- Transcriptional signals 5' to protein encoding regions
- RNA processing signals such as polyA tail
- Hard to translate these sequences if they have introns, but there are methods to do it
- Use cDNA sequence for translation, if available
- Breakup DNA sequence into regions such as upstream from ORF (promoter region) and downstream (RNA processing region) and protein encoding regions.
- Then do search for patterns (such as RNA polymerase or transcription factor recognition sites) or regions of similarity with other sequences

cDNA

- Translate into protein
- Analyze protein sequence

RNA genes such as ribosomal RNA, tRNA, etc.

- These fold into typical structures which can be predicted using energy minimization rules
- These do not encode proteins

21.3. GENOMIC ANALYSIS FOR PROTEIN SEQUENCES

Search database for similar sequence using BLAST, FASTA or DYNAMIC PROGRAMMING

- A close match can reveal function or biochemical activity
- Find relationship to protein families (for example, in the ENTREZ accessible protein databases)
- Search for similarity to protein of known 3D structure

Search the sequence for amino acid patterns already identified in related proteins and which determine a biochemical activity

- An active site can be identified in the PROSITE database
- Look for other patterns in the PROSITE families known as BLOCKS
- Check for protein transport or trafficking signals

Search for amino acid patterns defining a structural motif

- Hydrophobic membrane spanning regions
- Zinc fingers
- Leucine zippers
- Other motifs

Search for amino acid patterns present in this sequence and related sequences but not previously identified

- Find related sequences
- Perform a multiple sequence alignment
- Determine a consensus sequence to identify conserved amino acids, make profile
- Find the conserved regions which define motifs and conserved blocks of sequence using statistical methods (like HMMs)
- Search the sequence databases for more members defined by the profiles or motifs

Predict secondary structure of the protein from the amino acid sequence

- If a protein is related to another protein of known structure, predict approximate positions of amino acids in 3D structure
- Otherwise predict alpha helices, beta sheets and turns
- Predict protein class and search for complex patterns
- Look for amphiphobic regions (alternate hydrophobic and hydrophilic regions on alternate sides of structure - hydrophobic moment)

21.4. STRATEGIES AND OPTIONS FOR SIMILARITY SEARCH

Which program should be used to search a database? There is no easy and a single answer to this question. Many different similarity search programs are available. Several of these programs rely on shortcut algorithms that use a heuristic approach (based on a process of successive approximations). There is a tradeoff between sensitivity for detecting distantly related sequences versus the number of unrelated "false positives" that are found in a search.

Types of database searches

Type of search	Target database	Method	Type of query data	Programs that can be used	Output of the database search
Sequence similarity	Protein sequence or genomic sequence database	Search for database sequence that can be aligned with query sequence	Single sequence	FASTA, BLAST, WU-BLAST	List of database sequences having the most significant similarity scores
Alignment search with profile	Protein sequence database	Prepare profile from a MSA and align profile with database sequence	Profile representing gapped multiple sequence alignment	PROFILE SEARCH	List of database sequences that can be aligned with the profile
Search with PSSM representing ungapped sequence alignment (BLOCK)	Protein sequence database	Prepare PSSM from ungapped region of MSA or search for patterns of same length in unaligned sequences and then use for database search	PSSM representing ungapped alignment	MAST	List of database sequences with one or more patterns represented by PSSM but not necessarily in the same order
Iterative alignment search for similar sequences that starts with a query sequence, builds a gapped MSA, and then uses the alignment to augment the search	Protein sequence database	Uses initial matches to query sequence to build a type of scoring matrix and searches for additional matches to the matrix by an iterative search method	Build matches to query sequence	PSI-BLAST	PSI-BLAST finds a set of sequences related to each other by the presence of common patterns
Search query sequence for patterns representative of protein families	Database of patterns found in protein families	Search for patterns represented by scoring matrix or HMM	Single sequence	PROSITE, INTERPRO, PFAM, C DD/IMPA LA	List of sequence patterns found in query sequence

In general protein similarity searches are more sensitive than comparisons of DNA sequences. The DNA "alphabet" contains only 4 letters, while the amino acid alphabet has 20 letters, so the probability of chance matches is much greater with DNA-DNA comparisons. A pair of DNA bases can only be scored as a match or a mismatch, while two amino acids can share varying degrees of similarity based on their physical and chemical properties, similarity of DNA codons, and natural inter-mutation rates. The protein databanks are much smaller than the DNA databanks, so searches can be more sensitive without incurring too many false positives.

One of the first key decisions is whether you want to work on the Web, or in a custom program on your personal computer or an integrated environment like GCG. GCG gives the most flexibility to do further work with sequences that are found by the search, but may not be as simple as a Web server.

As a general strategy, it is best to start with the fastest tools. Initial searches should be done with both the BLAST and FASTA programs. You also need to decide whether to search protein or nucleotide databases. Generally if your query sequence is protein, you will search protein data, and with DNA sequence you will search nucleotide data (and this is the default for both BLAST and FASTA).

However, it is possible to automatically translate a DNA sequence into amino acids in all six reading frames (BLASTX) and compare it to protein databases, or to compare a protein sequence to the six reading frame translation of all DNA database sequences (TFASTA and TBLASTN). Searching translated databases uses a lot more computer power, so use this option sparingly - however, this is probably the best way to search the EST databases. Next, you need to decide what databases and what sections of those databases to search. Some researchers want to find every match to a given sequence, others may want to limit the search to humans or to mammals, or to the animal kingdom. The more you can restrict your search, the faster it will run and the fewer uninteresting hits you will have to sort through. Another important consideration is whether to search the EST, STS, and GSS and HTG (genomic survey sequence) databases. These "genome project" mass sequencing databases are very large, often unannotated and contain a lot of low quality "single pass sequence data". By leaving them out, your search will go significantly faster, and leave you with many fewer false matches to sort through. If you are starting with an essentially unknown sequence, then a match against an unannotated EST or genome fragment will probably not contribute much useful information. Once you have completed a search of the well-documented sections of the databases, you might run a separate search against the EST sections.

Framesearch

Framesearch is specifically designed for dealing with bad data. That is, it can find an alignment between a protein query and a nucleotide test sequence even if the latter contains frame-shifting gaps. There are a lot of sequences in the databases, primarily in the EST divisions, that contain many frame-shifts in the sequence. In a really junky sequence there might be multiple frame shifts, so that nothing is long enough to show up in BLAST or FASTA. Framesearch, unfortunately, is a very slow program, as it is an extended version of the Smith-Waterman method.

One thing that you might want to do, which is much less time consuming, is to run FRAMESEARCH directly against any EST hit you find with either FASTA or BLAST.

21.5. PRACTICAL CONSIDERATIONS IN SEQUENCE ANALYSIS

The following are some of the important issues and considerations for the analysis of sequences:

Predicting the protein structure

In general, protein three-dimensional (3D) structure can NOT be predicted from sequence. However, 3D structure can be predicted by homology modelling, i.e., by using a sequence homologue (>25% sequence identity) with an experimentally determined 3D structures. If no sequence homologue is found in PDB, there still is a chance to predict 3D structure by threading, i.e., by remote homology modelling (<25% sequence identity). However, correct 3D models -and even correct detection of remote homology - from threading are rare. But, theory can assist by predicting one-dimensional (1D) aspects of 3D structure, e.g., secondary structure, solvent accessibility, transmembrane helices, binding sites, sequence motifs, and aspects of protein function.

More than 30% pairwise sequence identity

Sequence analysis usually starts by searching homologues in databases. The success of alignment programs grounds on evolutionary connections between homologous proteins: if 24 out of 80 aligned residues (i.e. 30%; more for shorter matches) are identical between two naturally evolved proteins, the two have similar 3D structures and similar functions. The level of sequence identity significant for homology is much higher for smaller regions; for very short motifs (e.g. 'RGD', 'KDEL') homology can NOT be inferred from sequence identity.

Higher values for sequence similarity

If similarity scores (physico-chemical properties: D->E = 1) rather than identity scores (D->E =0; D->D = 1) are used to select homologues, the pairwise similarity, usually, has to be higher than 30% to be significant. A rule of thumb for true homologues is that for these similarity levels, scores are higher than identity scores. Similarity scores depend on the particular similarity metric used. Thus, results cannot be compared directly between different methods.

Constraints to significant identity: composition bias and gaps

There are two possible errors in inferring homology from a given level of pairwise sequence identity:

1. *Composition bias* : if the two aligned proteins have regions with a high composition of certain amino acids (e.g. ARG rich regions in DNA binding proteins) such regions may be important for protein function - and in many cases are indicative of functional class - but may be misleading for homology searches. Thus, composition biased regions should be ignored when compiling sequence identity, and be used only to confirm presence of similar composition bias in identified homologues.
2. *Many gaps* : if an alignment between two proteins contains too many insertions (gaps) even a relative high value of sequence identity may not suffice to ascertain homology (typical structure alignments contain up to 10% gaps).

Evolutionary patterns crucial for successful prediction of function

A typical mistake is to predict function by putative homology based on an over-interpreted level of sequence similarity. Functional and structural constraints are translated into sequence conservation in a particular way that depends on the particular protein structure and its evolution. The level of similarity required for identifying functionally equivalent proteins in two species depends on the overall divergence of the species and on the particular protein family.

Some databases use more reliable annotations than others

When predicting function based on similarity to proteins of known function (as annotated in databases), it is important to be aware of incomplete or wrong annotations. The annotations for the putative homologue ought to be verified in the original sources of the functional assignments (a more reliable database is SWISS-PROT). A similar problem arises for errors in sequences, such as frame-shifts or sequencing errors (very frequent in EST's).

Quality of alignment

Despite the central role that alignment programs play in sequence analysis, a thorough analysis of the quality of methods based on statistically significant numbers of proteins has yet to be accomplished. In general, alignments are more likely to be correct for higher levels of pairwise sequence identity; and are less likely to be correct in more variable regions.

Stability of alignment

Say you find three proteins you want to use to build a multiple alignment for your sequence of the unknown structure (U). In experiment A , you align them in the order 1-U (1 to U), 2-U, 3-U; in experiment B you inverse the order 3-U, 2-U, 1-U. The alignments of A and B may differ in detail.

Is it because of an error in the program? Not necessarily, the reason may, as well, be that the alignment is just not unique, i.e., the best and the second best solution to the alignment problem may have similar scores. In such cases the alignment is less reliable in regions where the results from A and B differ.

Sequence alignments reveal underlying evolutionary processes

Aligning protein sequences may appear to be purely a problem of matching letters. However, sequence alignments unravel information about structural and functional relations between residues in different proteins. Obviously it is not trivial to map the complexity of factors determining protein structure and function onto 1D relations between letters.

Evolutionary divergence within sequence families

In general, regions with many insertions and deletions in the alignment are less informative. For example, protein has 333 residues, 22 sequences are aligned in the N-terminal region, and only two near the C-term. One cannot draw firm conclusions about function and/or structure from the conservation patterns at the C-term. Do 20 sequences suffice for an informative alignment? Not necessarily. The information contained in a multiple alignment is determined rather by the divergence of the aligned sequences than by the number. Ideally, the entire range between 30-90% sequence identity should be covered, with preferably many sequences at lower levels (30-50%).

Extending local sequence motifs to entire folds

The goal of database searches is to find a good alignment for a full folding domain. This task is often very difficult in absence of 3D information. If you found a local motif (e.g. by a BLAST search), try to extend the alignment to cover the full core of the proteins. A good indication for a correct match is that motifs (or local hits from the BLAST search) appear in the same order in the final alignment.

Aligning entire families rather than subsets of sequences

Another helpful criterion indicative of true homologues is that the alignment rather than just a subset of sequences describe the 'full' protein family. In practice, searches often identify initially a few members of a given family. The aligned regions should then be investigated thoroughly: are local motifs compatible with the entire family? Are there other motifs that could be used to uncover further homologues by restricting the search to such motifs?

Is the pattern symmetrical, i.e., if protein U has been aligned to, e.g., the protein kinase family based on strong local motifs: do other patterns relevant for the kinase family match in U ? Incomplete family alignments are often indicative of a misleading local pattern and of falsely having aligned unrelated proteins.

Profile alignments may intrude into the grey area

In the twilight zone (20-30% pairwise sequence identity), sequence alignments become tricky. Only methods using profiles derived from the sequence family of protein U may reliably intrude into that zone. The quality of such alignments depends crucially on the information contained in the alignment, i.e., the size (number of sequences) and divergence (levels of pairwise sequence identity) of the sequence family. In sparse regions (less sequences) alignments are generally less reliable.

Predictions of protein structure in 1D

70% correct implies 30% incorrect. The most accurate methods for predicting secondary structure or solvent accessibility are based on multiple alignment information and reach levels of about 70% accuracy. This level of accuracy suffices to render useful predictions. However, in interpreting the predictions it is often instructive to spot the 30% of the residues you suspect to be falsely predicted.

Spread of prediction accuracy

An expected accuracy of 70% does NOT imply that for protein U 70% of all residues are correctly predicted. Instead, values published for prediction accuracy are averaged over hundreds of unique proteins. An expected accuracy of $70 \pm 10\%$ (one standard deviation) implies that, on average, for two thirds of all proteins between 60 and 80% of the residues will be predicted correctly. Thus, prediction accuracy can be higher than 80% or lower than 60% for protein U.

Special classes of proteins

Prediction methods are usually derived from knowledge contained in subsets of proteins from databases. Consequently, they should not be applied to classes of proteins that have not been included in the subsets. For example, methods for predicting helices in globular proteins are likely to fail when applied to predict transmembrane helices. In general, results should be taken with caution for proteins with unusual features, such as proline-rich regions, unusually many cysteine bonds, or for domain interfaces.

Better alignments yield better predictions

Multiple alignment-based predictions are substantially more accurate than single sequence-based predictions. How many sequences do you need in your alignment to expect an improvement; and how sensitive are prediction methods with respect to errors in the alignment? The more divergent sequences contained in the alignment, the better (two distantly related sequences often improve secondary structure predictions by several percentage points). Regions with few aligned sequences yield less reliable predictions. The sensitivity to alignment errors depends on the methods, e.g., secondary structure prediction is less sensitive to alignment errors than accessibility prediction.

1D structure may or may not be sufficient to infer 3D structure

Say you obtain as prediction for regular secondary structure: helix-strand-strand-helix-strand-strand (H-E-E-H-E-E). Assume, you find a protein of known structure with the same motif (H-E-E-H-E-E). Can you conclude that the two proteins have the same fold? Yes and no, your guess may be correct, but there are various ways to realise the given motif by completely different structures. For example, the secondary structure motif 'H-E-E-H-E-E' is contained in, at least, 16 structurally unrelated proteins.

Predicting 3D structure

A common mistake in using homology derived models of 3D structure is that the model is taken too literally. In general, accuracy of homology modelling decreases with lower levels of pairwise sequence identity between the sequence and the target structure. Models accurate enough to simulate ligand binding in detail require levels of above 90% pairwise sequence identity. Furthermore, successful applications of homology modelling may be hampered by two other difficulties.

1. Loop regions are, in general, less reliable.
2. Accurate predictions for regions with insertions or deletions, i.e., regions where the template structure does not match the sequence, are the exceptions.

Remote homology modelling (threading) is highly judgemental

One problem of homology modelling for lower levels of pairwise sequence identity is to get the alignment between a sequence U and the template structure T correct. But even if the alignments were correct, a major limitation is that T and U just do NOT have identical 3D structures. This problem is particularly fatal for remote homology modelling (threading), i.e., prediction of 3D structure based on less than 25% pairwise sequence identity. However, current threading methods are even more limited: getting the alignment correct is the exception rather than the rule.

21.6. FLOWCHART FOR PROTEIN STRUCTURE PREDICTION

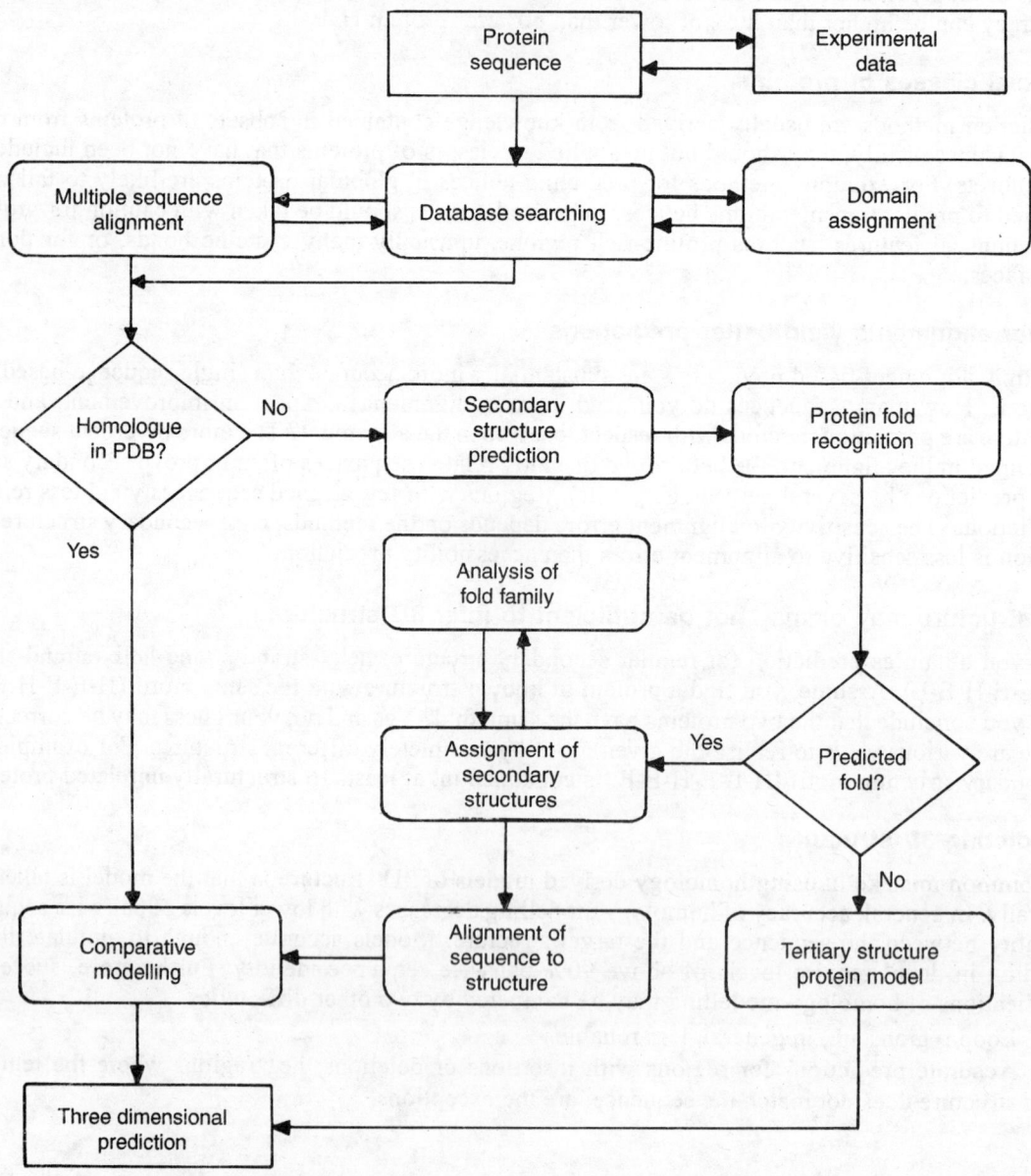

21.7. ILLUSTRATIONS : SOME PROBLEMS AND SOLUTIONS

1. You have an unknown protein sequence and you would like to know whether it contains regions similar to known proteins or protein domains

One of the possible approaches to this problem is as follows :

1. GenQuest E-Mail server or WWW site. GENQUEST is an integrated sequence comparison server which allows users to make use of a wide variety of sequence comparison methods and target databases. The purpose of the system is to allow rapid and sensitive comparison of DNA and protein sequences to existing DNA and protein sequence databases. The databases which can be accessed from the GENQUEST server include: GSDB, SWISSPROT, PROSITE, PDB, BLOCKS and dbEST.

2. ScanProsite tool, compare your sequence to PROSITE database. PROSITE is a method of determining what is the function of uncharacterized proteins translated from genomic or cDNA sequences. It consists of a database of biologically significant sites, patterns and profiles that help to reliably identify to which known family of protein (if any) a new sequence belongs.

3. BLOCKS database. Compare your protein or DNA sequences to a database of highly conserved protein regions.

4. PRODOM, A Protein Domain Database. The ProDom database is a comprehensive collection of protein families. It was constructed by clustering all complete protein sequences in Swiss-prot by the clustering algorithm Domainer. The novelty of ProDom is that the modular arrangement of proteins has been taken into account and whenever domain boundaries were detected the sequences were cut to produce consistent families of domains. The domain families produced by Domainer are stored both as multiple alignments and consensus sequences. To compare your sequence to PRODOM database go to the section "Search ProDom with blast".

5. PRINTS, Protein Motif Fingerprint Database. PRINTS is a compendium of protein fingerprints. A fingerprint is a group of conserved motifs used to characterise a protein family; Usually the motifs do not overlap, but are separated along a sequence, though they may be contiguous in 3D-space. Fingerprints can encode protein folds and functionalities more flexibly and powerfully than can single motifs: the database thus provides a useful adjunct to PROSITE.

6. Pfam, a high-quality comprehensive collection of protein domain families.

2. You have an unknown DNA sequence and you would like to analyse it for the existence of known consensus sequences

1. GRAIL. The current e-mail implementation of GRAIL provides analysis of protein coding potential of a DNA sequence, and an option for protein sequence database searches of putative coding regions.

2. GRAIL browser. This is freely distributed software for sequence analysis that runs on Unix systems.

3. How would you search for transcription factor binding sites in an unknown DNA sequence

Possibly use the following :

MatInspector, Search for potential binding sites in the sequence.

- TESS, Transcription Element Search Software. A set of software for locating and displaying transcription factor binding sites in DNA sequence. TESS uses the Transfac database as its store of transcription factors and their binding sites.

4. There is a list of ESTs of which the gene origin and biological function are unknown. How can we find homologous sequences in the nucleotide and protein databases, given the GenBank accession numbers of these ESTs?

1. Retrieve the GenBank entry for the EST
   - In the "Search Field" field, choose "Accession" (instead of "All Fields").
   - Enter the Accession Number in the text box.
   - Press on "Search".
   - In the resulting page, press on "Retrieve 1 Document".
   - In the resulting page, press on the blue link to "GenBank Report".
2. Perform a BLAST search against GenBank
   - In the field that starts with the words "Enter here your input data as:" choose "Accession or GI" (instead of "Sequence in FASTA format").
   - Enter the Accession Number in the box below.
   - Press on "Submit Query".
3. Search Unigene
   - In the Unigene database, ESTs are clustered to form a unique Human Gene Sequence Collection.
   - Enter the Accession Number in the text box.
   - In the resulting page, press on the blue/purple link(s).
4. Perform a Smith-Waterman search using the Bioccelerator
   - Search nucleotide and protein databases using the Bioccelerator if no satisfactory results were obtained in the previous searches.

5. How can you find all open reading frames in a given sequence?

Use ORF Finder at NCBI. The ORF Finder is a graphical analysis tool that finds all open reading frames of a selectable minimum size in a user's sequence or in a sequence already in the database. This tool identifies all open reading frames using the standard or alternative genetic codes. The deduced amino acid sequence can be saved in various formats and searched against the sequence database using the BLAST. The ORF Finder should be helpful in preparing complete and accurate sequence submissions. It is also packaged with the Sequin sequence submission software.

6. How do we find a restriction map of a given DNA sequence?

Use the following :
- WebCutter, an on-line tool for restriction mapping nucleotide sequences.
- TACG - restriction enzyme analysis and mapping.
- SeqPup, a biological sequence editor and analysis program which you will have to copy to your computer

7. Align the following sequences (using BLOSUM80):

Sequence 1: DALTNA
Sequence 2: DLLVAQTNAMSDA
Use the overlap matches method and use gap penalty of –5

	D	A	L	T	N	A
A						
D						
S						
M						
A						
N						
T						
Q						
A						
V						
L						
L						
D						

Use the result from your matrix to determine what would be the alignment if the two sequences were:
Sequence1: DALTNA
Sequence2: DLLVA

8. Align the following sequences use Threshold of 12:

Sequence 1: DALTNA
Sequence 2: DLLVAQTNAMSDA
Use repeated match method (using BLOSUM80)
Use repeated match method (using BLOSUM35)
Use global method (using BLOSUM80) with a gap penalty of -8

BLOSUM80

```
      A   R   N   D   C   Q   E   G   H   I   L   K   M   F   P   S   T   W   Y   V   B   Z   X
A     7  -3  -3  -3  -1  -2  -2   0  -3  -3  -3  -1  -2  -4  -1   2   0  -5  -4  -1  -3  -2  -1
R    -3   9  -1  -3  -6   1  -1  -4   0  -5  -4   3  -3  -5  -3  -2  -2  -5  -4  -4  -2   0  -2
N    -3  -1   9   2  -5   0  -1  -1   1  -6  -6   0  -4  -6  -4   1   0  -7  -4  -5   5  -1  -2
D    -3  -3   2  10  -7  -1   2  -3  -2  -7  -7  -2  -6  -6  -3  -1  -2  -8  -6   6   6   1  -3
C    -1  -6  -5  -7  13  -5  -7  -6  -7  -2  -3  -6  -3  -4  -6  -2  -2  -5  -5  -2  -6  -7  -4
Q    -2   1   0  -1  -5   9   3  -4   1  -5  -4   2  -1  -5  -3  -1  -1  -4  -3  -4  -1   5  -2
E    -2  -1  -1   2  -7   3   8  -4   0  -6  -6   1  -4  -6  -2  -1  -2  -6  -5  -4   1   6  -2
G     0  -4  -1  -3  -6  -4  -4   9  -4  -7  -7  -3  -5  -6  -5  -1  -3  -6  -6  -6  -2  -4  -3
H    -3   0   1  -2  -7   1   0  -4  12  -6  -5  -1  -4  -2  -4  -2  -3  -4   3  -5  -1   0  -2
I    -3  -5  -6  -7  -2  -5  -6  -7  -6   7   2  -5   2  -1  -5  -4  -2  -5  -3   4  -6  -6  -2
L    -3  -4  -6  -7  -3  -4  -6  -7  -5   2   6  -4   3   0  -5  -4  -3  -4  -2   1  -7  -5  -2
K    -1   3   0  -2  -6   2   1  -3  -1  -5  -4   8  -3  -5  -2  -1  -1  -6  -4  -4  -1   1  -2
M    -2  -3  -4  -6  -3  -1  -4  -5  -4   2   3  -3   9   0  -4  -3  -1   3  -3   1  -5   3  -2
F    -4  -5  -6  -6  -4  -5  -6  -6  -2  -1   0  -5   0  10  -6  -4  -4   0   4  -2  -6  -6  -3
P    -1  -3  -4  -3  -6  -3  -2  -5  -4  -5  -5  -2  -4  -6  12  -2  -3  -7  -6  -4  -4  -2  -3
S     2  -2   1  -1  -2  -1  -1  -1  -2  -4  -4  -1  -3  -4  -2   7   2  -6  -3  -3   0  -1  -1
T     0  -2   0  -2  -2  -1  -2  -3  -3  -2  -3  -1  -1  -4  -3   2   8  -5  -3   0  -1  -2  -1
W    -5  -5  -7  -8  -5  -4  -6  -6  -4  -5  -4  -6  -3   0  -7  -6  -5  16   3  -5  -8  -5  -5
Y    -4  -4  -4  -6  -5  -3  -5  -6   3  -3  -2  -4   3   4  -6  -3  -3   3  11  -3  -5  -4  -3
V    -1  -4  -5  -6  -2  -4  -4  -6  -5   4   1  -4   1  -2  -4  -3   0  -5  -3   7  -6  -4  -2
B    -3  -2   5   6  -6  -1   1  -2  -1  -6  -7  -1  -5  -6  -4   0  -1  -8  -5  -6   6   0  -3
Z    -2   0  -1   1  -7   5   6  -4   0  -6  -5   1  -3   6  -2  -1  -2  -5  -4  -4   0   6  -1
X    -1  -2  -2  -3  -4  -2  -2  -3  -2  -2  -2  -2  -2  -3  -3  -1  -1  -5  -3  -2  -3  -1  -2
```

A	5	17	12	7	11	23
D	10	5	2	9	16	11
S	-1	-1	7	14	9	12
M	-5	4	12	7	5	17
A	-3	9	4	-1	10	22
N	2	-3	-7	1	15	10
T	-2	-1	-6	6	3	8
Q	-1	-3	-2	3	8	10
A	-3	2	3	8	10	15
V	-5	-1	8	13	8	3
L	0	2	13	8	3	-2
L	5	7	11	6	1	-1
D	10	5	0	-2	2	-3
	D	A	L	T	N	A

The resulting alignment is:

```
DLLVAQTNMSDA
.......DALTNA
```

Use the result from your matrix to determine what would be the alignment if the two sequence were:

Sequence1:DALTNA

Sequence2:DLLVA

The resulting alignment would be:

```
DALTNA
DLLV-A
```

BLOSUM35

```
     A   R   N   D   C   Q   E   G   H   I   L   K   M   F   P   S   T   W   Y   V   B   Z   X
A    5  -1  -1  -1  -2   0  -1   0  -2  -1  -2   0   0  -2  -2   1   0  -2  -1   0  -1  -1   0
R   -1   8  -1  -1  -3   2  -1  -2  -1  -3  -2   2   0  -1  -2  -1  -2   0   0  -1  -1   0  -1
N   -1  -1   7   1  -1   1  -1   1   1  -1  -2   0  -1  -1  -2   0   0  -2  -2  -2   4   0   0
D   -1  -1   1   8  -3  -1   2  -2   0  -3  -2  -1  -3  -3  -1  -1  -1  -3  -2  -2   5   1  -1
C   -2  -3  -1  -3  15  -3  -1  -3  -4  -4  -2  -2  -4  -4  -4  -3  -1  -5  -5  -2  -2  -2  -2
Q    0   2   1  -1  -3   7   2  -2  -1  -2  -2   0  -1  -4   0   0   0  -1   0  -3   0   4  -1
E   -1  -1  -1   2  -1   2   6  -2  -1  -3  -1   1  -2  -3   0   0  -1  -1  -1  -2   0   5  -1
G    0  -2   1  -2  -3  -2  -2   7  -2  -3  -3  -1  -1  -3  -2   1  -2  -1  -2  -3   0  -2  -1
H   -2  -1   1   0  -4  -1  -1  -2  12  -3  -2  -2   1  -3  -1  -1  -2  -4   0  -4   0  -1  -1
I   -1  -3  -1  -3  -4  -2  -3  -3  -3   5   2  -2   1   1  -1  -2  -1  -1   0   4  -2  -3   0
L   -2  -2  -2  -2  -2  -2  -1  -3  -2   2   5  -2   3   2  -3  -2   0   0   0   2  -2  -2   0
K    0   2   0  -1  -2   0   1  -1  -2  -2  -2   5   0  -1   0   0   0   0  -1  -2   0   1   0
M    0   0  -1  -3  -4  -1  -2  -1   1   1   3   0   6   0  -3  -1   0   1   0   1  -2  -2   0
F   -2  -1  -1  -3  -4  -4  -3  -3  -3   1   2  -1   0   8  -4  -1  -1   1   3   1  -2  -3  -1
P   -2  -2  -2  -1  -4   0   0  -2  -1  -1  -3   0  -3  -4  10  -2   0  -4  -3  -3  -1   0  -1
S    1  -1   0  -1  -3   0   0   1  -1  -2  -2   0  -1  -1  -2   4   2  -2  -1  -2   0   0   0
T    0  -2   0  -1   1   0  -1  -2  -2  -1   0   0   0  -1   0   2   5  -2  -2   1  -1  -1   0
W   -2   0  -2  -3  -5  -1  -1  -1  -4  -1   0   0   1   1  -4  -2  -2  16   3  -2  -3  -1  -1
Y   -1   0  -2  -2  -5   0  -1  -2   0   0   0  -1   0   3  -3  -1  -2   3   8   0  -2  -1  -1
V    0  -1  -2  -2  -2  -3  -2  -3  -4   4   2  -2   1   1  -3  -1   1  -2   0   5  -2  -2   0
B   -1  -1   4   5  -2   0   0   0   0  -2  -2   0  -2  -2  -1   0  -1  -3  -2  -2   5   0  -1
Z   -1   0   0   1  -2   4   5  -2  -1  -3  -2   1  -2  -3   0   0  -1  -1  -2  -2   0   4   0
X    0  -1   0  -1  -2  -1  -1  -1  -1   0   0   0   0  -1  -1   0   0  -1  -1   0  -1   0  -1
```

Global   gap =   -8

A	-104	| -86 / -71	| -60	| -50	| -34	/ or | -19
D	-96	/ -78 | -63	| -52	| -42	| -26	| -11
S	-88	| -70 | -55	| -44	/ -34	| -18	| -3
M	-80	| -62 | -47	/ -36	| -27	| -10	| 5
A	-72	| -54 / -39	/ -34	| -19	| -2	/ 13
N	-64	| -46 | -31	| -26	| -11	/ 6	-- -2
T	-56	| -38 | -23	/ -18	/ -3	/ -3	/ 5
Q	-48	| -30 | -15	/ -11	| -3	/ 5	/ 8
A	-40	| -22 / -7	| -3	/ 5	/ 10	/ 12
V	-32	| -14 / -7	| 5	/ 13	-- 5	/ -4
L	-24	| -6 / -1	/ 13	/ 5	-- -3	/ -11
L	-16	| 2 / 7	/ 8	-- 0	-- -8	-- -16
D	-8	/ 10 -- 2	-- -6	-- -14	-- -22	-- -30
		-8	-16	-24	-32	-40	-48
		D	A	L	T	N	A

Alignment: DLLVAQTNAMSDA or   DLLVAQTNAMSDA
           D---ALTN----A   D---ALTNA----

Repeat Match   gap =   -8   Threshold = 12

BLOSUM80

15							
15	A	15	15	15	15	15	15
15	D	15	15	15	15	15	15
15	S	15	15	15	15	15	
15	M	15	15	15	15	15	| 19
8	A	8	/ 9	8	8	| 12	/ 27
1	N	/ 2	1	1	| 3	/ 20	-- 12
1	T	1	1	1	/ 11	-- 3	/ 5
1	Q	1	1	/ 3	1	/ 5	/ 8
1	A	1	/ 7	1	| 5	/ 10	/ 12
1	V	1	1	| 5	/ 13	-- 5	1
0	L	0	0	/ 13	/ 5	0	0
0	L	| 2	/ 7	/ 8	-- 0	0	0
0	D	/ 10	-- 2	0	0	/ 2	0
		D	A	L	T	N	A

Alignment: DLLVAQTNAMSDA

DALTALTNA....

BLOSUM35

8							
8	A	8	/ 13	8	8	8	/ 17
8	D	/ 8	8	8	8	/ 12	8
8	S	8	8	8	/ 11	8	8
8	M	8	8	/ 9	8	8	| 12
3	A	3	/ 6	3	3	| 7	/ 20
0	N	/ 1	0	0	0	/ 15	-- 7
0	T	0	0	0	/ 8	0	/ 5
0	Q	0	0	/ 3	0	/ 5	/ 11
0	A	0	/ 5	0	| 4	/ 11	/ 9
0	V	0	0	| 3	/ 12	-- 4	0
0	L	0	0	/ 11	/ 5	0	0
0	L	0	/ 6	/ 5	0	0	0
0	D	/ 8	0	0	0	/ 1	0
0		D	A	L	T	N	A

Alignment: DLLVAQTNAMSDA

....ALTNA....

9. Imagine you want to calculate the shortest common super-sequence, i.e. the shortest sequence to which all sequences can be aligned without mismatches. Which cost/ weight scheme can you use?

Despite its name, the shortest common super-sequence cannot be shorter than the longest of the sequences. Cast the problem "columns first", and imagine how the cost of a column should be defined. If you do it right, there will be a simple relation between the cost of the whole > multiple alignment and the length of the super-sequence. The cost of a column is simply the number of distinct symbols from the alphabet A that appear in a column. Then the overall cost is the length of the super-sequence. E.g., the shortest common super-sequence of ECDEAECEC, CDEECAC, and CEC is ECDEAECEAC, and one possible "alignment" of cost 10 is as follows, ECDEAECE-C -CDE-EC-AC ———CE-C. (Note that (E,-) is not a mismatch, but a deletion.)

10. Write a perl program to convert a nucleotide (DNA or RNA) sequence to an amino acid sequence according to the genetic code. It should have options that support different reading frames, reversing the sequence, and complementing the sequence

The possible program is as follows :

```
#!/usr/bin/perl
#         genetic_translation - a perl program
#         syntax : genetic_translation -c -r -f[1-3] -i "inputfile" -o "outputfile"
#
#         Options:
#                 -c        complement the nucleotide sequence before conversion
#                 -r        reverse the nucleotide sequence before conversion
#                 -f[1-3]   specifies reading frame 1, 2, or 3
#                 -i        "inputfile" name the nucleotide (input) file; defaults to STDIN
#                 -o        "outputfile" name the amino acid (output) file; defaults to STDOUT
#                 -dna      takes the sequence to be a DNA sequence
#                 -rna      takes the sequence to be an RNA sequence
####################################################################
# Start with important constants
$DEBUG = 0;       # Set level for debug information: 0 none and on up
$prg_name = "genetic_translation";
$frame = 1;       # Frame defaults to 1
@base_list_DNA = ("T","C","A","G");       # Typical order of DNA bases for a table
@base_list_RNA = ("U","C","A","G");       # Typical order of RNA bases for a table
&build_genetic_code();
if ($DEBUG >= 6) {
   print STDERR &genetic_code_table(3);
}
####################################################################
#   Supported nucleic acid codes:
#         A —> adenosine              M —> A C (amino)
#         C —> cytidine               S —> G C (strong)
#         G —> guanine                W —> A T (weak)
#         T —> thymidine              B —> G T C
#         U —> uridine                D —> G A T
#         R —> G A (purine)           H —> A C T
#         Y —> T C (pyrimidine)       V —> G C A
#         K —> G T (keto)             N —> A G C T (any)
#                                     - gap of indeterminate length
```

```
#    These come from the FASTA format.
################################################################################
@nucleic_acid_codes = ("A","C","G","T","U","R","Y","K","M","S","W","B","D","H","V","N","-");
$nucleic_acid_string = join("",@nucleic_acid_codes);
################################################################################
#    Supported amino acid codes:
#         A  alanine                      P  proline
#         B  aspartate or asparagine      Q  glutamine
#         C  cystine                      R  arginine
#         D  aspartate                    S  serine
#         E  glutamate                    T  threonine
#         F  phenylalanine                U  selenocysteine
#         G  glycine                      V  valine
#         H  histidine                    W  tryptophan
#         I  isoleucine                   Y  tyrosine
#         K  lysine                       Z  glutamate or glutamine
#         L  leucine                      X  any
#         M  methionine                   *  translation stop
#         N  asparagine                   -  gap of indeterminate length
#    These come from the FASTA format.
################################################################################
@amino_acid_codes = ("A","B","C","D","E","F","G","H","I","K","L","M","N","P","Q","R","S","T","U","V","W",
                     "Y","Z","X","*","-");
$amino_acid_string = join("",@amino_acid_codes);
################################################################################
#         Start processing
################################################################################
# Open a log file
open(LOG,">$prg_name.log") ||progress_log("FATAL","log file $prg_name.log cannot be opened");
# Process command line arguments
while ($argument = shift(@ARGV)) {
   if ($argument eq "-c") {
        $complement_sequence = 1;
        progress_log("NORMAL","Complement sequence option in force.");
   } elsif ($argument eq "-r") {
        $reverse_sequence = 1;
        progress_log("NORMAL","Reverse sequence option in force.");
   } elsif ($argument =~ m/^-f([1-3])/) {
        $frame = $1;
        progress_log("NORMAL","Using reading frame $frame.");
   } elsif ($argument =~ m/^-dna$/i) {   # A DNA sequence
        $dna_flag_command_line = 1;
        progress_log("NORMAL","Have an RNA sequence.");
   } elsif ($argument =~ m/^-rna$/i) {   # An RNA sequence
        $rna_flag_command_line = 1;
        progress_log("NORMAL","Have an RNA sequence.");
   } elsif ($argument eq "-i") {
        $input_file = shift(@ARGV);
        progress_log("NORMAL","Input file is $input_file.");
```

```
      } elsif ($argument eq "-o") {
             $output_file = shift(@ARGV);
             progress_log("NORMAL","Output file is $output_file.");
      } else {
             progress_log("FATAL","Argument <$argument> invalid or not recognized");
      }
}
if ($dna_flag_command_line && $rna_flag_command_line) {
      progress_log("FATAL","Cannot have both -dna and -rna flags");
}
if ($input_file eq "") {
      progress_log("NORMAL","Taking input from STDIN");
      $input_file_handle = STDIN;
      $input_file = "standard input";
      progress_log("NORMAL","Input taken from standard input.");
} elsif (open(NUCLEOTIDE,$input_file)) {
      progress_log("NORMAL","Ready to process nucleotide file $input_file");
      $input_file_handle = NUCLEOTIDE;
} else {
      progress_log("FATAL","Unable to open nucleotide file $input_file");
}
if ($output_file eq "") {
      progress_log("NORMAL","Sending output to STDOUT");
      $output_file_handle = STDOUT;
      $output_file = "standard output";
      progress_log("NORMAL",
             "Send aa sequence to standard output.");
} elsif (open(AAS,">$output_file")) {
      progress_log("NORMAL","Send output to aa file $output_file");
      $output_file_handle = AAS;
} else {
      progress_log("FATAL","Unable to open aa file $output_file");
}
#   Retrieve one nucleotide sequence from the input file and verify the syntax
#          Lower case is converted to upper case.
#          The file must contain only the 5 allowed bases, N (any base),and white space.  White space is removed.
$nucleotide_sequence = "";  # string for accumulating the input sequence
while ($line = <$input_file_handle>) {
      $line_number++;
      if ($line =~ m/-/) {
             progress_log("FATAL","Gap character - not allowed in $input_file" .
                " line $line_number");
      }
      chomp($line);
      $line =~ s/\s_//g;              # Remove all white space
      $line =~ tr/[a-z]/[A-Z]/;
```

```perl
        if ($line =~ m/([^ACTGUN])/) {
            progress_log("FATAL","Invalid character <$1> found in $input_file" .
                " line $line_number");
        }
        if ($line =~ m/T/) {
            $dna_flag = 1;              # Contains T, must be DNA
            if ($rna_flag_command_line) {
                progress_log("FATAL","-rna on the command line, but a T" .
                    " in $input_file");
            }
        }
        if ($line =~ m/U/) {
            $rna_flag = 1;              # Contains U, must be RNA
            if ($dna_flag_command_line) {
                progress_log("FATAL","-dna on the command line, but a U" .
                    " in $input_file");
            }
        }
        $nucleotide_sequence .= $line;      # Accumulate the sequence
    }
    if ($dna_flag && $rna_flag) {
        progress_log("FATAL","$input_file contains both T and U.");
    }
    if ($complement_sequence) {
        if ($rna_flag) {    # Alternate translation for RNA
            $nucleotide_sequence =~ tr/[ACGUN]/[UGCAN]/;
        } else {            # Default translation is for DNA
            $nucleotide_sequence =~ tr/[ACGTN]/[TGCAN]/;
        }
    }
    if ($reverse_sequence) {
        $nucleotide_sequence = reverse($nucleotide_sequence);
    }
    print $nucleotide_sequence, "\n";
    #   Generate the output amino acid file
    progress_log("NORMAL","Creating amino acid file $output_file");
    $nucleic_sequence_length = length $nucleotide_sequence;
    if ($frame == 1) {  # Translation starts exactly at the beginning!
        $AA_sequence = "";
    } else {    # One or two untranslated nucleotides at the beginning!
        $AA_sequence = "X";
    }
    for ($index = $frame-1; $index+3 <= $nucleic_sequence_length; $index += 3) {
        # translate a codon to an amino acid
        $codon = substr($nucleotide_sequence,$index,3);
        if ($codon =~ m/N/) {       # codon contains an unknown base
            $one_letter = "X";
```

```
    } else {
        $one_letter = $codon2one_letter{$codon};
    }
    $AA_sequence .= $one_letter;
    if (DEBUG > 0) {
        progress_log("NORMAL","Translated codon \"$codon\" to $one_letter");
    }
}
if ($index != $nucleic_sequence_length) {          # Something at the end!
    $AA_sequence .= "X";
}
print $output_file_handle "$AA_sequence\n";
progress_log("NORMAL","Successful creation of amino acid sequence");
#          &progress_log(type,message);
#
# This subroutine logs messages of different general categories with respect to the progress of the parsing and
# later processing. The log type is one of "NORMAL", "WARNING", "SERIOUS", and "FATAL", in increasing
# order of distress.seriousness
sub progress_log {
    my $type = $_[0];
    my $message = $_[1];
if ($type eq "NORMAL") {
    print LOG "$prg_name: $message\n";
} elsif ($type eq "WARNING") {
    print LOG "$prg_name: WARNING ", ++$warnings, ": $message\n";
} elsif ($type eq "SERIOUS") {
    print LOG "$prg_name: SERIOUS ERROR ", ++$serious, ": $message\n";
} else {
    print LOG "$prg_name: FATAL ERROR: $message\n";
    die "$prg_name: FATAL ERROR: $message\n";
}
}
#   build_genetic_code() Subroutine to build the genetic code hashes, which are:
#                  AA2three_letter          amino acid name to 3-letter amino acid
#                  AA2one_letter            amino acid name to 1-letter amino acid
#                  one_letter2AA            1-letter amino acid to amino acid
#                  three_letter2AA          3-letter amino acid to amino acid
#                  three_letter2one_letter  3-letter to 1-letter amino acid
#                  one_letter2three_letter  1-letter to 3-letter amino acid
#                  codon2AA                 3 bases to amino acid
#                  codon2one_letter   3 bases to one-letter amino acid
#                  codon2three_letter 3 bases to three-letter amino acid
sub build_genetic_code {
# Initialize global hashes so we can run this more than once
```

```perl
%AA2three_letter = ();
%AA2one_letter = ();
%three_letter2AA = ();
%one_letter2AA = ();
%three_letter2one_letter = ();
%one_letter2three_letter = ();
%codon2AA = ();
%codon2one_letter = ();
%codon2three_letter = ();


my $amino_acid_codes =
"A        Alanine  Ala\
C        Cystine  Cys\
D        Aspartic acid     Asp\
E        Glutamic acid     Glu\
F        Phenylalanine     Phe\
G        Glycine  Gly\
H        Histidine His\
I        Isoleucine        Ile\
K        Lysine            Lys\
L        Leucine  Leu\
M        Methionine        Met\
N        Asparagine        Asn\
P        Proline           Pro\
Q        Glutamine         Gln\
R        Arginine Arg\
S        Serine            Ser\
T        Threonine         Thr\
V        Valine            Val\
W        Tryptophan        Trp\
Y        Tyrosine Tyr\
X        Any               Any\
*        Translation stop  End\
-        Gap of indeterminate length  Gap\n";

@amino_acid_lines = split(/\n/,$amino_acid_codes);
while ($line = pop @amino_acid_lines) {
    ($one_letter,$amino_acid_name,$three_letter) = split(/\t+/,$line);
    $AA2three_letter{$amino_acid_name} = $three_letter;
    $AA2one_letter{$amino_acid_name} = $one_letter;
    $three_letter2AA{$three_letter} = $amino_acid_name;
    $one_letter2AA{$one_letter} = $amino_acid_name;
    $three_letter2one_letter{$three_letter} = $one_letter;
    $one_letter2three_letter{$one_letter} = $three_letter;
}
```

```
my $codon_to_AA =
"TTT    F\
TCT    S\
TAT    Y\
TGT    C\
TTC    F\
TCC    S\
TAC    Y\
TGC    C\
TTA    L\
TCA    S\
TAA    *\
TGA    *\
TTG    L\
TCG    S\
TAG    *\
TGG    W\
CTT    L\
CCT    P\
CAT    H\
CGT    R\
CTC    L\
CCC    P\
CAC    H\
CGC    R\
CTA    L\
CCA    P\
CAA    Q\
CGA    R\
CTG    L\
CCG    P\
CAG    Q\
CGG    R\
ATT    I\
ACT    T\
AAT    N\
AGT    S\
ATC    I\
ACC    T\
AAC    N\
AGC    S\
ATA    I\
ACA    T\
AAA    K\
AGA    R\
ATG    M\
ACG    T\
AAG    K\
AGG    R\
```

```
GTT      V\
GCT      A\
GAT      D\
GGT      G\
GTC      V\
GCC      A\
GAC      D\
GGC      G\
GTA      V\
GCA      A\
GAA      E\
GGA      G\
GTG      V\
GCG      A\
GAG      E\
GGG      G\n";

@codon_lines = split(/\n/,$codon_to_AA);
while ($line = pop @codon_lines) {
    ($codon,$one_letter) = split(/\t+/,$line);
    $codon2AA{$codon} = $one_letter2AA{$one_letter};
    $codon2one_letter{$codon} = $one_letter;
    $codon2three_letter{$codon} = $one_letter2three_letter{$one_letter};
}

if ($DEBUG >= 7) {
    print STDERR "$prg_name: Dumping amino acid name to 3-letter code:\n";
    foreach $amino_acid_name (keys(%AA2three_letter)) {
        print STDERR "$amino_acid_name\t$AA2three_letter{$amino_acid_name}\n";
    }
    print STDERR "$prg_name: Dumping amino acid name to 1-letter code:\n";
    foreach $amino_acid_name (keys(%AA2one_letter)) {
        print STDERR "$amino_acid_name\t$AA2one_letter{$amino_acid_name}\n";
    }
    print STDERR "$prg_name: Dumping 3-letter code to amino acid name:\n";
    foreach $three_letter (keys(%three_letter2AA)) {
        print STDERR "$three_letter\t$three_letter2AA{$three_letter}\n";
    }
    print STDERR "$prg_name: Dumping 1-letter code to amino acid name:\n";
    foreach $one_letter (keys(%one_letter2AA)) {
        print STDERR "$one_letter\t$one_letter2AA{$one_letter}\n";
    }
    print STDERR "$prg_name: Dumping 3-letter code to 1-letter code:\n";
    foreach $three_letter (keys(%three_letter2one_letter)) {
        print STDERR "$three_letter\t$three_letter2one_letter{$three_letter}\n";
    }
    print STDERR "$prg_name: Dumping 1-letter code to 3-letter code:\n";
    foreach $one_letter (keys(%one_letter2three_letter)) {
        print STDERR "$one_letter\t$one_letter2three_letter{$one_letter}\n";
```

```perl
    }
    print STDERR "$prg_name: Dumping codon to amino acid name:\n";
    foreach $codon (keys(%codon2AA)) {
        print STDERR "$codon\t$codon2AA{$codon}\n";
    }
    print STDERR "$prg_name: Dumping codon to 1-letter code:\n";
    foreach $codon (keys(%codon2one_letter)) {
        print STDERR "$codon\t$codon2one_letter{$codon}\n";
    }
    print STDERR "$prg_name: Dumping codon to 3-letter code:\n";
    foreach $codon (keys(%codon2three_letter)) {
        print STDERR "$codon\t$codon2three_letter{$codon}\n";
    }
}
}
#   genetic_code_table($dimensions) subroutine to build the typical 3-dimensional table of the genetic code that
#   maps codons to amino acids or a simple one-dimensional version.
sub genetic_code_table {
my $dimensions = $_[0];
my @base_list = @base_list_DNA;
my $base_list_last = $base_list_DNA - 1;
my $table = "";
if ($dimensions == 1) {
  foreach $base1 (@base_list) {
        foreach $base2 (@base_list) {
            foreach $base3 (@base_list) {
                $codon = $base1 . $base2 . $base3;
                $table .= "$codon\t$codon2AA{$codon}\t" .
                  "($codon2three_letter{$codon})\t" .
                  "[$codon2one_letter{$codon}]\n";

            }
        }

    }
} elsif ($dimensions == 3) {
  foreach $base1 (@base_list) {
        foreach $base3 (@base_list) {
            foreach $base2 (@base_list) {
                $codon = $base1 . $base2 . $base3;
                $table .= "$codon\t$codon2AA{$codon} " .
                  "($codon2three_letter{$codon}) " .
                  "[$codon2one_letter{$codon}]";
                if ($base2 ne $base_list[$base_list_last]) {
                    $table .= "\t";
                } else {
                    $table .= "\n";
                }
            }
        }
    }
```

```
} else {
    progress_log("FATAL","genetic_code_table asked to build a table " .
        "of $dimensions dimensions\n");
}
return $table;
}
```

11. There is a small protein R and it has been determined that its sequence is :
    rrmiptsfsskfqgvlsmnaveddrgsstgdaigv
    1. What are four DNA sequences that could be the open reading frame from which the mRNA for protein R was transcribed? (Assume there are no introns.) Be sure to include a stop codon in each sequence.
    2. There are many coding sequences that could be the open reading frame for protein R (again, assuming no introns). How would you compute the number of sequences, and what is the number?

There are infinite, but a large number of ORFs that could be the one that gave the particular protein R. A convenient way to get at these possible ORFs is to build a reverse genetic table that gives for each code in a protein (including the Stop code *) a list of those codons from which it might arise through translation. Here is such a table:

	Amino Acid Code	All Codons for that Amino Acid
	A	gct, gcc, gca, gcg
C	tgt, tgc	
D	gat, gac	
E	gaa, gag	
F	ttt, ttc	
G	ggt, ggc, gga, ggg	
H	cat, cac	
I	att, atc, ata	
K	aaa, aag	
L	tta, ttg, ctt, ctc, cta, ctg	
M	atg	
N	aat, aac	
P	cct, ccc, cca, ccg	
Q	caa, cag	
R	cgt, cgc, cga, cgg, aga, agg	
S	tct, tcc, tca, tcg, agt, agc	
T	act, acc, aca, acg	
V	gtt, gtc, gta, gtg	
W	tgg	
Y	tat, tac	
	* (Stop)	taa, tag, tga

Using the table, it is easy to come up with four different ORFs for the protein R:
MRRMIPTSFSSKFQGVLSMNAVEDDRGSSTGDAIGV*

Here are some possibilities:
atgcgaaggatgatacccacaagttttttcctcgaagttccaaggagtactttctatgaat
gcagttgaagatgatcggggctcatcgacaggtgacgcgattggggtgtaa

atgcgccgtatgatacccacaagttttttcctcgaagttccaaggagtactttctatgaat
gcagttgaagatgatcggggctcatcgacaggtgacgcgattggggtgtga

atgcgccgtatgatacccacaagttttttcctcgaagttccaaggagtactttctatgaac
gcagttgaagatgatcggggctcatcgacaggtgacgcgattggggtgtag

atgcgccgtatgatacccacaagtttcagttcgaagttccaaggagtactttctatgaac
gcagttgaagatgatcggggctcatcgacaggtgacgcgattggggtgtag

For each amino acid or Stop code x in a protein sequence, let $c(x)$ be the number of codons in the table for x. For example, $c(I)=3$. Extending the definition to sequences of codes, it is easy to see that c is a multiplicative function; that is, if x and y are any string of codes from the first column of the table, then the number of DNA sequences that translate to xy is just $c(xy)=c(x)c(y)$.

Hence, the number of DNA sequences that translate to protein R is just this product

c (MRRMIPTSFSSKFQGVLSMNAVEDDRGSSTGDAIGV*)

$$
\begin{aligned}
= \quad & c(M)*c(R)*c(R)*c(M)*c(I)*c(P)*c(T)*c(S)*c(F)*c(S)*c(S)* \\
& c(K)*c(F)*c(Q)*c(G)*c(V)*c(L)*c(S)*c(M)*c(N)*c(A)*c(V)* \\
& c(E)*c(D)*c(D)*c(R)*c(G)*c(S)*c(S)*c(T)*c(G)*c(D)*c(A)* \\
& c(I)*c(G)*c(V)*c(*) \\
= \quad & 1*6*6*1*3*4*4*6*2*6*6* \\
& 2*2*2*4*4*6*6*1*2*4*4* \\
& 2*2*2*6*4*6*6*4*4*2*4* \\
& 3*4*4*3 \\
= \quad & 14023813415445725184
\end{aligned}
$$

12. Let S_1 = AATTCGCGTA and S_2 = TATCGCTACA.

   1. Build the complete dynamic programming table for these strings.
   2. What is the edit distance between S_1 and S_2?
   3. List all optimal global alignments between S_1 and S_2.

The dynamic table is as follows :

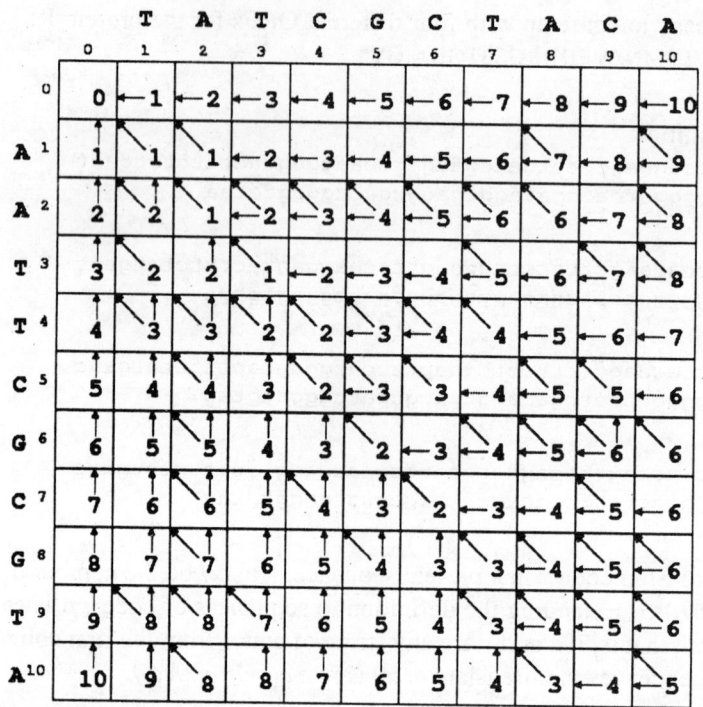

The edit distance between S_1 and S_2 is $D(10,10) = 5$.

All optimal global alignments between S_1 and S_2 can be found by considering only the traceback, as shown in the following table:

		T	**A**	**T**	**C**	**G**	**C**	**T**	**A**	**C**	**A**
	0	1	2	3	4	5	6	7	8	9	10
0	0	1	2	3	4	5	6	7	8	9	10
A 1	1	1	1	2	3	4	5	6	7	8	9
A 2	2	2	1	2	3	4	5	6	6	7	8
T 3	3	2	2	1	2	3	4	5	6	7	8
T 4	4	3	3	2	2	3	4	4	5	6	7
C 5	5	4	4	3	2	3	3	4	5	5	6
G 6	6	5	5	4	3	2	3	4	5	6	6
C 7	7	6	6	5	4	3	2	3	4	5	6
G 8	8	7	7	6	5	4	3	3	4	5	6
T 9	9	8	8	7	6	5	4	3	4	5	6
A 10	10	9	8	8	7	6	5	4	3	4	5

In summary, there are five paths from $(10,10)$ to $(7,6)$; one path from $(7,6)$ to $(4,3)$; two paths from $(4,3)$ to $(2,2)$; and one path from $(2,2)$ to $(0,0)$. Taking the product, we find that there are 10 optimal global alignments between S_1 and S_2. They are given explicitly in this table:

```
A  A  T  T  C  G  C  -  G  T  A
T  A  T  -  C  G  C  T  A  C  A

A  A  T  T  C  G  C  G  -  T  A
T  A  T  -  C  G  C  T  A  C  A

A  A  T  T  C  G  C  G  T  -  A
T  A  T  -  C  G  C  T  A  C  A

A  A  T  T  C  G  C  G  T  -  -  A
T  A  T  -  C  G  C  -  T  A  C  A

A  A  T  T  C  G  C  G  T  A  -  -
T  A  T  -  C  G  C  -  T  A  C  A

A  A  T  T  C  G  C  -  G  T  A
T  A  -  T  C  G  C  T  A  C  A

A  A  T  T  C  G  C  G  -  T  A
T  A  -  T  C  G  C  T  A  C  A

A  A  T  T  C  G  C  G  T  -  A
T  A  -  T  C  G  C  T  A  C  A

A  A  T  T  C  G  C  G  T  -  -  A
T  A  -  T  C  G  C  -  T  A  C  A

A  A  T  T  C  G  C  G  T  A  -  -
T  A  -  T  C  G  C  -  T  A  C  A
```

13. Take the following to be the weight table defining the weight function $W(i,j)$.

	-	A	C	G	T
-	5000	4	4	4	4
A	4	0	3	3	
C	4	3	0	2	3
G	4	3	2	0	3
T	4	2	3	3	0

Let S_1 = AATTCGCGTA and S_2 = TATCGCTACA.

1. Build the complete dynamic programming table for the weighted edit distance problem.

2. What is the weighted edit distance between S_1 and S_2?

3. List all optimal global alignments between S_1 and S_2 for the weighted edit distance problem.

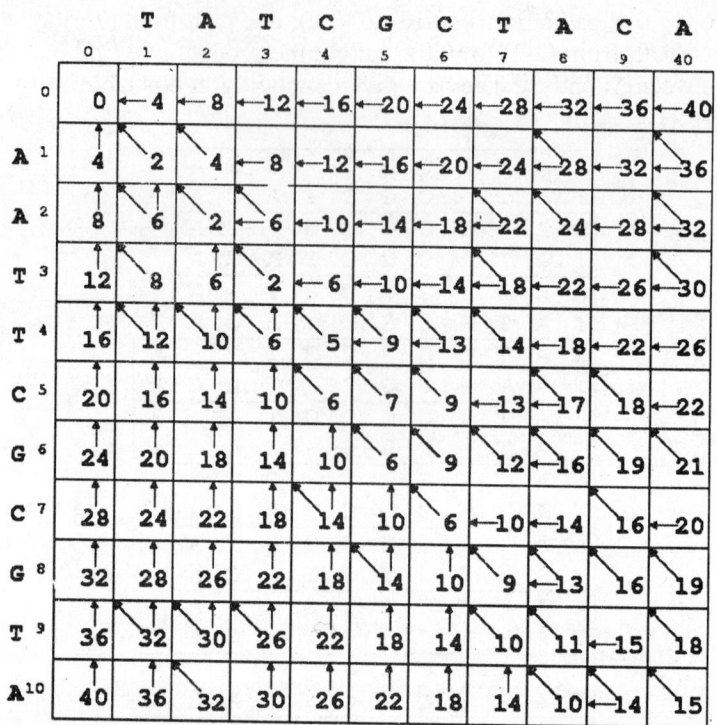

The weighted edit distance between S_1 and S_2 is $W(10,10) = 15$.

All optimal global alignments between S_1 and S_2 can be found by considering only the traceback arrows, as shown in the following table:

		T	A	T	C	G	C	T	A	C	A
	0	1	2	3	4	5	6	7	8	9	40
	0	0	4	8	12	16	20	24	28	32	36	40
A	1	4	2	4	8	12	16	20	24	28	32	36
A	2	8	6	2	6	10	14	18	22	24	28	32
T	3	12	8	6	2	6	10	14	18	22	26	30
T	4	16	12	10	6	5	9	13	14	18	22	26
C	5	20	16	14	10	6	7	9	13	17	18	22
G	6	24	20	18	14	10	6	9	12	16	19	21
C	7	28	24	22	18	14	10	6	10	14	16	20
G	8	32	28	26	22	18	14	10	9	13	16	19
T	9	36	32	30	26	22	18	14	10	11	15	18
A	10	40	36	32	30	26	22	18	14	10	14	15

In summary, there is one path from (10,10) to (4,3); two paths from (4,3) to (2,2); and one path from (2,2) to (0,0). Taking the product, we find that there are 2 optimal global alignments between S_1 and S_2. They are given explicitly in this table:

A	A	T	T	C	G	C	G	T	-	A
T	A	T	-	C	G	C	T	A	C	A
A	A	T	T	C	G	C	G	T	-	A
T	A	-	T	C	G	C	T	A	C	A

22

Problems for Self Assessment

1. Briefly discuss the "central dogma" of molecular genetics.
2. What are the main components of a gene?
3. How many introns are removed as the primary transcript is processed?
4. At what specific bases does the start codon appear? At what specific base does the stop codon appear? Which of the three stop codons is used?
5. Describe at least two differences between DNA and RNA molecules.
6. Define the following terms:
    a. Transcription
    b. Translation
    c. Intron
    d. Exon
    e. Pseudogene
    f. Genetic code
    g. Reading Frame
7. Give 3 examples of post-translational modifications that can affect intracellular protein activity.
8. What kind of information gives us the comparison between gene density and CpG islands regarding specific human chromosomes?
9. What is the field of proteomics designed to measure? Why are proteomics studies often more complex than genomics studies?
10. How is MALDI-TOF mass spectroscopy used as a diagnostic tool in proteomics?
11. How is tandem mass spectroscopy (mass spec/mass spec) used as a diagnostic tool in proteomics?
12. Find all possible amino acid sequences that might be produced from the following double stranded DNA sequence. Assume that transcription starts within the given sequence. Any of the two strands can act as coding strand. (Hint : Transcription always happens from the 3' to the 5' direction. Translation always starts from an 'AUG', and ends in one of the three stop codons.)
    3'-CTTAGATGGATGGATGCAGCTTACTATAACTGACTAGCAT-5'
    5'-GAATCTACCTACCTACGTCGAATGATATTGACTGATCGTA-3'

13. Compute the number of distinct genes (DNA sequences) that will produce the following, amino acid sequence: MEPVFTYILH. You need to refer to the genetic code. You can ignore stop codons.

14. Translate the following DNA sequence into an amino acid sequence, starting the translation at the start codon.

    aacctccagt ttgtgtcaag gtccagtttg aatgaccgct ttcagctggt gaagacatga

    cgaccctgga ctccaataac aacacaggtg gtgttatcac ctacattggc tctagtggct

15. Compare and contrast the PAM & BLOSUM amino acid substitution matrices. Include comments about how they are constructed, assumptions they make, and situations when they are useful.

16. Using the two DNA sequences, tttgga and ttgaa perform
    a. A global sequence alignment using the Needleman-Wunsch algorithm
    b. A local sequence alignment using the Smith-Waterman algorithm

    Use a score of +2 for a match, -1 for a mismatch, and −2 for a gap penalty. Show an optimal alignment and the resulting dynamic programming matrix for each algorithm.

17. Create a random sequence of 100 amino acids. Do a BLAST search. Are any matches with statistically significant scores recovered? Provide the BLAST output for the best match and interpret the results.

18. Using BioPerl, write a Perl script that performs a BLAST search on the non-redundant database with the following query sequence.

    GGGAGATGATCAACAAGATCGGAGTCCCCCTCATGACCTGAGGTCCACTTTCGA
    TGGCGG

    Retrieve the subject sequence for the first HSP. Using that sequence, perform a local alignment with the subject sequence of each of the next 4 HSPs and display the results of each in a reasonable fashion (including a score).

19. Retrieve the amino acid sequence for the human protein ACBP (acyl-CoA-binding protein, P07108, which has approximately 87 aa).

    Conduct the appropriate BLAST search of the nr database to find orthologues from *Drosophila melanogaster, C. elegans*, mouse, yeast, duck and cotton (*Gossypium hirsutum*). Conduct a multiple sequence alignment for these 6 sequences using ClustalW. Determine the consensus sequence of identical conserved amino acids.

20. Conduct a phylogenetic analysis of the 6 ACBP sequences using parsimony and neighbor joining. Compare the trees. Using the neighbor joining analysis, identify the 2 most closely related sequences.

21. Using the human sequence available from the course website, submit the sequence to a gene prediction tool and report on the gene(s) predicted in the sequence.

22. Construct a second-order HMM to model sequences dependent on the previous 2 nucleotides. Your model need to have 16 states. Label the transitions with the transition probabilities assuming every transition from a state is equally as likely. What is the sequence of states visited if the DNA sequence is CGTCTGA?

23. Apply the Smith-Waterman Algorithm without using a separate gap extension penalty to determine the best alignment for the following amino acid sequences.

    Sequence #1: IYGWPALK
    Sequence #2: YGPALGK
    Use a BLOSUM62 matrix for your match scores, and a gap penalty of 8.

24. What is the identifier for the *E. coli* MARA protein in the Swiss-Prot database? How many amino acids are there in the protein?

    How many domains does the MARA protein have? What are the identifiers for these domains? Approximately how many proteins are there in Swiss-Prot that have this domain?

25. What amino acids seem to be particularly important for this domain (converved in all or almost all members of the family)?

26. What is the PDB identifier for the MARA protein? What is the FSSP representative for this protein? What other proteins in the PDB database are similar? Do any of them have a similarity greater than Z score 4.0?

27. Mutations in the human BRCA1, BRCA2, and CHEK2 genes have been implicated in breast cancer. Use the MeSH Database on NCBI server to find all the papers related to this.

28. Search Entrez nucleotides to find the absolutely best non-contig sequence record (and only that record) available for the mouse leptin gene (LEP). What is the accession # for this best mouse leptin nucleotide sequence? What is the chromosome location for this gene in the mouse? The coding sequence begins and ends at which base positions?

29. Search for the human obesity gene OBS in Entrez Genes. What is the official gene name for this gene? What is the name of the protein that is encoded? What is the accession number of the best protein sequence link that could be retrieved from this Entrez Genes record?

30. Warfarin is an anticoagulant with a narrow therapeutic range. Variability in patient response (efficacy/toxicity) is due to a number of factors, including genetic variation in the enzyme CYP2C9. CYP2C9 plays a key role in warfarin metabolism. Use Entrez SNP to find records for variants in the CYP2C9 gene that have been mapped to a structure.

31. Predict the 3-D structure of the ribosome-inactivating protein: antiviral protein from *Mirabilis jalapa* (MAP). What 3-D structures did Swiss-Model find as possible structural templates for building MAP? List the sequence identity of the templates with the target protein.

32. How many protein structures have been deposited into PDB? Give number and date.

33. Retrieve PDB entry *1ahc* and answer the following questions:
    a. What type of protein is this?
    b. This crystal structure was solved at what resolution and what is the reported R factor?
    c. Give the title of the paper and reference where the structure was published.
    d. 1ahc contains how many residues?
    e. The structure contains how many crystal waters? Which water exhibits the lowest B factor? Report the value and units.
    f. Calculate the spatial distance between the C*alpha* atom of residue 3 and C*alpha* of residue 4. (Include proper units). What type of secondary structure element (SSE) contains both residues?
    g. Calculate the same C*alpha*-C*alpha* distance between residues 3 and 51. The latter residue is located in what type of SSE?
    h. What percent of non-glycine and non-proline residues are located in the most favorable *phi-psi* space? Is this structure adequately refined relative to other structures?
    i. Which residue exhibits unfavorable backbone dihedral angles? Print out of the Ramachandran plot. Compare a Ramachandran plot of Inorganic pyrosphosphatase (PDB 1pyp) with 1ahc.

34. Given the following sequences, obtain a multiple alignment using the center star alignment. Use the BLOSSUM62 alignment matrix.

Name   *Sequence*

ENGC_NITEU/88-236
    MFYRELGYPVLEISAKISVQPLIPLLSGQTSLLAQVLA

ENGC_PASMU/123-272
    RIYQQIGYQTLMISALSGENMEKLTALFDEGTSIFVQVIH

ENGC_PORGI/88-241
    AVYTAIGYPCCHVSAITGEGLPDLKSLLDGKLTLLAHVIA

ENGC_PROMA/97-245
    KKLQTWGYQPIPISIVNGEGIQKLSARLKSKLGVLCPVIY

ENGC_PSEAE/120-269
    NVYRTLGYPLIEVSAFNGLAMDELRGALDGHVSVFVQVVA

35. Semi-global alignment of two sequences is an alignment that ignores the end spaces which are spaces that appear before the first or at the end of the last character of the sequence in the sequences.

    For example, for the following alignment, the spaces in the second sequence are all end sequences whereas the space in the first sequence is not an end sequence.

    ```
    C A G C A – C T T G G A T T C T C G G
    – – – C A G C G T G G – – – – – – – –
    ```

    With the scoring scheme, match=+1, mismatch=-1 and space (insert or delete)=-2, this alignment gives a score of -19. But, the following alignment

    ```
    C A G C A  C T T G G A T T C T C G G
    C A G C – – – – – G – T – – – – G G
    ```

    gives a better global score of -12. But, the first alignment is a better one from biological point of view.

    Write a modified dynamic programming algorithm to obtain an optimal semi-global alignment.

36. Let P be a pattern of length n and T a text of length m. Let P^m be the concatenation of P with itself m times, so P^m has length mn. You need to compute a local alignment between P^m and T, which will assist in finding an interval in T that has the best global alignment (according to standard alignment criteria) with some tandem repeat of P.

    A problem arises in studying the secondary structure of proteins that form a *coiled coil*. In this context, P represents a *motif* or *domain* that can repeat in the protein an unknown number of times, and T represents the protein. Local alignment between P^m and T picks out an interval of T that "optimally" consists of tandem repeats of the motif. If P^m is explicitly created, then standard local alignment will solve the problem in $O(nm^2)$ time. But because P^m consists of identical copies of P, an $O(nm)$-time solution is possible. The method simulates what the dynamic programming algorithm for local alignment would do if it were executed with P^m and T explicitly. This method is outlined below :

    The dynamic Programming algorithm will fill an $m+1$ by $n+1$ table V. Here rows are numbered 0 to n, and columns are numbered 0 to m. Row 0 and column 0 are initialized to all 0 entries. Then in each row i, from 1 to m, the algorithm does the following:

    a. It executes the standard local alignment recurrences in row i; it sets $V(i,0)$ to $V(i,n)$; and then it executes the standard local alignment recurrences in row i again.

    b. After completely filling each row, the algorithm selects the cell with largest V value, as in the standard solution to the local alignment problem.

This algorithm takes $O(nm)$ time. Prove that it correctly finds the value of the optimal local alignment between P^m and T. Then give the details of the traceback to construct the optimal local alignment. Discuss why P was (conceptually) expanded to P^m and not a longer or shorter string.

37. We say that a string C is a merge of strings A and B, if it is obtained by merging the characters of A and B in their original relative order together. For example, string "FLOTILLA" is a merge of strings "FLO" and "TILLA", string "COMING" is a merge of strings "MON" and "CIMG". Develop a dynamic programming algorithm that takes three strings $A[1...n]$, $B[1...m]$ and $C[1...n+m]$ and tests whether C is a merge of A and B. What is the complexity?

38. Given the following sequence: PLSQETFSDLWKLLPENNVLSP use the Kyte/Doolittle Hydropathy scale and a sliding window of 7 amino acids to construct a hydropathy plot.

39. The p53 protein is known to have a certain number of conserved domains. Use the Dotter program and a series of p53 proteins from different species (at least 5 proteins) to determine the number of conserved domains and the boundaries of the conserved domains. In reporting the boundaries, use the human sequence number as the standard.

40. Use the FASTA search page to compare Drosophila glutathione transferase gtt1_drome (gi|121694) to the PIR Annotated protein sequence database.

    a. What is the highest scoring non-homolog? How would you confirm that your candidate non-homolog was truly unrelated? What happens to the length of the alignment as non-homologous sequences are aligned?

    b. Note that this drosophila glutathione transferase shares significant similarity with both sequences from *E. Coli* and mammals. How might you confirm that the *E. coli* stringent starvation protein is homologous to glutathione transferases?

    c. Compare the expectation (E()) values for the distant relationships between gtt1_drome and xurt8c (SwissProt gta3_rat) or xurtg4 (SwissProt gta1_rat). How would you demonstrate that gtt1_drome is homologous to xurtg4?

    d. Examine how the expectation value changes with different scoring matrices (BLOSUM62, BlastP62, PAM250) and different gap penalties. What happens to the E()-value for the highest scoring unrelated sequence with the different matrices?

41. Do a FASTA and blast2.0 search with leptin (**ob_rat / gi|1709436**). Try the same search with PSI-Blast. Are all statistically significant matches homologous?

42. Three proteins, hexokinase (**1hkb,hxkb_yeast**), actin (1atn) and HSP70 (DnaK, 1dkg) share statistically significant structural similarity.

43. Identify the genes encoded by y140_metja (mj0140) and y144_metja (mj0144).

44. Identify homologues to the intein (protein intron) sequence in rpa1_metja (mj1042).

45. Identify non-mammalian homologues of cli2_human.

46. Consider the following data:

    A : gtgttc

    B : taccgt

    C : gacatc

    D : tagcgc

    What is the most parsimonious tree(s)? What is the minimum distance tree(s)?

47. Consider the following data:

    A: taa

    B: aat

C: cgg

D: ggc

What is the most parsimonious tree? Now, suppose that the probability of a transversion (T) is half that of a transition (t) (P(t) = 2P(T)). Does the most parsimonious tree have the maximum likelihood?

48. Identify triosephosphate isomerase (tpis_ecoli) and glutatmate dehydrogenase (dhe4_human) in *Methanococcus jannaschii* and *Synechocystis*.

49. Is there a yeast, *C. elegans*, or bacterial homologue of p53_human? What is the most distant p53-homologue you can identify?

50. Are metaxin mtx2_human and/or yqjg_ecoli glutathione transferase homologs?

51. Is gtk1_rat homologous to other the soluble glutathione transferase family that includes gtt2_rat?

52. Demonstrate, if possible, that *S. griseus* protease A prta_strgr is homologous to bovine trypsin (try1_bovin) based on sequence similarity alone.

53. Use the fasta program to search the PIR1 database with grou_drome. Do the same search against the PIR1 (seg) database. Compare the E()-value of the highest scoring unrelated sequence and the GTP-binding regulatory protein RGFFBH. Do the same search with blast. Compare the results (high scoring sequences and homolog scores) with and without using the seg option.

54. Is the secretin receptor (scrc_human) related to the much larger class of G-protein coupled receptors that includes the beta adrenergic receptor b2ar_rat (/ecg/data/b2ar_rat.aa) and opsin opsd_human (/ecg/data/opsd_human.aa)?

55. Create a class called DataGrab that does the following : (a) parses a fasta file (def fasta_parse) and (b) stores the data in a dictionary (self.fasta_dic) with the key being the accession number and the value being the sequence.

56. Create a class called SeqSearch that has methods (class functions) that do the following :

 a. Identify whether a DNA motif exists in a particular sequence. The function, call it motif_search, should return a "true or false". For example, searching for the DNA motif "CATTGC" in the sequence "ATATATATAT" should return false.

 b. Counts the number of times the motif occurs in a particular sequence. Return the count.

 c. Does number (b) above for the reverse compliment of the motif ('CATT' becomes 'AATG').

57. Using the GenBank accession number V00519 as a starting point, answer the following questions: What GenBank sequence does the accession number specify? What does this sequence encode? How many bases of sequence are in the file? How many total in GenBank (as of this date)?

58. Use Medline to answer the following questions: How many amino acids are in the "precursor region?" In what organism has this protein been expressed? To what bacterial gene was the cDNA fused?

59. Run a basic BLAST search using the following sequence as a query. You may use the default settings but increase the number of shown alignments to 100 (from 50). You will have to choose a database and an algorithm. Run the search using an untranslated nucleotide query against a nucleotide database.

GTCCGGCCTGGGCGACAGAGCAAGACTCCGTCTCAAAAAAAAAAAAAAAAAAAA
AAAAAAAAA AAAAAA

Answer the following :

 a. Examine the output from the BLAST search. Did your search identify a single unique matching sequence in the database? Are the matches biologically relevant?

    b. Do all the matches correspond to DNA from one organism? Out of the sequences that match your query and are human, do they all correspond to sequences on the same chromosome?

    c. Formulate a hypothesis to account for these results.

60. Using the following nucleic acid sequence as a query, search the protein database using the algorithm Blastx.

acaggtaagc gcccctaaaa tccctttggg cacaatgtgt cctgagggga gaggcagcga cctgtagatg ggacgggggc actaaccctc aggtttgggg cttctgaatg agtatcgcca tgtaagccca gtatggccaa tctcagaaag ctcctggtcc ctggagggat ggagagagaa aaacaaacag ctcctggagc agggagagtg ctggcctctt gctctccggc tccctctgtt gccctctggt ttctccccag g

Examine the best matches to the query sequence above. What does the query sequence match best to in this search? Which reading frame of the query sequence was translated to align with the best matching protein sequence in the database? What was the percent identity between the two aligned sequences? What was the percent similarity? Do the identical and similar residues "cluster" in regions of the alignment or are they scattered? Given your answers to these questions, do you feel that the matches are "biologically relevant? Why or why not?

61. Do a BLAST search for the following human amino acid sequence (given in one letter code) :

MSTAVLENPGLGRKLSDFGQETSYIEDNCNQNGAISLIFSLKEEVGALAKVLRLFEEN DVNLTHIESRPSRLKKDEYEFFTHLDKRSLPALTNIIKILRHDIGATVHELSRDKKKDTVPW FPRTIQELDRFANQILSYGAELDADHPGFKDPVYRARRKQFADIAYNYRHGQPIPRVEYM EEEKKTWGTVFKTLKSLYKTHACYEYNHIFPLLEKYCGFHEDNIPQLEDVSQFLQTCTGFRLR PVAGLLSSRDFLGGLAFRVFHCTQYIRHGSKPMYTPEPDICHELLGHVPLFSDRSFAQFSQ EIGLASLGAPDEYIEKLATIYWFTVEFGLCKQGDSIKAYGAGLLSSFGELQYCLSEKPKLL PLELEKTAIQNYTVTEFQPLYYVAESFNDAKEKVRNFAATIPRPFSVRYDPYTQRI EVLDNTQQLKILADSINSEIGILCSALQKIK

    a. Identify the protein.

    b. Retrieve and examine the best matching sequence.

    c. What is the primary accession number of the sequence that best matches the query?

    d. What is the most common name of the protein?

    e. How close is the protein encoded by the cDNA sequence to the same protein from a rat? Express your answer by percentages, i.e., 23% identical and 44% similar.

    f. Does the enzyme require a co-factor to function? If so, what?

62. Use the Hierarchy Browser to find *Methylomonas scandinavica*. Does this organism belong to the domain Archaea or Bacteria? Which phylum does it belong to? Which class, order and family does it belong to? Where was this organism isolated from?

63. Are there regions of the sequence where Eukarya and Archaea (*Methanococcus*) have sequence in common but the Bacterial sequence (*E. coli*) is different? How about for Archaea and Bacteria? How about for Eukarya and Bacteria?

64. You have found a gene in *Arabidopsis thaliana* that is tightly linked to the copper/zinc superoxide dismutase gene CZSOD2 (or CSD2). You suspect, based on recombination data, that your clone is "south" of CZSOD2 at about 60 cM. Answer the following :

    a. CZSOD2 is located on which chromosome?

    b. Where is CZSOD2 located (in cM and Mbp)? Is it above or below the centromere?

    c. List the BAC clones in the contig in order from the BAC containing CZSOD2 to the BAC containing the SSLP marker nga361.

    d. What other molecular markers are located in the region of the chromosome contained in the above contig?

    e. What types of markers are mi54 and m283?

    f. How many clones are in the contig from the BAC containing mi54 to the BAC containing m283?

65. The following sequence is the coding sequence of the *HBB* (haemoglobin beta) gene in humans.

acatttgctt ctgacacaac tgtgttcact agcaacctca aacagacacc atggtgcacc tgactcctga ggagaagtct gccgttactg ccctgtgggg caaggtgaac gtggatgaag ttggtggtga ggccctgggc aggctgctgg tggtctaccc ttggacccag aggttctttg agtcctttgg ggatctgtcc actcctgatg ctgttatggg caaccctaag gtgaaggctc atggcaagaa agtgctcggt gcctttagtgatggcctggc tcacctggac aacctcaagg gcacctttgc cacactgagt gagctgcact gtgacaagct gcacgtggat cctgagaact tcaggctcct gggcaacgtg ctggtctgtg tgctggccca tcactttggc aaagaattca ccccaccagt gcaggctgcc tatcagaaag tggtggctgg tgtggctaat gccctggccc acaagtatca ctagctcgct ttcttgctgt ccaatttcta ttaaaggttc ctttgttccc taagtccaac tactaaactg ggggatatta tgaagggcct tgagcatctg gattctgcct aataaaaaac atttattttc attgc

Use this sequence to perform a BLAST search to find the *HBB* gene from other organisms. What organism are humans most related to based on the *HBB* gene alignment?

66. What is an E-value? You do a databank search using FASTA with an amino acid sequence as query. The only reported match has an E-value of 10. What does this mean for the similarity of the two sequences?

67. How would you recognize a duplication or a deletion in a dot plot?

68. You do protein BLAST searches of the Swiss Protein and the non-redundant databank using the same sequence as query. You get the same top hits, however, the E-values for the top hit are different. Why could this happen?

69. Two sequences A and B show significant similarity in a BLAST search. It is known that sequence B is homologous to sequence C. Which additional information would you require to conclude that sequence A is homologous to sequence C. (The P-value for the pairwise comparison of A with C is 0.12).

70. You use a protein-encoding genomic sequence to search a nucleotide database. Assume that there are proteins in the database that are homologous to the encoded protein. How might you infer that an intron is present in the genomic sequence?

71. What conclusion can you draw from finding that in Eukaryotes introns that separate protein domains are frequently in the same phase?

72. You do a PSI BLAST search using an uncharacterized ORF from a *Methanococcus* strain as a equerry. In the zero iteration you pick up a couple of hypothetical proteins form other Euryarchaeota, in the first iteration an rho termination factor form a Gram positve bacterium scores above the cut-off level, in the second iteration this and other termination factors score with E values below 10^{-24}. Does this prove that the ORF you used as a query is a homolog of the rho termination factors?

73. Assume you have calculated a molecular phylogeny. Describe at least three approaches that would allow you to assess if a single branch in this tree is significantly supported by the alignment from which this tree was calculated.

74. Consider the purely hypothetical tree shown in Fig. 22.1. This tree was calculated for homologs of enolase. In case an organism's genome encoded more than one homolog these are labeled a and b or 1 and 2. Answer the following :

    a. When did the gene duplication happen that gave rise to homologs *a* and *b* in fungi.

b. Would we expect to find homologs of a and b in other eukaryotes? If yes, in which groups?

c. What are possible explanation(s) for *Plasmodium* having paralogs 1 and 2?

75. Consider the tree given in Fig. 22.2. Answer the following questions :

a. Which type of protein appears to be the one labeled as extein? (bet: beta subunit of the F-ATPase, fl: flagellar assembly ATPase, ttf: transcription termination factor.

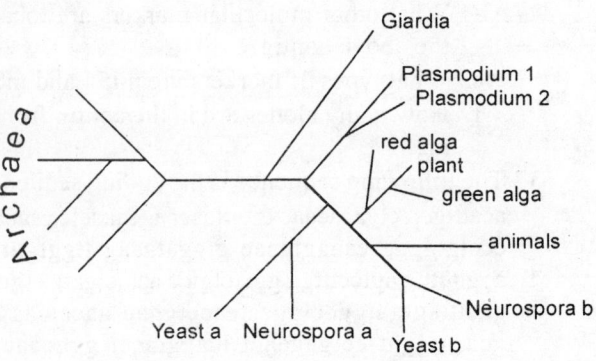

Fig. 22.1. Tree for problem 74.

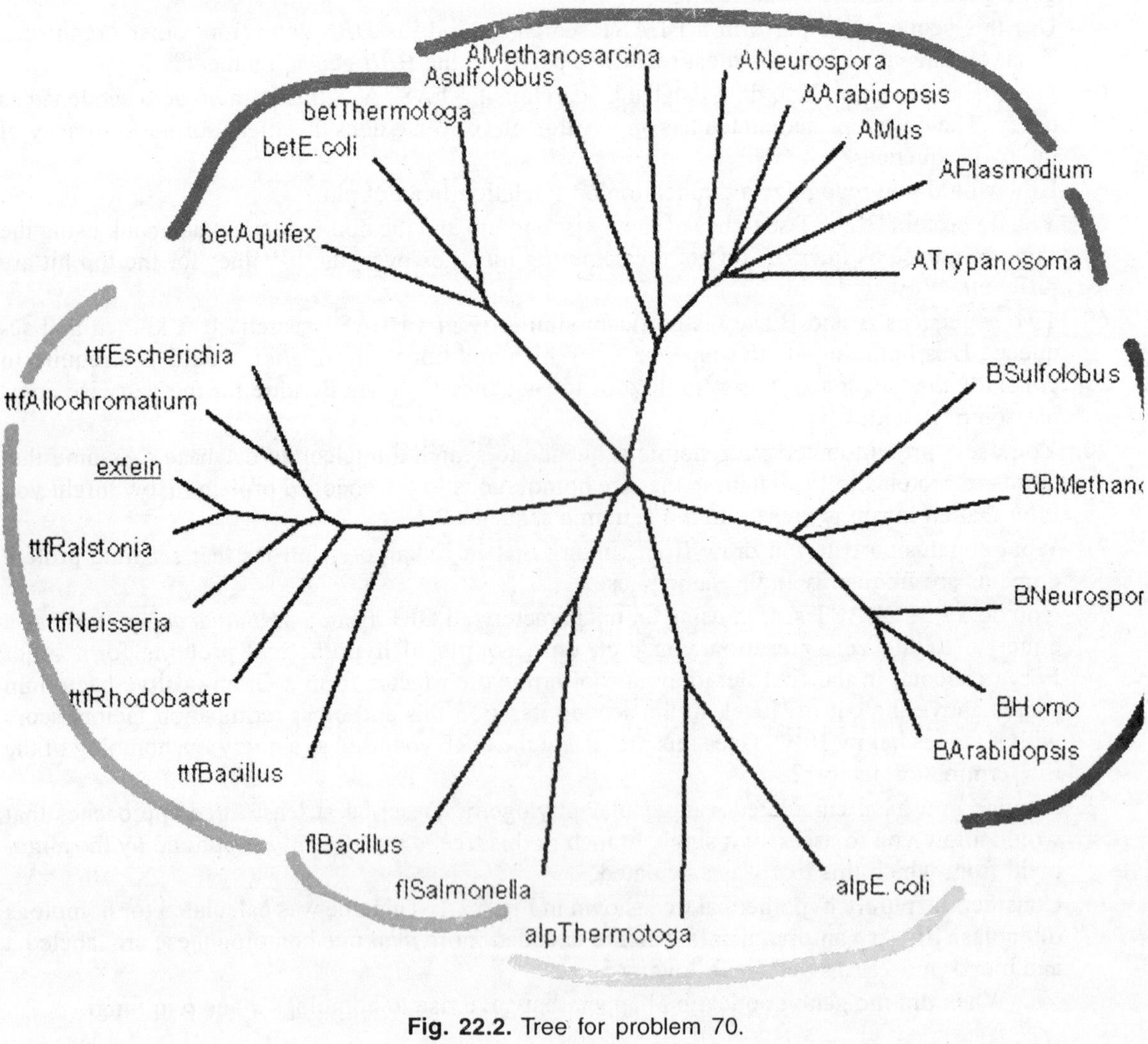

Fig. 22.2. Tree for problem 70.

b. Assuming that the extein sequence was obtained from *Burkholderia brasilensis*, is it possible that the extein might encode a paralog to the transcription termination factor?

76. A DNA microarray can be used to compare expression under two different conditions, or in two developmental stages. At what step are the fluorescent dyes introduced into the assay? How many dyes are usually used? Given the usual choices, what does yellow correspond to in the generated images?

77. The ratios (Ti) of red (Ri) to green (Gi) fluorescence intensity usually are given as logarithms to the base of 2. If the red fluorescence is 4 time more intense than the green fluorescence, what is the log(base2)Ti?

78. Imagine that you analyze the expression of 1000 mRNAs under two conditions. Assume that you perform sufficient replicates to assess the variance for each mRNA. A simple ANOVA test of the samples for a single mRNA allows you to decide if the difference between the two conditions is significant. If you were to apply this test to all 1000 mRNAs, how many false positives would you expect, if you were to perform your test at a significance level of 5%?

79. Why might co-evolution of two interacting subunits lead to clustering of the two encoding genes? Why does this mechanism not explain the evolution of all operons? Does this mechanism require the transfer of genetic information?

80. NCBI website contains a large set of information and tools.
   a. List what databases you can access through Entrez website.
   b. You are asked to collect information about "inositol 1,3,4,5-tetrakisphosphate (InsP4) binding proteins". Give a list of accession numbers and names for the proteins that are retrieved.

81. In PDB, what is current number of structures deposited in the database? How many of them are protein structures? When the structure for a newly crystallized protein is deposited, it is first used as query to search PDB database to see if similar folding is already in the database. What is the trend of number of "old folding" and "new folding" deposited in the recent years?

82. Find the optimal global alignment by constructing the DP matrix for the following strings: x = "A G C" and y = "A A A C". If there is more than one optimal alignment, derive all of them. Assign s(a,b) = 1 if a=b, -1 otherwise let gap penalty = -2. Show your dynamic programming matrix.

83. Find the local alignment(s) using the Smith-Waterman algorithm for the following strings: x = "T A C T A A" and y = "T A A T A". Use the same scoring method as in problem 77. Show dynamic programming matrix.

84. An affine gap penalty function is usually represented as shown below:
   w(k) = h + gk, k > 0;
   where h penalizes opening of a gap and is usually large (-12 or so), and g penalizes extension of a gap (usually -2 or -3)...
   Sketch a DP algorithm for the affine gap penalty case.

85. What are the steps used in FASTA and where are the init1, initn, and opt scores calculated? With respect to FASTA :
   a. Determine initial diagonals using lookup table
   b. Rescore all positions in top 10 diagonals using (init1 score)
   c. Connect diagonals into longer regions (initn score)
   d. Calculate optimal SW alignment in band around diagonals (opt score)
   e. Fit statistical distribution and calculate statistics

86. Describe the differences in how BLAST and FASTA calculate significance? What are the advantages of each approach?

87. What is a log-odds scoring system and how does it related to the Dayhoff PAM250 scoring table?

88. What are the basic energy terms used in Zuker's minimum free energy approach to RNA secondary structure prediction? Explain what each means and note which are positive and which are negative.

89. Explain the basic principal used to predict RNA structures using a covariance approach?

90. Use the global alignment algorithm to align: ACCTGT and CCATGAAT. What is the score of the optimal alignment?

91. In unix shell, how would count the number of lines in a file that contain the substring "AAA"?

92. What does the following command do: "sort -k 2 exam_scores | head -n 10"?

93. What does the following command do: "ls *.big | grep "not needed" | rm -rf' ?

94. What is the difference between a scoring matrix, such as BLOSUM62 and a position-specific scoring matrix (PSSM)?

95. Comparison of DNA sequences of homologous chromosomes in different people show that, on the average, 1 of every 700 bp of non-coding DNA is different. 95% of the genome is non-coding. Estimate the number of polymorphisms in the human genome to give some idea of the number of possible DNA markers.

96. Find the approximate size of the West Nile viral genome, the microbial *Escherichia coli* K12 genome, the *Caenorhabditis elegans* haploid genome, the haploid human genome.

97. The *Rate of Nucleotide Substitution* can be defined as the number of substitutions per site per year and can be calculated by dividing the number of substitutions per site between two homologous sequences (K) by 2T, where T is the time of divergence between the two sequences, so r = K / (2T). The number of substitution per site k = $- (3/4) \ln [1 - (4/3)D]$. D=number of differences per site

The influenza type A virus has a substitution rate for the HA1 region of the haemagglutinin gene of 5.7×10^{-3} substitutions per nucleotide site per year. If two flu viruses isolated this year differ at 10% of their nucleotide sites, approximately when did the viruses last share a common ancestor?

98. It is estimated that the human immune system can produce 10^{15} antibodies. Would it be possible for such a large number of proteins each to be encoded entirely by a separate gene, the diversity arising from gene duplication and divergence? A typical gene for an IgG molecule is about 2000 bp long.

99. Align the string A=TTGACAT and B=GTTGTACTT, according to the simple scoring scheme: match=0, mismatch=20, insertion and deletion=25, using dynamic programming. Show the optimal global alignment as well as the matrix that score all possible alignments.

100. Consider 4 species characterized by homologous sequence ATCC, ATGC, TTCG, and TCGG. Taking the number of differences as a measure of the dissimilarity between each pair of species, use a simple clustering procedure to derive a phylogenic tree.

Selected References

Computational biology books

1. Eddy,S., A. Krogh, G. Mitchison and Richard Durbin. 1999. Biological sequence analysis : probabalistic models of proteins and nucleic acids. Cambridge University Press.
2. Gusfield, Dan. 1997. Algorithms on strings, trees, and sequences : computer science and computational biology. Cambridge University Press.
3. Ewens, W.J. and G.R. Grant. 2001. Statistical Methods in Bioinformatics: An Introduction. Springer-Verlag, New York.
4. Setubal, J. and J. Meidanis. 1997. Introduction to Computational Molecular Biology. PWS Publishing Company, Boston.

General bioinformatics and applications books

1. Baldi,Pierre and Soren Brunak. 1998. Bioinformatics : The Machine Learning Approach (Adaptive Computation and Machine Learning). MIT Press
2. Baxevanis, A.D. and D.F. Fancis Ouellette (Eds). 2001. Bioinformatics: A Practical Guide to the Analysis of Genes and Proteins. 2nd Ed. Wiley-Interscience, New York.
3. Cantor, C.R. and C.L. Smith. 1999. Genomics: The Science and Technology Behind the Human Genome Project. Wiley-Interscience, New York.
4. Gibas, C. and P. Jambeck. 2001. Developing Bioinformatics Computer Skills. O'Reilly and Associates, Sebastopol, California.
5. Misener, S. and S.A. Krawetz (Eds). 2000. Bioinformatics Methods and Protocols. Volume 132: Methods in Molecular Biology. Humana Press, Towota, New Jersey.
6. Mount, David. 2001 Bioinformatics: Sequence and Genome Analysis. Cold Spring Harbor Laboratory Press.
7. Rashidi, Hooman and Lukas K. Buehler. 1999. Bioinformatics Basics Applications in Biological Science and Medicine. CRC Press.

Molecular evolution and population genetics books:

1. Cantor,Charles, Cassandra L. Smith, 1999. Human Genome Project. Genomics : the science and technology behind the Human Genome Project. John Wiley & Sons, Inc.
2. Doolittle, Russel. 1990. Molecular evolution : computer analysis of protein and nucleic acid sequences. Academic Press.
3. Graur, D. and W.-H. Li. 2000. Fundamentals of Molecular Evolution. Second Edition. Sinauer Associates, Sunderland, Massachusetts.
4. Hartl, D.L. and A.G. Clark. 1997. Principles of Population Genetics. Third Edition. Sinauer Associates, Sunderland, Massachusetts.
5. Hillis, D.M., C. Moritz and B.K. Mable (Eds). 1996. Molecular Systematics. Second Edition. Sinauer Associates, Sunderland, Massachusetts.
6. Li, W.-H. 1997. Molecular Evolution. Sinauer Associates, Sunderland, Massachusetts.
7. Nei, M. and S. Kumar. 2000. Molecular Evolution and Phylogenetics. Oxford University Press, Oxford.
8. Patthy, L. 1999. Protein Evolution. Blackwell Science, Oxford.
9. Page, R.D.M. and E.C. Holmes. 1998. Molecular Evolution: A Phylogenetic Approach. Blackwell Science, Oxford.
10. Weir, B.S. 1996. Genetic Data Analysis II: Methods for Discrete Population Genetic Data. Sinauer Associates, Sunderland, Massachusetts.

Programming and Computer Books

1. Goodrich, Michael and Roberto Tamassia. 2001. Algorithm Design: Foundations, Analysis, and Internet Examples. John Wiley & Sons. New York
2. Peek,Jerry, Grace Todino and John Strang. 2001. 5th ed. Learning the Unix Operating System, A Concise Guide for the New User. O'Reilly and Associates, Sebastopol, California.
3. Tisdall, James. 2001. Perl for Bioinformatics. O'Reilly and Associates, Sebastopol, California.

Glossary

Accession number : An identifier supplied by the curators of the major biological databases upon submission of a novel entry that uniquely identifies that sequence (or other) entry.

Affine gap penalty : A gap penalty score that is a linear function of gap length, consisting of a gap opening penalty and a gap extension penalty multiplied by the length of the gap. Using this penalty scheme enhances the performance of DP methods for sequence alignment.

Agents : Independent, autonomous, software modules that can search the Internet for data or content pertinent to a particular application, such as a gene, protein, or biological system.

Algorithm : A series of steps defining a procedure or formula for solving a problem, that can be coded into a programming language and executed. Bioinformatics algorithms typically are used to process, store, analyze, visualize and make predictions from biological data.

Alignment : The result of a comparison of two or more gene or protein sequences in order to determine their degree of base or amino acid similarity. Sequence alignments are used to determine the similarity, homology, function or other degree of relatedness between two or more genes or gene products.

Alignment score : An algorithmically computed score based on the number of matches, substitutions, insertions and deletions within an alignment. Scores for matches and substitutions are derived from a scoring matrix such as the PAM and BLOSUM matrices for proteins, and affine gap penalties suitable for the matrix are chosen. Alignment scores are in log odd units, often bit units. Higher scores denote better alignments.

Allele : A given form of a gene that occupies a specific position or locus on a chromosome. Variant forms of genes occurring at the same locus are said to be alleles of one another.

Alternative splicing : One of the alternate combinations of a folded protein that are possible due to by recombination of multiple gene segments during mRNA splicing that occurs in higher organisms.

Alternative splice-form : One of the possible alternate combinations of exons into a folded protein that are possible by recombining multiple gene segments during mRNA splicing in higher organisms.

Alu family : A common set of dispersed DNA sequences found throughout the human genome; each is about 300 bases long and they are repeated at least 500,000 times. Alu sequences are speculated to have originated from viral RNA sequences that integrated into human DNA thousands of years ago.

Amino acid : One of the 20 chemical building blocks that are joined by amide (peptide) linkages to form a polypeptide chain of a protein.

Analogy : Reasoning by which the function of a novel gene or protein sequence may be deduced from comparisons with other gene or protein sequences of known function. Identifying analogous or homologous genes via similarity searching and alignment is one of the chief uses of Bioinformatics. (See also alignment, similarity search).

Annotation : A combination of comments, notations, references, and citations, either in free format or utilizing a controlled vocabulary, that together describe all the experimental and inferred information about a gene or protein. Annotations can also be applied to the description of other biological systems. Batch, automated annotation of bulk biological sequence is one of the key uses of Bioinformatics tools. The elucidation and description of biologically relevant features in the sequence is essential in order for genome data to be useful. The quality with which annotation is done will have direct impact on the value of the sequence. At a minimum, the data must be annotated to indicate the existence of gene coding regions and control regions. Further annotation activities that add value to a genome include finding simple and complex repeats, characterizing the organization of promoters and gene families, the distribution of G + C content, and tying together evidence for functional motifs and homologs. Annotation can be manual (as in SWISS- PROT) or automated (as in TrEMBL). Since annotation is highly skilled and labor intensive, efforts are being made to automate the process, at least for preliminary data. Related term: curated databases.

Anticodon : The triplet of contiguous bases on tRNA that binds to the codon sequence of nucleotides on mRNA. Example: GGG codes for Glycine.

Antigen : Any foreign molecule that stimulates an immune response in a vertebrate organism. Many antigens are proteins such as the surface proteins of foreign organisms.

Antisense : DNA or RNA composed of the complementary sequence to the target DNA/RNA. Also used to describe a therapeutic strategy that uses antisense DNA or RNA sequences to target specific gene DNA sequences or mRNA implicated in disease, in order to bind and physically inhibit their expression by physically blocking them.

Assay : A method for measuring a biological activity. This may be enzyme activity, binding affinity, or protein turnover. Most assays utilize a measurable parameter such as color, fluorescence or radioactivity to correlate with the biological activity.

Assembly : Compilation of overlapping sequences from one or more related genes that have been clustered together based on their degree of sequence identity or similarity. Sequence assembly may be used to piece together "shotgun" sequencing fragments (see shotgun sequencing) based upon overlapping restriction enzyme digests, or may be used to identify and index novel genes from "single-pass" cDNA sequencing efforts.

Autoradiography : A method used to locate radioisotope-labeled materials which have been separated in gels or are present in blots. The location of the radiolabeled material is determined by overlaying the test material with a photographic film that is sensitive to the radioisotope.

Bacterial artificial chromosome (BAC) : Cloning vector that can incorporate large fragments of DNA. (see YACS)

Bacteriophage : A virus that infects bacteria. The bacteriophage DNA has served as a basis for cloning vectors, and is also utilized to create phage libraries containing human or other genes.

Baculovirus : An insect virus which forms the basis of a protein expression system.

Base pair : A pair of nitrogenous bases (a purine and a pyrimidine), held together by hydrogen bonds, that form the core of DNA and RNA i.e the A:T, G:C and A:U interactions.

Base Analogue : A chemical compound which is sufficiently similar to one of the nitrogenous bases normally found in DNA, that it can replace it. Base analogues may cause mutations, or be used in a modified PCR reaction (e.g. when sequencing)

Bioinformatics : The field of endeavor that relates to the collection, organization and analysis of large amounts of biological data using networks of computers and databases (usually with reference to the genome project and DNA sequence information)

Bit units : A bit denotes the amount of information required to distinguish between equally likely possibilities. The number of bits of information, N, required to convey a message that has M possibilities is $\log_2 M = N$ bits.

Bivalent : Having two binding sites; having 2 free electrons available for binding.

BLAST : A set of programs, used to perform fast similarity searches. Nucleotide sequences can be compared with nucleotide sequences in a database using BLASTN, for example. Complex statistics are applied to judge the significance of each match. Reported sequences may be homologous to, or related to the query sequence. The BLASTP program is used to search a protein database for a match against a query protein sequence. There are several other flavours of BLAST.

BLAST2 : A newer release of BLAST. Allows for insertions or deletions in the sequences being aligned. Gapped alignments may be more biologically significant.

Beta sheet : A three dimensional arrangement taken up by polypeptide chains that consists of alternating strands linked by hydrogen bonds. The alternating strands together form a sheet that is frequently twisted. This is one of the secondary structural elements characteristic of proteins.

Biock : Conserved ungapped patterns approximately 3-60 amino acids in length in a set of related proteins.

Blunt-end (ligation) : The joining of DNA fragments that contain no overhang at both ends and consequently no DNA bases available for hybridization.

Bootstrap analysis : A method for testing how well a particular data set fits a model. For example, the validity of the branch arrangement in a predicted phylogenetic tree can be tested by resampling columns in a multiple sequence alignment to create many new alignments. The appearance of a particular branch in trees generated from these resampled sequences can then be measured. Alternatively, a sequence may be left out of an analysis to determine how much the sequence influences the results of an analysis.

Browser : Program used to access sites on the World Wide Web. Hypertext markup language (HTML) enables browsers to represent a Web page the same way regardless of computer platform.

Carboxyl group : The -COOH functional group, acidic in nature, found in all amino acids

cDNA (complementary DNA) : A DNA strand copied from mRNA using reverse transcriptase. A cDNA library represents all of the expressed DNA in a cell.

cDNA library : A set of DNA fragments prepared from the total mRNA obtained from a selected cell, tissue or organism.

Cell : The basic unit of any living organism.

Cell Cycle : The life cycle of a cell which is marked by cell division which is separated into four phases: G1, S, G2, and M. DNA replication is confined to the S(synthesis) phase, and chromosomal separation in the M (mitotic) phase.

Characters and character states : In phylogenetics, characters are homologous features in different organisms. The exact condition of that feature in a particular individual is the character state. For example, the character "hair colour" might have the character states "gold", "red", and "yellow". In molecular biology, the character states can be one of the four nucleotides (A, C, T, G) or one of the 20 amino acids., Some authors define "character" to mean the character state as defined here.

Chimeric clone : A cloning artifact created by a foreign gene being inserted into a vector in an incorrect orientation resulting in the expression of a protein consisting of a fusion of two different gene products.

Chromat : Data file output from most popular DNA sequencers. Chromat files consist of the fluorescent traces generated by the sequencer for each of the four chemical bases, A, C, G, and T, together with the sequence and measures of the error in the traces at each sequence position.

Chromatin : The chromosome as it appears in its condensed state, composed of DNA and associated proteins (mainly histones).

Chromosome : The structure in the cell nucleus that contains the cellular DNA together with a number of proteins that compact and package the DNA.

Client : A computer, or the software running on a computer, that interacts with another computer at a remote site (server). Note the differences between client and user.

Clinical trials : Research studies that involve patients. Biotechnology companies typically use clinical trials to assess the efficacy and safety of new therapies and to answer scientific questions. Typically, there are 3 phases during a clinical trial. Phase I is designed to evaluate the safety of the product in humans; phase II analyses the effects of dose escalation, and phase III definitively evaluates the clinical efficacy of the product.

Clone : A population of genetically identical cells or DNA molecules.

Cloning : The formation of clones or exact genetic replicas.

Cloning Vector : A molecule that carries a foreign gene into a host, and allows/facilitates the multiplication of that gene in a host. When sequencing a gene that has been cloned using a cloning vector (rather than by PCR), care should be taken not to include the cloning vector sequence when performing similarity searches. Plasmids, cosmids, phagemids, YACs and PACs are example types of cloning vectors.

Cluster : The grouping of similar objects in a multidimensional space. Clustering is used for constructing new features which are abstractions of the existing features of those objects. The quality of the clustering depends crucially on the distance metric in the space. In bioinformatics, clustering is performed on sequences, high-throughput expression and other experimental data. Clusters of partial or complete gene sequences can be used to identify the complete (contiguous) sequence and to better identify its function. Clustering expression data enables the researcher to discern patterns of co-regulation in groups of genes.

Cobbler : A single seuqnce that represents the most conserved regions in a multiple sequence alignment. The BLOCKS server uses the cobbler sequence to perform a database similarity search as a way to reach sequences that are more divergent than would be found using the single sequences in the alignment for searches.

Coding regions (CDS) : The portion of a genomic sequence bounded by start and stop codons that identifies the sequence of the protein being coded for by a particular gene.

Codon : A sequence of three adjacent nucleotides that designates a specific amino acid or start/stop site for transcription.

COG : Clusters of orthologous groups in a set of groups of related sequences in micro-organisms and yeast. These groups are found by whole proteome comparisons and includes paralogues and orthologues.

Combinatorial chemistry : The use of chemical methods to generate all possible combinations of chemicals starting with a subset of compounds. The building blocks may be peptides, nucleic acids or small molecules. The libraries of compounds formed by this methodology are used to probe for new pharmaceutical reagents (see high-throughput screening).

Complementary determining region (CDR) : The hypervariable regions of an antibody molecule, consisting of three loops from the heavy chain and three from the light chain, that together form the antigen-binding site.

Complexity (of gene sequence) : The term "low complexity sequence" may be thought of as synonymous with regions of locally biased amino acid composition. In these regions, the sequence composition deviates from the random model that underlies the calculation of the statistical significance (P-value) of an alignment. Such alignments among low complexity sequences are statistically but not biologically significant, i.e., one cannot infer homology (common ancestry) or functional similarity.

Configuration : The complete ordering and description of all parts of a software or database system. Configuration management is the use of software to identify, inventory and maintain the component modules that together comprise one or more systems or products.

Conformation : The precise three-dimensional arrangement of atoms and bonds in a molecule describing its geometry and hence its molecular function.

Consensus sequence : A single sequence delineated from an alignment of multiple constituent sequences that represents a "best fit" for all those sequences. A "voting" or other selection procedure is used to determine which residue (nucleotide or amino acid) is placed at a given position in the event that not all of the constituent sequences have the identical residue at that position.

Constitutive synthesis (expression) : Synthesis of mRNA and protein at an unchanging or constant rate regardless of a cell requirements.

Context-free grammars : A recursive set of production rules for generating patterns of strings. These consist of a set of terminal characters that are used to create strings, a set of non-terminal symbols that correspond to rules and act as placeholders for patterns that can be generated using terminal characters, a set of rules for replacing non-terminal symbols with terminal characters and a start symbol.

Contig : A length of contiguous sequence assembled from partial, overlapping sequences, generated from a "shotgun" sequencing project. Contigs are typically created computationally, by comparing the overlapping ends of several sequencing reads generated by restriction enzyme digestion of a segment of genomic DNA. The creation of contigs in the presence of sequencing errors, ambiguities and the presence of repeats is one of the most computationally challenging aspects of the role of Bioinformatics in genome analysis.

Convergence : The end-point of any algorithm that uses iteration or recursion to guide a series of data processing steps. An algorithm is usually said to have reached convergence when the difference between the computed and observed steps falls below a pre-defined threshold.

Cosmids : DNA vectors that allow the insertion of long fragments of DNA (up to 50 kbases).

Crystal structure : Term used to describe the high resolution molecular structure derived by x- ray crytallographic analysis of protein or other biomolecular crystals.

Curated databases : Often less complete than primary databases, but they have less redundancy and the added value of scientific annotation; therefore, a biologically significant sequence should be easier to find in such a database and of greater value. Naturally, the degree of redundancy and annotation in such a database depends on the experience, skills, aims, and devotion of its curators. The only proper way to curate databases is the way groups like those that developed OMIM, SWISS-PROT and most commercial databases have done it—that is, through making scientific judgments as data are cleaned up and merged(under the supervision of a curator). Examples of curated databases are LocusLink, OMIM (Online Mendelian Inheritance in Man), RefSeq, SGD (*Saccharomyces cerevisae* Genome Database) and SWISS- PROT

Cytoplasm : The medium of the cell between the nucleus and the cell membrane.

Databases : Collections of data in machine-readable form, which can be manipulated by software to appear in varying arrangements and subsets. Genetic information is stored in different ways in different databases, which makes it hard to compare their holdings. So while computational biologists are trying to improve the quality of the databases, they are also working to build bridges between them. Each database has its own Web site with unique navigation tools and data storage formats that make such searching difficult - programs can't easily recognize data that are not stored in a uniform way.

Descriptor : Information about a sequence or set of sequences whose scope depends on its placement in a record. A descriptor is placed on a set of sequences to reduce the need to save multiple redundant copies of information.

Dendogram : A form of a tree that lists the compared objects in a vertical order and joins related ones by levels of branches extending to one side of the list.

Distance in sequence analysis : The number of observed changes in an optimal alignment of two sequences, usually not counting gaps.

DNA Sequencing : The experimental process of determining the nucleotide sequence of a region of DNA. This is done by labelling each nucleotide (A, C, G or T) with either a radioactive or fluorescent marker which identifies it. There are several methods of applying this technology, each with their advantages and disadvantages. For more information, refer to a current text book. High throughput laboratories frequently use automated sequencers, which are capable of rapidly reading large numbers of templates. Sometimes, the sequences may be generated more quickly than they can be characterised.

Domain name : Refers to one of the levels of organization of the Internet; used to both classify and identify host machines. Top-level domain names indicate the type of site or the country in which the host is located.

Dot Matrix : Dot matrix diagrams provide a graphical method for comparing two sequences. One sequence is written horizontally across the top of the graph and the other along the left-hand side. Dots are placed within the graph at the intersection of the same letter appearing in both sequences. A series of diagonal lines in the graph indicate regions of alignment. The matrix may be filtered to reveal the most-alike regions by scoring a minimal threshold number of matches within a sequence window.

Download : To transfer a file from a remote host to a local machine via FTP.

Downstream : Toward the 3' end of a nucleotide sequence.

Dynamic programming : A DP algorithm solves a problem by combining solutions to sub-problems that are computed once and saved in a table or matrix. DP is typically used when a problem has many possible solutions and an optimal one needs to be found. This algorithm is used for sequence alignments, given a scoring system for sequence comparisons.

EBI : The European Bioinformatics Institute, an outstation of EMBL in the UK.

e-mail : Electronic mail. Refers to messages that can be composed on the computer and transmitted via the Internet to a remote location within seconds.

EMBL : The European Molecular Biology Laboratory in Heidelberg, Germany.

EST : Expressed sequence tag. ESTs are usually short (300-500 bp) single reads from mRND (cDNA) which are usually produced in large numbers. They represent a snap-shot of what is expressed in a given tissue, and/or at a given developmental stage. They represent tags of expression for a given cDNA library. These records usually are very poor in annotation and have only library and BioScource information. They are represented in a variety of databases, notably DDBJ/EMBL/GenBank, dbEST, and Unigene.

E-value : For a given score, the number of hits in a database search that we expect to see by chance with this score or better. The E-value takes into account the size of the database that was searched. The lower the E-value, the more significant the score is. See also P-value.

False negative : A negative data point collected in a data set that was incorrectly reported due to a failure of the test in avoiding negative results.

False positive : A positive data point collected in a data set that was incorrectly reported due to a failure of the test. If the test had correctly measured the data point, the data would have been recorded as negative.

FAQ : A computer file of frequently asked questions. Exactly what it sounds like: a compiled list of questions and answers intended for new users of a computer-based resource, such as a mailing list or a newsgroup.

Feature : Annotation on a specific location on a given sequence.

Federated databases : An integrated repository data from of multiple, possibly heterogeneous, data sources presented with consistent and coherent semantics. They do not usually contain any summary data, and all of the data resides only at the data source (i.e. no local storage).

Filtering : During pair-wise sequence analysis using the dot matrix method, random matches can be filtered out by using a sliding window to compare the two sequences. Rather than comparing a single sequence position at a time, a window of adjacent positions in the two sequences is compared and a dot, indicating a match, is generated only if a certain minimal number of matches occur.

Firewall : Refers to the separation of a company or organization's internal network from the public part, if any, of the same network. Intended to prevent unauthorized access to private computer systems.

Flat files : Pure text documents that are totally unstructured. This type of file generally does not provide very specific search answers, but it is the most popular type of file on the Web and is now a bit easier to search, thanks to the use of hyperlinks.

FTP : File transfer protocol. The method by which files are transferred between hosts.

Functional genomics : Assessment of the function of genes identified by between-genome comparisons. The function of a newly identified gene is tested by introducing mutations into the gene and then examining the resultant mutant organism for an altered phenotype.

Gap : Mismatch in the alignment of two sequences caused by either an insertion in one sequence or a deletion in the other.

Gap penalty is the numeric score used in sequence alignment to penalize the presence of gaps within an alignment. The value of a gap penalty affects how often gaps appear in alignments produced by the algorithm. Most alignment programs suggest gap penalties that are appropriate for particular scoring matrices.

Gene family : Two or more genes that are related by divergent evolution from a common ancestor, either by speciation of gene duplication.

Genome : The genetic material of an organism, contained in one haploid set of chromosomes.

Gopher : A document delivery system allowing the retrieval and display of text-based files.

Graphical user interface : Software that allows a user to interact via "user-friendly" menu and mouse-drive commands, as is typical of Macintosh and Windows applications, and less common for UNIX applications; as opposed to a "command line interface" of typed or scripted commands.

GSS : Genome survey sequences. This DDBJ/EMBL/GenBank division is similar in nature to the EST division, except that its sequences are genomic in origin, rather than cDNA 9MRNA). The GSS division contains (but will not be limited to) the following types of data: random "single-pass read" genome survey sequences; single-pass reads from cosmid/BAC/YAC ends (these could be chromosome specific, but need not be); exon-trapped genomic sequences; Alu PCR sequences.

GUI : Graphical user interface. Refers to software front ends that rely on pictures and icons to direct the interaction of users with the application.

Heuristic alogirthm : An economical strategy for deriving a solution to a problem for which an exact solution is computationally impractical or intractable. Consequently, a heuristic approach is not guaranteed to find the optimal or "true" solution.

HGMP (Human Genome Mapping Project) : The UK HGMP Resource Centre is an academic institution in the UK which provides a number of services, including access to databases, mirrors of databases, and access to extensive services/software for registered academic users.

Hidden Markov model : A kind of formal probablistic model that is well suited to providing a mathematical framework for multiple sequence alignment and finding periodic patterns in a single sequence, representing, for example, patterns found in the exons of a gene and doing profile analysis. In a model of multiple sequence alignments, each column of symbols in the alignment is represented by a frequency distribution of the symbols called a state, and insertions and deletions by other states. One then moves along the model on a particular path from state to state trying to match a given sequence. The next matching symbol is chosen from each state, recording its probability (frequency) and also the probability of the given sequence.

Homologous : In phylogenetics, describing particular features in different individuals that are genetically descended from the same feature in a common ancestor. In molecular biology, often "homologous" simply means similar, regardless of genetic relationship.

Homoplasy : Similarity that has evolved independently and is not indicative of common phylogenetic origin.

Host : Any computer on the Internet that can be addressed directly through a unique IP address.

HTGS (HTG) : High-throughput genome sequences (HTG is the HTGS division in DDBJ/EMBL/GenBank). Various genome sequencing centers worldwide have begun the large-scale sequencing of human and other higher eukaryotic genomes. The databases have deemed it beneficial to put the unfinished sequences that are the result of such sequencing efforts in a separate division. These unfinished records, in most cases, are notable for important numbers of gaps in the nucleotides, low accuracy, and no annotations on the record. These sequences do not achieve the high standard expected DDBJ/EMBL/GenBank records.

HTML : Hypertext markup language. The standard, text-based language used to specify the format of World Wide Web documents. HTML files are translated and rendered through the use of Web browsers.

Hyperlink : A graphic or text within a World Wide Web document that can be selected by means of a mouse. Clicking on a hyperlink transports the user to another part of the same Web page or to another Web page, regardless of location.

Hypertext : Within a Web page, text that is differentiated by colour or by underlining and functions as a hyperlink.

Indel : Acronym for "Insertion of DELetion". Applied to length-variable regions of a multiple alignment when it is not specified whether sequence length differences have been created by insertions or deletions.

Integrated databases : Integration [of databases] typically is accomplished by creating small, object-oriented software elements, or "wrappers" that let a single overlaying, often browser like, desktop application interact with all the pieces. The original separate systems are intact and functional, and new ones can be added, while the underlying complexity is transparent to users. There are still many challenges, but computing environments are becoming more unified, flexible and expandable

Integrative Bioinformatics :_High-Throughput Interpretation of Pathways and Biology. Study of information content and information flow in biological systems and processes-the bridge between observations (data) in diverse biologically- related disciplines and the derivations of understanding (information) about how the systems or processes function.

Internet : A system of linked computer networks used for the transmission of files and messages between hosts. A network of networks.

Intranet : Intranets use Internet technology and protocols over a private network. They are often not connected to the Internet or are protected from the Internet by a firewall.

Intron : Non-coding region of DNA.

IP address : The unique, numeric address of a computer host on the Internet.

Iterative search : A search procedure that is repeated, usually with increasing sensitivity in each round. For instance, taking all the significant hits from an initial BLAST search and using each of them as a query for a new round of BLAST searches would be one form of iterative search.

Java : A programming language developed by Sun Microsystems that allows small programs (applets) to be run on any computer. Java applets are typically invoked when a user clicks on a hyperlink on a Web page.

LAN : Local area network. A network that connects computers in a small, defined area, such as the offices in a single wing or a group of buildings.

Linux : A freely available but commercial-strength clone of the UNIX operating system. Easily installed alongside Windows on a PC, so the same machine can be booted into either Linux of Windows.

Memory-mapped data structures : In this approach [to data- level integration without semantic cleaning] subsets of data from various sources are collected, normalized, and integrated in memory for quick access. While this approach performs actual data integration and addresses the problem of poor performance in the federated approach, it requires additional calls to traditional relational databases to integrate descriptive data. While data cleaning is being performed on some of the data sources, it is not being done across all sources or in the same place. This makes it difficult to quickly add new data sources.

Memory mapped data structures interoperability : The ability of different types of computers, networks, operating systems, and applications to work together effectively, without prior communication, in order to exchange information in a useful and meaningful manner.

Metadata : One of the major issues of the World Wide Web as it exists today is that it is really hard to automate any tasks which one has to perform on the web. So far, the web is mainly built as a forum for human interaction; because most web documents are written for human consumption, the only available form of searching on the web (for example) is to simply match words or sentences contained in documents. Anyone who has used a web search service like AltaVista or HotBot knows that typing in a few keywords and receiving a couple of thousand "hits" is not necessarily very useful. A lot of manual "weeding" of information has to happen after that; it may also happen that the keywords for which you are searching are not prominent in the relevant document itself. A possible solution for the search problem - and for the general issue of letting automated "agents" roam the web performing useful tasks - is to provide a mechanism which allows a more precise description of things on the web. This, in turn, could elevate the status of the web from machine-readable to something we might call machine- understandable. Metadata is "data about data" or specifically in our current context "data describing web resources." The distinction between "data" and "metadata" is not an absolute one; it is a distinction created primarily by a particular application ("one application's metadata is another application's data").

MMDB : Molecular Modelling Database. A taxonomy assigned database of PDB (see PDB) files, and related information.

Molecular clock : The hypothesis that nucleotide or amino acid substitutions occur at more or less fixed rat over evolutionary time, like the slow ticking of a clock. It has been proposed that given a calibration data and a constant molecular clock, the amount of sequence divergence can be used to calculate the time that has elapsed since two molecules diverged.

Multiple alignment : An alignment of three or more sequences, with gaps (spaces) inserted in the sequences such that residues with common structural positions and/or ancestral residues are aligned in the same column of the multiple alignment.

Mutation studies : In Sequin, a set of sequences for the same gene in the same species, perhaps the same individual, in which several different induced mutations are isolated and sequenced.

NCBI : The US National Center for Biotechnology Information.

NIH : The US National Institute of Health.

Object- Protocol Model (OPM) : Developed initially by members of the Data Management Research and Development Group at Lawrence Berkeley National Laboratory. Aim to support rapid development of complete database systems, construction of powerful system- independent query interfaces on top of relational and flat- file data resources, integration of heterogeneous data resources and applications into a common object- oriented framework, deployment of configurable Web- based query interfaces for single or multiple databases.

Open Bioinformatics Foundation OPEN-BIO : The purpose of the foundation is to act as an umbrella organization for the various bio*.org projects that grew out of the original BioPerl project. The goal of the foundation is to provide financial, administrative and technical assistance for our various open source life science projects.

Ontology : An ontology is a classification methodology for formalizing a subject's knowledge or belief system in a structured way (typically for consumption by a computer database). Dictionaries and encyclopaedias are examples of ontologies, as are many Web- based entities, such as Yahoo or Excite, and so is the schema for a database.

ORF : Open Reading Frame. A series of codons (base triplets) which can be translated into a protein. There are six potential reading frames of an unidentifed sequence; TBLASTN (see BLAST) transalates a nucleotide sequence in all six reading frames, into a protein, then attempts to align the results to sequeneces in a protein database, returning the results as a nucleotide sequence. The most likely reading frame can be identified using on-line software (e.g. ORF Finder).

Orthologous : Homolgous sequences are said to be orthologous when they are direct descendants of a sequence in the common ancestor (i.e without having undergone a gene duplication event).

PAM matrix : PAM (percent accepted mutation) and BLOSUM (blocks substitution matrix) are matrices that define scores for each of the 210 possible amino acid substitutions. The scores are based on empirical substitution frequencies observed in alignments of database sequences and in general reflect similar physicochemical properties (eg a substitution of leucine for isoleucine, two amino acids of similar hydrophobicity and size, will score higher than a substitution of leucine for glutamate).

Paralogous : Two homologous sequences (eg sequences that share a common evolutionary ancestor) that diverged by gene duplication, as opposed to orthologs, which diverged by speciation. A gene family within a single organism is necessarily composed only of paralogs (barring horizontal transmission of genes from another species).Homologous sequences in two organisms A and B that are descendants of two different copies of a sequence that was created by a duplication event in the genome of the common ancestor. Paralogs diverged by gene duplication, as opposed to orthologs, which which diverged by speciation.

PDB : Brookhaven Protein Data Bank. A database and format of files which describe the 3D structure of a protein or nucleic acid, as determined by X-ray crystallography or nuclear magnetic resonance (NMR) imaging. The molecules described by the files are usually viewed locally by dedicated software, but can sometimes be visualised on the world wide web.

Phylogenetic studies : In Sequin, a set of sequences for the same gene in individuals of different species. The presumption is that the individuals cannot interbreed. Sequin does not allow a single organism name, but expects the organism to be encoded in the Definition line. It does, however, present a control for setting the proper genetic codes.

PIR : A database of translated GenBank nucleotide sequences. PIR is a redundant (see Redundancy) protein sequence database. The database is divided into four categories:

PIR1 - Classified and annotated.

PIR2 - Annotated.

PIR3 - Unverified.

PIR4 - Unencoded or untranslated.

Platform : Properly, the operating system running software on a computer (eg Unix or Windows95). More often used to refer to the type of computer, such as a Macintosh or PC-compatible.

Population studies : In Sequin, a set of sequences for the same gene in individuals of a single species. The presumption is that the individuals can interbreed. Sequin allows entry of a single organism name, through some distinguishing source information, such as strain, clone, or isolate, must be entered for each sequence if the program is to function properly.

Profile : A linear model of the consensus of a multiple alignment For each column of a protein alignment, a profile assigns 20 residue scores (one per amino acid), and one or more gap penalties for insertions of extra residues adjacent to this column or a deletion of the consensus residue at this column. Profiles are also called " position specific scoring matrices" (PSSMs). Profiles that don't allow insertions and deletions are also called "weight matrices".

Protein description : In a sequence record, used if the protein name is not known.

Protein name : In a sequence record, the preferred field for a Protein feature.

P-value : Like an E-value, but a P-value is the probability of a hit occurring by chance with this score or better, as opposed to the expected number of hits. A P-value has a maximum of 1.0, while an E-value has a maximum of the number of sequences in the database that was searched. For small (significant) P-values, P and E are approximately equal, so the choice of one or the other in a software package is arbitrary. NCBI BLAST 2.0, FASTA, and HMMER report E values. WU-BLAST 2.0 reports P-values.

Redundancy : The presence of more than one identical item represents redundancy. In bioinformatics, the term is used with reference to the sequences in a sequence database. If a database is described as being *redundant*, more than one identical (redundant) sequence may be found. If the database is said to be *non-redundant* (nr), the database managers have attempted to reduce the redundancy. The term is ambiguous with reference to genetics, and as such, the degree of non-redundancy varies according to the database manager's interpretation of the term. One can argue whether or not two alleles of a locus defines the limit of redundancy, or whether the same locus in different, closely related organisms constitutes redundency. Non-redundant databases are, in some ways, superior, but are less complete. These factors should be taken into consideration when selecting a database to search.

Server : A computer that processes requests issued from remote locations by client machines.

Site : An individual column of residues in an amino acid or nucleotide alignment. The residues at a site are presumed to be homologous.

Spam : Postings to newsgroups or mail broadcast to a large number of e-mail accounts that usually are irrelevant or not of interest to the recipients. Analogous to postal junk mail.

STS : Sequences tagged site. STSs are operationally unique sequences that identify the combinations of primer pairs used in PCR assays that generate mapping reagents, each of which maps to a single position within the genome. Variations on this definition are also present in this division. This division of GenBank is intended to facilitate cross-comparison of STSs with sequences in other divisions for the purpose of correlating map positions of anonymous sequences with known genes.

SWISS-PROT : A non-redundant protein sequence database. Thoroughly annotated and cross referenced. A subdivision is TrEMBL.

Telnet : An Internet protocol or application that allows users to connect to computers at remote locations and use these computers as if they were physically operating the remote hardware.

Training Set : A collection of trusted sequences (amino acid or nucleotide) from which a multiple sequence alignment, profile or profile-HMM is built.

URL : Uniformed resource locator. Used Web browsers, URLs specify both the type of site being accessed (FTP, Gopher, or Web) and the address of the Web site.

Word Wide Web : A document delivery system capable of handling non-text-based media of various types.

Index

Affinity chromatography, 53
Algorithm, definition, 407
Algorithm for sequencing fragment, 298
Aligning amino acids and nucleotides, 201
Aligning contigs, 299
Alignment, 148-172
    end-free space alignment, 150-151
    gap penalty, 148, 151-152
    global, 148-152
    local, 148, 151, 167
    methods of, 152-153
    optimal, 164
Alignment construction, 217
    methods of, 218
Alignment of multiple sequences, 191-205
Alignment of sequences, 148-172
    analogous, 148-149
    homologous, 148-149
    identical, 148
    lookup tables, 155
    models of, 149
    orthologous, 148-149
    paralogous, 148
    scoring matrices, 155-158
    sequence analysis of data, 148
Alignment tools for sequencing, 173-190, 297-298
    finding overlaps, 298
    general methods, 298
    sequence assembly process, 298
Amino acids, 43-46
    classification of, 46

physical properties of, 47
    structure of, 44-46
Ancient conserved region (ACR), 228
Applications of bioinformatics, 23-26
    defining gene function, 26
    DNA level, 24-25
    monitoring level, 25
    multiple sequence alignment of proteins, 25
    protein shapes, 25
    RNA level, 25
Apoptosis, 338
Awk, nawk, gawk, 66-67

Bacterial artificial chromosome, 223
Bacterial chromosome, 37
BAC, 223
BAC clones, 294
Basis of gene prediction, 224
Baum-Welch algorithm, 231
Baye's theorem, 345
BCM gene finder, 232
Beta sheet, 249
Bioinformatics, 1-17
    analytical tools, 16-17, 320, 330
    applications of, 3, 23-26
    careers in, 12
    data analysis, 12-14
    data integration, 11
    definition of, 2, 409
    introduction to, 1

kind of data analysed, 4
list of databases, 5-9
major databases in, 5-7
objectives of, 3
resources, 17
tools for function analysis, 16-17
tools and resources, 14-16
BIOCORBA, 131
BIOJAVA, 131
BIOPERL, 106-108, 131
using bioperl, 107-108
Biological databases, 129-147
flatfile databases, 132-133
hypertext, 137
relational databases, 133
types of, 132
BIOPYTHON, 131
BIRCH system, 217-218
BLAST (Basic Local Alignment Search Tool), 157, 167,
173, 179
algorithms, 180-182
considerations, 181
databases, 183
filtering in, 183-184
gapped, 183, 185-186
programs in, 182
results, 181
BLASTN program, 182, 185
BLASTP search, 185
BLAST searches, 183
BLASTX, 185, 229
BLOCKS, 276
BLOCKS databases, 203, 225
BlockMaker, 199
BLIMPS program, 203
BLOSUM (blocks amino acid substitution matrices), 160-
162
Bootstrap & Jacknife replicates, 215-216

CATH database, 9, 256-257
CDD (conserved domain data search), 254
Central BLAST, 186
Central dogma, 18, 20-21
Central limit theorem, 144
CG islands, 230
Chebychev's inequality, 142
Chou-Fasman method, 280
Chromatin, 23, 37
Chromosomal theory of inheritance, 19

Clade, 207
Client server interface, 134-137
CLUSTAL, 196
CLUSTAL programme, 196
CLUSTALX, 218
CLUSTALW, 199
Clone mapping, 291
Clone library, 291
Cloning methodology, 38-39
Cloning vehicles, 38
Cluster analysis, 327-328
Cn3D, 252
Computational tools for DNA sequencing, 297
GCG fragment assembly, 297
sequencher, 297-298
Conducting MSA, 199-201
CONSENSE programme, 218
Constructing alignments and phylogenies, 217
Contigs aligning, 299
Contigs building, 298
CORBA, 130-131

DART (domain architectural retrieval tool), 255
Data acquisition, 305
Data analysis, 12-14
Data mining, 143-145
Database searches, 14
Database, types of, 110-123, 124-131
cell stock databases, 110
flat file database, 110
object-oriented databases, 124-131
relational databases, 111-119
Data integration, 11, 138
Databases for FASTA, 178-179
Dendrogram, definition, 412
Dialysis, 53
Distance sequence analysis, definition, 412
DNA cloning, 38-39, 41
cloning vehicles, 38-39
methodology of, 38-39
DNA, 22-31
chemistry of, 28
components of, 27-31
replication of, 32
structure of, 29-31
DNA fingerprinting, 291-292
DNA microarrays, 301-312
data acquisition, 303, 305
definition of, 301

data analysis, 304
  cDNA probes, 303
  double label, 303
  experimental design, 304-305
  exploratory techniques, 308
  filter arrays, 302
  normalisation, 306
  uses of, 302
  working of, 302
DNA sequencing, 39, 293-299
  clone based, 294
  computer tools for, 297-301
  error probabilities in, 296-297
  Maxam-Gilbert method, 40
  methodologies, 294
  primer walking, 295
  problems in, 295
  Sanger's method, 39-40
Domain, definition, 412
Dot matrices, 154-155
  applications, 154-155
  using lookup tables, 15
Dot plots, 153-154
Dynamic programming for global sequence, 163-167
Dynamic programming, definition, 412

EBI, 9, 133
  definition, 412
E-cell, 339-340
  applications, 340
  concept of, 339
  primary databases, 6
  using, 340
EMBL, 1, 7, 9-10
Ensemble, 131, 138, 139
Entrez system, 11, 136, 150
ESTs (expressed sequence tags), 163, 197-198, 228, 369, 412
EST sequences, 177, 300-301
Evaluating phylogenies, 215
  jumbling sequence order, 215
Exon, 35, 224, 226
Exon prediction, 226
Exon trapping, 226
Expectation maximization algorithm, 230
Extensions of FASTA, 177-178
  LFASTA, 177-178
  PL FASTA, 177
  TFASTA, 173, 177

FASTA, 3, 148, 167, 173-190
  matches, 176
  search, 176
  tools, 173
File input and output, 91-108
Find-find files, 63
FIND PATTERNS, 271
Fingerprints, 272
Fitch-Margoliash method, 211-214
FRAMES program, 228

Gapped blast, 185
Gap penalty, 152-153
GEN lang, 232
GenBank, 9, 133, 150
Gene, 22-26, 34, 223
  eukaryotic, 35
  exons, 35
  functional elements, 34
  introns, 35
  organization, 36
  prokaryotic, 35, 37
  structure of, 36, 223
Genetic code, 34
Gene census, 10
Gene expression, 10, 22, 35
Gene ID, 227
GeneMark, 229
Gene mapping, 287-308
  applications, 290
  clone mapping, 291
  DNA fingerprinting, 291
  human, 289
  meiotic recombination, 288
  physical, 290
  PQ tree algorithm, 293
  STS mapping, 291-293
Gene parser, 227, 232
Gene prediction, 223-234
  basis of, 224
  feature-based approaches, 225-228
  homology-based, 228-229
  lab-based approaches, 225-226
  method of, 225
  pattern searching, 224
  problems in, 224
Gene prediction tools, 232-234
  BCM gene finder, 232
  exon prediction, 232

GenLang, 232
gene parser, 232
GRAIL, 232
poly-A site prediction, 233
procrustes, 232
Gene regulation, 23
Genetranscription network, 332
Gene works, 228
Genetic mapping, 286-308
human, 289
Genetic networks, 317
Genome, 21, 299-301
analysing, 299
comparison, 300
sequences, 8
Genomic analysis, 365
for DNA, 365
for protein, 213
Genomic elements, 323
Genomic on-line database (GOLD), 287
Glycolysis pathway, 335
GOR method, 280
GRAIL, 227, 232
Graphic similarity comparisons, 148

Hashes, 88-91
Hidden Markov Model, definition, 2, 414
Hidden Markov Models (HMMs), 230, 280
HMM approaches, 229, 357
HMM, 230-231
Homology based gene prediction, 228
Homology modelling, 261, 263
Hybridization, 41

Imperfect data, 293
Information molecules, 27-42
Integrated databases, definition, 45
Internet, definition, 415
Introns, 35, 221, 224
Intron, definition, 415
Interproscan, 277
Isoelectric focussing, 318-319
Iterative search, definition, 415

Java, definition, 415
Java applets, 128-129
Java language, 128
Java, uses of, 128

JIPID, 7
Java virtual machine (JVM), 128-129

KEGG, 331, 333-338
KEGG database, 335-338
Kinemags, 253

LAMA, 203
LAN, definition, 415
LAN and internet exploration tools, 58
LINUX, definition, 55, 415
Linux operating system, 55-73
advantages of, 55-56
basics of, 56
common commands, 58
directories, 59-60
file system, 58
graphical interface, 56
linking files, 61
networking, 57
Shell account, 57
Shell programmes, 68-73
speed, 56
software, 56
text processing, 63-66
wild cards, 61
working with files, 62
Lookup tables, 155

MACAW programme, 199
MAGE, 253
MALDI, 315
Managing biological databases, 132-147
curation of, 134
database integration, 137-143
databases of networks, 134-137
Data mining, 143-144, 145
client-server interface, 134
data submission, 133
management of workflow, 146-147
Map, 288
Mapping, 287-308
applications, 290
physical, 290
MAPVIEWER, 126
Mass spectrometry, 54
MAST programme, 203
Maximum likelihood (ML), 214-215

Maximum parsimony (MP), 212-214
Medical information, 2
Meiotic recombination, 288
Metabolic pathways, 332-343
   analytical methods of, 333-338
   E-cell simulation, 341-342
   signaling networks, 338-339
   signaling pathways database (SPAD), 340-342
   simulation of cellular metabolism, 340-343
Methods for alignments, 169
MEME 99
Microarrays, 2, 301-312
MMDB (molecular modelling database), 253
Molecular biology, 18, 20-21, 22-26
   central dogma of, 18, 20-21
   definition of, 21
Models of sequence analysis, 167
   ends-free space alignment, 167-168
   gap penalty, 168-169
   global alignment, 167
   local alignment, 167
Motif search, 272
Multiple alignments, 191-205
Multiple sequence alignment, 191-205, 358
   application of, 201
   bioinformatics approach, 192
   global, 193
   local, 193
   methods for, 191-194, 197
   motivation, 191
   sequence detection, 204-205
   sreps in, 197
   tools for, 193
   viewing, 204
MSA (multiple sequence alignment), 191-205
MSA viewing, 204
Multiplicity of data, 6
   redundancy in, 6
Mutation, 149
MySQL, 119-122
   commands of, 121

National centre for biotechnology information (NCBI), 11, 179, 243, 244
NCBI genomic biology website, 133
NCBI structure database, 253-254
Nearest neighbour method, 280
Networks and databases, 131
Northern blots, 226

Nucleic acids, 27-42
Nuclease mapping, 227
Nucleotide sequence databases, 183

Optimal alignment methods, 148, 163-167
   dynamic programming, 163
Object request broker (ORB), 130
ORFs (open reading frames), 227, 228, 233, 287

Pairwise alignment, 148-172, 191
   Brute force, 169
   definitions, 166
   dot matrix, 154
   dot plots, 154, 170
   dynamic programming, 169
   ends free-space, 167
   gap penalty, 152
   graphic similarity, 153-158
   global alignment, 150
   heuristic methods, 169
   local alignment, 151, 167
   methods of alignment, 169
   optimal alignments, 164-169
   PAM & BLOSUM, 164
   PAM vs. BLOSUM, 163-164
   scoring metrices, 155, 162
   sensitivity, 168, 204
   similarity and difference, 166
   similarity vs. distance, 158
   similarity ys. homology, 158
PAM, 158, 173
PAM matrices, 158-160, 173
Paralogous, 148
Parsimony, maximum (MP), 212-213
Patterns to predict genes, 224
Pattern searching, 224, 225
PCR (polymerase chain reaction), 39, 40-42, 201-227
PCR, primer design, 203-206
PDB (protein data bank), 3, 8-9, 253, 255
   NCBI database, 253-254
PDB sum, 255
Perl language, 74-108
   applications of, 94-106
   control structure, 82-85
   conventions, 75
   functions, 80-82
   operators, 77-80
   priming strings, 76
   programming, 74-94
   variables, 76

Perl programming, 74-76, 86, 379-382
  operations with arrays, 88-91
  illustrations of, 86-88
  processing regular expressions, 99-106
  writing of, 379-382
Perl-DBI-MySQL interface, 122
PFAM, 275
PHYLIP (phylogenetic inference package), 214, 218
  bootstrap analysis, 215-216
  jumbling sequence addition order, 215
PHYLIP DANAPARS programme, 213
Phylogenetic analysis of trees, 206-222, 358
  alignment strategies, 209
  character-based method, 208, 212
  distance method, 208
  distance matrix method, 209-210
  Fitch-Margoliash method, 211-212
  Jukes-Canter method, 210
  maximum likelihood method, 208, 214-218
  maximum parsimony method, 208-213
  neighbour-joining method, 210-211
  scoring method, 209
Phylogenies, evaluation of, 215
  bootstrap method, 215-216
  jumbling sequence, 215-216
Phylogenetic trees, 207-222
  construction of, 219
  heuristics for tree construction, 219-221
  three-way alignment, 221-222
PILE Up method, 196-197
PIMA (pattern induced multiple alignment), 194-195
P-node, 293
PIMA (pattern induced multiple alignment), 194
PRINTS database, 255
Problems for self-assessment, 394-404
Predicting protein sequence, 368
  3D structure, 283, 368
  ID structure, 368
PROCHECK, 255
PROMOTIF, 255
PROSITE, 255
Problem solving in bioinformatics, 365-393
Problems and solutions, 373-393
Procrustus, 232
Procrustus scan databases, 228

Proteins, 43-54
  amino acid sequence in, 48
  domains of, 50
  folding, 51
  folds and motifs, 49-50
  α-helix, 49
  loops and turns, 49
  peptide bonds, 46
  primary structure, 47
  quaternary structure, 51
  secondary structure, 48
  structure of, 46
PROSITE, 8, 202, 275
Protein classification, 256-257
  methodology, 256
  tools, 256-257
Protein data bank (PDB), 8-9, 253
Protein databases, 6-9
  composite, 8
  primary, 7
  structural, 8
Protein information resource, 7
Protein fingerprinting, 313, 316
Protein function prediction, 284
  accuracy in, 284-285
Protein profiles, 271
Protein profile search, 272-273
Protein patterns, 271
Protein-protein interaction, 321-328
  nonhomology methods, 325
Protein sequence alignments, 262-265
  alignment, 262-263
  database search, 262
  multiple alignments, 263
Protein structure, 46
Protein structure prediction, 257-285
  folding, 257
  homology modelling, 258
  in 1D, 258, 266
  in 2D, 259, 278
  in 3D, 259, 283
Protein structure prediction and visualization tools, 248-285
Proteomics, 309-331
  definition, 309
  analysis, 311
Proteome analysis, 311-312
  tools for, 312-315

PSI-BLAST, 187-189, 190
    search for, 188
    scoring metrices, 188

Quaternary structure of proteins, 51, 250
Querry mechanisms, 129

RasMol scripts, 252
Relational databases, 109-123
    creating, 119
    design of, 113-114
    flat file, 110-111
    relational, 111-113
    types of, 110
    using, 114-119
Remote homology modelling (threading), 261, 264-265
Restriction enzymes, 37, 42
Restriction fragments (R. fragments), 37
RNA, 22, 31-33
    primers, 33
    structure of, 31-32
RNA structure prediction, 235-247
    assumptions, 237
    bulge loops, 237
    grammer for palindromes, 245-247
    hairpin loops, 236
    interior loops, 237
    kissing hairpins, 237
    methods of, 238-244
    secondary structure, 236
    tertiary structure, 237
    transformational grammers, 244
tRNA gene prediction, 234
RT-PCR, 226-227
SAPS, 270
SCOP (structural classification of proteins), 11, 256
Scoring matrices, 155-158, 188
    for nucleic acid, 162
Search motifs, 188
Searching for CG islands, 230
Secondary structure prediction tools, 281
Sequence alignments,
    alignment, 262
    database search, 262
    HMM algorithms, 263
    homology modelling, 263
    multiple alignment, 263-264
    threading tools, 263
    tools for, 173

Sequence alignment, 148-152, 262
    brute force, 152
    dot matrix, 152, 157
    dynamic, 152
    extensions of FASTA, 177
    FASTA, 173-179
    FASTA search, 176
    FASTA matches, 176
    gap penalty, 151, 165
    global, 149
    local, 149
Sequence analysis, 148
    analogy, 149
    analysis models, 149
    homology, 149
    of biodata, 149
    similarity, 149
Sequence detection efficiency measures, 204-205
Sequence assembly, 298
Sequence retrieval system (SRS), 11
Sequence targeted site (STS), 291
Sequencher, 297-298
Shell programmes, 68-73
    control commands for, 71
SIB (Swiss institute of bioinformatics), 7
Signatures, 229
Signal scan programme, 229
Signalling networks, 338
Similarity comparisons, 153-158
    BLAST, 157
    block-indel model, 157
    BLOSUM, 166-167
    dot plots, 153
    PAM, 158
    PAM matrices, 158-159
    scoring matrices, 153-156, 165
    similarity vs. homology, 157
    similarity vs. distance, 156
Similarity search, 229
Southern blot, 301
SPAD, 340
Splice site prediction, 234
Splicing, 224
Statistical analysis, 344-364
    Bayes' theorem, 345
    clustering, 363
    F-test, 354
    filtering, 362
    Goodness of fit test, 352

Kruskal-Wallis test, 354
normalisation, 362
normal distribution, 348
population and samples, 349-352
probability theory, 345
tools for, 355-357
types of data, 346-348
types of variables, 344
STS mapping, 291
Structure alignments, 253-269
Structure prediction methods, 266-285
    identification using EXPASy, 268
    predicting transmembrane helices, 267
    prediction in ID, 266
    solvent accessibility, 266
Structural genomics, 2
SSEARCH, 262
SWISS-MODEL, 264, 283
SEISS-PROT, 7, 9, 268

Taq polymerase, 227
TATA signalling, 233
TBLASTIN programme, 368
TBLASTIN search, 368
TBLASTX programme, 368
Test code, 228
Text processing, 63-66
    commands, 63-66
Threading, 261
TFASTA, 173
TIGR microbial database, 287
TrEMBL, 7
Training HMMs, 230-231
Transcription factors, 23
Tree-building, 206-207, 208-222
    concept, 206
    evaluation, 207
    phylogenetic, 207-222
    properties, 207

Tree building methods, 207-222
    additive, 219
    additive metrices, 219
    character-based, 208
    distance-based, 208-210
    heuristic, 219
    three-way alignment, 220
tRNA gene prediction, 234
Types of matches, 225

URL, 418
UPGMA, 198, 359

VAST (vector alignment search tool), 254
Vast search, 254
Vector sequences, 299
View save alignments, 254
Visualization tools for protein structure, 248-285
    chemscape chime, 252
    Cn3D, 252
    Mage, 253
    protein explorer, 252
    prowl, 239
    RasMol, 239
Viterbi algorithm, 230-231
VRML browser, 255

Workflow management, 146-147
Working with phylogenetic trees, 219
    additive metrices, 219
    heuristic, 219-222
    reconstruction, 219
Writing Perl program, 379-387

Y2H (yeast two hybrid system), 323

Zinc fingers, 366
Zippers, leucine, 366
Zooblots, 226